School Mental Health

Editors

MARGARET M. BENNINGFIELD
SHARON HOOVER STEPHAN

CHILD AND ADOLESCENT PSYCHIATRIC CLINICS OF NORTH AMERICA

www.childpsych.theclinics.com

Consulting Editor
HARSH K. TRIVEDI

April 2015 • Volume 24 • Number 2

ELSEVIER

1600 John F. Kennedy Boulevard • Suite 1800 • Philadelphia, Pennsylvania, 19103-2899

http://www.theclinics.com

CHILD AND ADOLESCENT PSYCHIATRIC CLINICS OF NORTH AMERICA Volume 24, Number 2
April 2015 ISSN 1056–4993, ISBN-13: 978-0-323-37013-4

Editor: Joanne Husovski
Developmental Editor: Stephanie Wissler

Child and Adolescent Psychiatric Clinics of North America (ISSN 1056-4993) is published quarterly by Elsevier Inc., 360 Park Avenue South, New York, NY 10010-1710. Months of issue are January, April, July, and October. Business and Editorial Offices: 1600 John F. Kennedy Boulevard, Suite 1800, Philadelphia, PA 19103-2899. Periodicals postage paid at New York, NY and additional mailing offices. Subscription prices are $310.00 per year (US individuals), $491.00 per year (US institutions), $155.00 per year (US students), $360.00 per year (Canadian individuals), $598.00 per year (Canadian institutions), $200.00 per year (Canadian students), $430.00 per year (international individuals), $598.00 per year (international institutions), and $200.00 per year (international students). International air speed delivery is included in all *Clinics* subscription prices. All prices are subject to change without notice. **POSTMASTER:** Send address changes to *Child and Adolescent Psychiatric Clinics of North America*, Elsevier Health Sciences Division, Subscription Customer Service, 3251 Riverport Lane, Maryland Heights, MO 63043. **Customer Service: 1-800-654-2452 (U.S. and Canada); 314-447-8871 (outside U.S. and Canada). Fax: 314-447-8029. E-mail: JournalsCustomer Service-usa@elsevier.com (for print support) or journalsonlinesupport-usa@elsevier.com (for online support).**

Reprints. For copies of 100 or more of articles in this publication, please contact the Commercial Reprints Department, Elsevier Inc., 360 Park Avenue South, New York, New York 10010-1710 Tel.: 212-633-3874; Fax: 212-633-3820, E-mail: reprints@elsevier.com.

Child and Adolescent Psychiatric Clinics of North America is covered in *MEDLINE/PubMed (Index Medicus), ISI, SSCI, Research Alert, Social Search, Current Contents,* and *EMBASE/Excerpta Medica.*

Contributors

CONSULTING EDITOR

HARSH K. TRIVEDI, MD, MBA
Executive Director and Chief Medical Officer; Behavioral Health Vice Chair for Clinical Affairs; Associate Professor of Psychiatry, Vanderbilt University School of Medicine, Nashville, Tennessee

CONSULTING EDITOR EMERITUS

ANDRÉS MARTIN, MD, MPH

FOUNDING CONSULTING EDITOR

MELVIN LEWIS, MBBS, FRCPSYCH, DCH

EDITORS

MARGARET M. BENNINGFIELD, MD, MSCI
Assistant Professor of Psychiatry and Pediatrics, Department of Psychiatry, Vanderbilt University, Nashville, Tennessee

SHARON HOOVER STEPHAN, PhD
Associate Professor, Center for School Mental Health, Division of Child and Adolescent Psychiatry, University of Maryland School of Medicine, Baltimore, Maryland

AUTHORS

BLAISE A. AGUIRRE, MD
Massachusetts General Hospital, Harvard Medical School, Boston, Massachusetts

ALEXA BAGNELL, MD, FRCPC
Interim Chief, Child and Adolescent Psychiatry; Associate Professor, Department of Psychiatry, IWK Health Centre, Dalhousie University, Halifax, Nova Scotia, Canada

PAUL BAN, PhD
Director Outreach, Child and Family Behavioral Health Office, Medical Command, United States Army, Tacoma, Washington

MAURA BARSTEAD, BA
Research Assistant in Child and Adolescent Psychiatry, Lucile Packard Children's Hospital at Stanford University, Palo Alto, California

KIMBERLY D. BECKER, PhD
Assistant Professor, Division of Child and Adolescent Psychiatry, University of Maryland School of Medicine, Baltimore, Maryland

MARGARET M. BENNINGFIELD, MD, MSCI
Assistant Professor of Psychiatry and Pediatrics, Department of Psychiatry, Vanderbilt University, Nashville, Tennessee

ANGELA M. BLIZZARD, BA
Research Assistant, Division of Child and Adolescent Psychiatry, University of Maryland School of Medicine, Baltimore, Maryland

JILL HAAK BOHNENKAMP, PhD
Assistant Professor, Division of Child and Adolescent Psychiatry, University of Maryland School of Medicine, Baltimore, Maryland

JEFF Q. BOSTIC, MD, EdD
Child Psychiatry, Massachusetts General Hospital, Harvard Medical School, Boston, Massachusetts

NICOLE EVANGELISTA BRANDT, PhD
Instructor, Department of Psychology, Columbus State Community College, Columbus, Ohio

SARA L. BUCKINGHAM, MA
Doctoral Candidate, Human Services Psychology Program, University of Maryland, Baltimore County, Baltimore, Maryland

GABRIELLE L. CHAPMAN, PhD
Research Associate, Peabody Research Institute, Vanderbilt University, Nashville, Tennessee

ELIZABETH CONNORS, PhD
University of Maryland School of Medicine, Baltimore, Maryland

JON S. EBERT, PsyD
Assistant Professor of Clinical Psychiatry, Department of Psychiatry, Vanderbilt University School of Medicine, Nashville, Tennessee

SARAH EDWARDS, DO
Assistant Professor, Division of Child and Adolescent Psychiatry, University of Maryland School of Medicine, Baltimore, Maryland

RICHARD A. EPSTEIN, PhD, MPH
Associate Professor, Department of Psychiatry, Vanderbilt University School of Medicine, Nashville, Tennessee

MICHAEL E. FARAN, MD, PhD
Chief, Child and Family Behavioral Health Office, Medical Command, United States Army, Tacoma, Washington

LOIS T. FLAHERTY, MD
Lecturer on Psychiatry, Department of Psychiatry, Cambridge Health Alliance, Harvard Medical School, Cambridge, Massachusetts

TRACY GLASCOE, LCSW
Department of Psychiatry, Vanderbilt University, Nashville, Tennessee

KATHY A. GRACEY, MEd
Department of Psychiatry, Vanderbilt University School of Medicine, Nashville, Tennessee

SAMANTHA N. HARTLEY, BA
Clinical and Research Coordinator, School Mental Health Team, Lucile Packard Children's Hospital at Stanford University, Stanford, California

L. ELLIOT HONG, MD
Department of Psychiatry, Maryland Psychiatric Research Center, University of Maryland School of Medicine, Baltimore, Maryland

STEPHEN HYDON, MSW
Clinical Professor, Field Education, University of Southern California School of Social Work, Los Angeles, California

PATTI L. JOHNSON, PhD
Deputy Chief, Child and Family Behavioral Health Office, Medical Command, United States Army, Tacoma, Washington

SHASHANK V. JOSHI, MD, FAAP
Associate Professor of Psychiatry, Pediatrics and Education, Stanford University School of Medicine, Stanford; Director of Training in Child and Adolescent Psychiatry, Lucile Packard Children's Hospital at Stanford University, Palo Alto, California

SHERYL H. KATAOKA, MD, MSHS
Associate Professor, Department of Psychiatry and Biobehavioral Sciences, UCLA, Los Angeles, California

MOIRA KESSLER, MD
Fellow in Child and Adolescent Psychiatry, Lucile Packard Children's Hospital at Stanford University, Palo Alto, California

TARAH M. KUHN, PhD
Assistant Professor of Clinical Psychiatry, Department of Psychiatry, Vanderbilt University School of Medicine, Nashville, Tennessee

STAN KUTCHER, MD, FRCPC, FCAHS
Professor, Department of Psychiatry, Sun Life Financial Chair in Adolescent Mental Health; Director, WHO Collaborating Centre, IWK Health Centre, Dalhousie University, Halifax, Nova Scotia, Canada

AUDRA K. LANGLEY, PhD
Associate Professor, Department of Psychiatry and Biobehavioral Sciences, UCLA, Los Angeles, California

NANCY LEVER, PhD
University of Maryland School of Medicine, Baltimore, Maryland

COURTNEY McMICKENS, MD, MPH
Child and Adolescent Psychiatry Fellow, Department of Psychiatry, Cambridge Health Alliance, Harvard Medical School, Cambridge, Massachusetts

MICHAEL D. NEVAREZ, MD
Massachusetts General Hospital, Harvard Medical School, Boston, Massachusetts

WILLIAM S. POLLACK, PhD, FAACP
Associate Clinical Professor (Psychology), Department of Psychiatry, Harvard Medical School, Newton Center; Senior Consultant/Research Director, Mental Health of Men and Boys, Department of Psychiatry, Cambridge Health Alliance, Cambridge, Massachusetts

MONA P. POTTER, MD
McLean Psychiatric Hospital, Harvard Medical School, Boston, Massachusetts

JEFFERSON B. PRINCE, MD
Massachusetts General Hospital, Harvard Medical School, Boston, Massachusetts; North Shore Medical Center, Salem, Massachusetts

NANCY RAPPAPORT, MD
Director of School-Based Programs; Associate Professor of Psychiatry, Department of Psychiatry, Cambridge Health Alliance, Harvard Medical School, Cambridge, Massachusetts

GLORIA REEVES, MD
Division of Child and Adolescent Psychiatry, Department of Psychiatry, University of Maryland School of Medicine, Baltimore, Maryland

PAULA RIGGS, MD
Professor; Director of the Division of Substance Dependence, Department of Psychiatry, School of Medicine, Aurora, Colorado

JASON SCHIFFMAN, PhD
Department of Psychology, University of Maryland, Baltimore County, Baltimore, Maryland

SARAH E.O. SCHWARTZ, PhD, MEd
Post-Doctoral Clinical Research Fellow in Psychology, Department of Psychiatry, Cambridge Health Alliance, Harvard Medical School, Cambridge, Massachusetts

TRACY SHUE, MS
Program Manager, Child and Family Behavioral Health Office, Medical Command, United States Army, Tacoma, Washington

BRADLEY D. STEIN, MD, PhD
Senior Natural Scientist, RAND Corporation, Pittsburgh, Pennsylvania

SHARON HOOVER STEPHAN, PhD
Associate Professor, Center for School Mental Health, Division of Child and Adolescent Psychiatry, University of Maryland School of Medicine, Baltimore, Maryland

GEORGE SUGAI, EdD
University of Connecticut, Storrs, Connecticut

TIERRA SYDNOR-DIGGS, LCSW
Health Educator, Division of Child and Adolescent Psychiatry, University of Maryland School of Medicine, Baltimore, Maryland

COURTNEY VAUGHAN, LCSW-C
Health Educator, Division of Child and Adolescent Psychiatry, University of Maryland School of Medicine, Baltimore, Maryland

YIFENG WEI, MEd
PhD Candidate, School Mental Health Lead, Sun Life Financial Chair in Adolescent Mental Health Team, IWK Health Centre, Dalhousie University, Halifax, Nova Scotia, Canada

CATHARINE L. WEISS, PhD
Clinical Assistant Professor, Division of Child and Adolescent Psychiatry, University of Maryland School of Medicine, Baltimore, Maryland

MARK D. WEIST, PhD
Professor, Department of Psychology, University of South Carolina, Columbia, South Carolina

MARLEEN WONG, PhD
Clinical Professor and Associate Dean, Field Education, University of Southern California School of Social Work, Los Angeles, California

Contents

> To fully realize the potential of mental health supports in academic settings, it is essential to consider how to effectively integrate the mental health and education systems and their respective resources, staffing, and structures. Historically, school mental health services have not effectively spanned a full continuum of care from mental health promotion to treatment, and several implementation and service challenges have evolved. After an overview of these challenges, best practices and strategies for school and community partners are reviewed to systematically integrate mental health interventions within a school's multitiered system of student support.

> Mental health literacy is an integral component of health literacy and has been gaining increasing attention as an important focus globally for mental health interventions. In Canada, youth mental health is increasingly recognized as a key national health concern and has received more focused attention than ever before within our health system. This article outlines 2 unique homegrown initiatives to address youth mental health literacy within Canadian secondary schools.

> Developmentally sensitive efforts to help students learn, practice, and regularly use mindfulness tactics easily and readily in and beyond the classroom are important to help them manage future stresses. Mindfulness emphasizes consciously focusing the mind in the present moment, purposefully, without judgment or attachment. Meditation extends this to setting aside time and places to practice mindfulness, and additionally, yoga includes physical postures and breathing techniques that enhance mindfulness and meditation. Several mindfulness programs and techniques have been applied in schools, with positive benefits reported. Some elements of these programs require modifications to be sensitive to the developmental state of the children receiving mindfulness training.

> Teachers can be vulnerable to secondary traumatic stress (STS) because
> of their supportive role with students and potential exposure to students'
> experiences with traumas, violence, disasters, or crises. STS symptoms,
> similar to those found in posttraumatic stress disorder, include night-
> mares, avoidance, agitation, and withdrawal, and can result from second-
> ary exposure to hearing about students' traumas. This article describes
> how STS presents, how teachers can be at risk, and how STS can manifest
> in schools. A US Department of Education training program is presented,
> and thoughts on future directions are discussed.

> Students with emerging psychosis often experience delays in diagnosis
> and treatment that impact mental health and academic outcomes. School
> systems have tremendous potential to improve early identification and
> treatment of adolescent psychosis. As a community-based resource,
> schools can support outreach, education, and screening for adolescents
> with psychosis and engage identified students and their families for treat-
> ment. The concept of duration of untreated psychosis (DUP; the gap
> between symptom onset and treatment initiation) in adolescent psychosis
> and the potential role of schools in reducing DUP are reviewed. Future
> directions for clinical care and research needed to support school-based
> interventions are proposed.

> Suicide is a leading cause of preventable death in youth, and numerous
> curricula and other prevention and intervention programs have been
> developed in the last 15 years. Comprehensive suicide prevention plan-
> ning should include the 4 components of health promotion, prevention/
> education, intervention, and postvention. School-based suicide preven-
> tion and mental health education programs have become more common
> as an efficient and cost-effective way to reach youth. Process consider-
> ations that are based on the principles of therapeutic engagement with
> patients and families can provide mental health professionals with strate-
> gies that can assist education professionals, students, and the larger
> school community simultaneously.

> The School Transition Program (STP) is a 3-month intervention developed to
> address the unique needs of youth transitioning back to school from an
> inpatient psychiatric hospitalization. The STP focuses on promoting com-
> munication across school, home, and hospital. It includes psychoeducation,

emotional support for caregivers, and the creation of transition plans in collaboration with school staff and families. Matching interventions to the academic, social, emotional/behavioral needs of these youth and increasing support to their caregivers has the potential to ease stress, reduce challenges and promote success during and after the transition period.

In this article, an overview is provided of strategies to engage youth and their families in school mental health (SMH) services throughout the course of treatment. Resources are outlined to help SMH providers determine which strategies are most suitable for youth and their families, based on outcomes desired, barriers to engagement, and stage of treatment. Four case vignettes are presented to describe implementation of these strategies.

Evidence-based assessment (EBA) has been shown to improve clinical outcomes, but this practice is frequently not implemented in school mental health practice. This article reviews potential barriers to implementation and offers practical strategies for addressing these challenges. Several valid and reliable tools for assessment are reviewed, and information is provided on clinical use. Case examples of EBA implementation in school mental health settings are provided to illustrate how these tools can be used in everyday practice by school mental health clinicians.

The US Army has developed an innovative School Behavioral Health (SBH) program, part of the Child and Family Behavioral Health System, a collaborative, consultative behavioral health care model that includes SBH, standardized training of primary care providers in treatment of common behavioral health problems, use of tele-consultation/tele-behavioral health, optimizing community outreach services, and integration with other related behavioral health services. In this article, the needs of military children, adolescents, and families are reviewed, a history of this initiative is presented, key themes are discussed, and next steps in advancing this evolving, innovative system of health care featuring SBH are described.

CHILD AND ADOLESCENT PSYCHIATRIC CLINICS

FORTHCOMING ISSUES

Family Based Treatment in Child Psychiatry
Michelle Rickerby and
Thomas Roesler, *Editors*

Global Mental Health
Paramjit Joshi and Lisa Cullins,
Editors

RECENT ISSUES

January 2015
Top Topics in Child and Adolescent Psychiatry
Harsh K. Trivedi, *Editor*

October 2014
ADHD: Non-Pharmacologic Interventions
Stephen V. Faraone and
Kevin M. Antshel, *Editors*

July 2014
Alternative and Complementary Therapies for Children with Psychiatric Disorders, Part 2
Deborah R. Simkin and
Charles W. Popper, *Editors*

RELATED INTEREST

Juvenile Offenders: Competence to Stand Trial (Pages 837–854)
Soulier M, *Author*
in
Psychiatric Clinics of North America, December 2012 (Vol. 35, No. 4, Pages 757–982)
Forensic Psychiatry
Scott CL, *Editor*

AACAP Members: Please go to www.jaacap.org for information on access to the Child and Adolescent Psychiatric Clinics. *Resident* Members of AACAP: Special access information is available at www.childpsych.theclinics.com.

DOWNLOAD
Free App!

Review Articles
THE CLINICS

NOW AVAILABLE FOR YOUR iPhone and iPad

Preface

Integrating Mental Health into Schools to Support Student Success

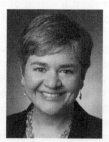 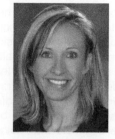

Margaret M. Benningfield, MD, MSCI   Sharon Hoover Stephan, PhD
Editors

Schools represent arguably the most critical venue for promoting child and adolescent mental health and for identifying and addressing mental illness early and effectively. Most children in the United States attend school for thousands of hours over the course of their development, thereby offering an unparalleled location for identification and implementation of mental health supports. While schools are predominantly focused on academic success (eg, grades, attendance, test scores), they must also attend to student mental health to promote student success. This is for two reasons: (1) academic success is contingent on health, both physical and mental health; and (2) schools are ultimately responsible not just for promoting good readers, writers, and mathematicians but also for producing well-rounded, well-adjusted citizens prepared to live happy, meaningful lives and to contribute successfully to society.

The mental health field, including child psychiatry, has an important role to play in promoting student success in school. Historically, child psychiatry has most often been accessed by schools to address tertiary care needs of individual students with severe problems that negatively impact schooling. We would argue against simply engaging mental health professionals when students become ill or when there are complex mental health problems to address. Rather, schools and students will most benefit by utilizing the science and practice of psychiatry to inform all levels of a continuum of student mental health supports, from universal promotion and prevention to tertiary intervention. We are at a critical juncture with respect to the integration of education and mental health, with a growing science and practice base in the areas of brain development, intervention development, and implementation. The literature and our experience would suggest that successful integration of mental health into education systems requires an intentional partnering of all those invested in student mental health, including mental health professionals, educators, and youth and families.

Child Adolesc Psychiatric Clin N Am 24 (2015) xv–xvii
http://dx.doi.org/10.1016/j.chc.2014.12.005
1056-4993/15/$ – see front matter © 2015 Published by Elsevier Inc.

childpsych.theclinics.com

This issue reflects state-of-the-art efforts to meaningfully integrate mental health into education across a multitiered system of support for students. In the first article of the volume, Stephan, Sugai, Lever, and Connors describe the landscape of the educational system in a post-No-Child-Left-Behind era that emphasizes test scores as a primary measure for student success. The authors make the case that integrating mental health services into a multitiered system of support is key factor to optimizing learning environments. Furthermore, schools may represent one of our best opportunities to facilitate an integrated implementation of mental health practices and systems to provide for the needs of all children. Next, we present a series of articles focused on universal applications of mental health to schools. Effective mental health promotion in school systems begins with increasing mental health literacy. Kutcher, Bagnell, and Wei report on two initiatives designed to engage students and educators using technology to improve mental health awareness, reducing stigma, and improving health-related decision-making. Next, Bostic Nevarez, Potter, Prince, Benningfield, and Aguirre describe specific strategies for promoting mental health in schools through mindfulness practice. Mindfulness—the practice of attending nonjudgmentally to the present moment—can be incorporated into the regular school day; emerging evidence suggests that doing so improves cognitive performance and resilience to stress. Benningfield, Potter, and Bostic then describe the neurobiology related to emotional and cognitive integration, making the case for the incorporation of social and emotional learning within academic programming to promote student success. The authors argue that the brain's organization makes it impossible to segregate cognitive processes from emotional ones.

The next collection of articles describes specific mental health interventions and programming to support students with a variety of concerns. In an article on Safety Assessments in Schools, Rappaport, Pollack, Flaherty, Schwartz, and McMickens highlight key components of a thorough evaluation of a student's risk of harm to self or others. The authors emphasize the role of the consultant in establishing rapport with the identified student of concern and the family in evaluating threat. Clinical vignettes illustrate the principles discussed. Next, we consider schools as an important setting for prevention and treatment of substance use disorders (SUD), which are highly prevalent and present a significant public health burden. Several prevention programs have been found to be effective at delaying the onset of alcohol and drug use. Individual treatment for SUD is effective at decreasing substance use as well as substance-related harm, but few studies to date have tested whether these programs can be effectively delivered in school settings. Benningfield, Riggs, and Stephan review the literature and propose components of school-based treatment of SUD. Requests for assistance with management of disruptive behaviors are some of the most common reasons for school mental health consultation. Kuhn, Ebert, Gracey, Chapman, and Epstein review effective interventions for dealing with disruptive behaviors in adolescents, noting that effective implementation is a key factor to success. The stress encountered in school settings can take a significant toll on teachers who witness traumas, violence, disasters, or crises. Secondary traumatic stress (STS) describes a constellation of symptoms similar to those of posttraumatic stress disorder that can result from hearing about students' traumas. Hydon, Wong, Langley, Stein, and Kataoka describe a US Department of Education training program that promotes education and interventions to prevent STS in teachers. Psychotic illness can have a devastating impact on those affected. One factor linked to the severity of illness and ultimate quality of life is the length of time between onset of symptoms and proper treatment. Schools have the potential to decrease the duration of untreated psychosis by providing education, screening, and access to early intervention.

Schiffman, Stephan, Hong, and Reeves review the concept of duration of untreated psychosis and evaluate the data that support screening and early intervention for psychotic disorders in schools. Suicide accounts for more deaths among youth and young adults in the United States than do all natural causes combined. Joshi, Hartley, Kessler, and Barstead provide up-to-date recommendations for suicide prevention in schools and identify areas of active research in the field. Because most deaths by suicide occur in people who have had mental health conditions, prevention efforts must focus on school-based mental health education and promotion. When youth require inpatient treatment for psychiatric illness, the transition at discharge can be quite challenging. Limited family support and lack of coordination with school personnel may increase the risk for hospital readmission. Weiss, Blizzard, Vaughan, Sydnor-Diggs, Edwards, and Stephan have developed an innovative School Transition Program that supports students, families, and school personnel for up to 3 months after hospital discharge. Through improving communication, coordinating of services, and identifying the individual needs of youth returning to school, this program has the potential to significantly improve clinical outcomes.

Finally, we close with three articles to help guide school mental health program implementation. Family engagement is often a challenging component of successful mental health treatment in schools and is the focus of the contribution from Becker, Buckingham, and Brandt. In this article, the authors provide practical strategies school mental health providers can employ to improve family involvement in treatment. Next, we present an article reviewing methods for evidence-based assessment (EBA). While evidence-based treatments have gained in popularity, an emphasis on assessment has lagged behind. Accurately defining the challenges faced by an individual student as well as a population of students is essential to providing quality care. Bohnenkamp, Glascoe, Gracey, Epstein, and Benningfield review common instruments available for EBA and describe the methods employed in two well-established school mental health programs. To close the issue, Faran, Johnson, Ban, Shue, and Weist provide a description for one model of integrated mental health services in the US Army School Behavioral Health program. Their review of this unique program identifies potential barriers and describes their solutions and may serve as a blueprint for other systems that wish to implement integrated mental health services.

Margaret M. Benningfield, MD, MSCI
Vanderbilt University
Department of Psychiatry
1601 23rd Avenue South, #3068C Nashville, TN 37212, USA

Sharon Hoover Stephan, PhD
Center for School Mental Health
Division of Child and Adolescent Psychiatry
University of Maryland School of Medicine
737 W. Lombard Street, 426
Baltimore, MD 21201, USA

E-mail addresses:
meg.benningfield@Vanderbilt.edu (M.M. Benningfield)
sstephan@psych.umaryland.edu (S.H. Stephan)

Strategies for Integrating Mental Health into Schools via a Multitiered System of Support

Sharon Hoover Stephan, PhD[a],*, George Sugai, EdD[b],
Nancy Lever, PhD[a], Elizabeth Connors, PhD[a]

KEYWORDS

- Mental health-education integration • Multitiered systems of support
- Positive behavior interventions and supports • Response to intervention

KEY POINTS

- Historically, school mental health services have not effectively spanned a full continuum of care, from mental health promotion to treatment, and several implementation and service challenges have evolved.
- To fully realize the potential of mental health supports in academic settings, it is essential to consider how to effectively integrate the mental health and education systems and their respective resources, staffing, and structures.
- It is essential that the community mental health workforce is prepared to engage with and work in schools, and educators and other school professionals are similarly prepared to address student mental health and to integrate community professionals into their systems of care for students.
- It is critical to integrate mental health and education teams into unified teams that consider the "whole child," addressing academic as well as social-emotional-behavioral considerations.
- Education and mental health systems should consider using implementation science to more effectively integrate a full continuum of evidence-based mental health practices into schools.

Disclosure: See last page of article.
[a] Department of Psychiatry, University of Maryland School of Medicine, Baltimore, MD 21201, USA; [b] University of Connecticut, Neag School of Education, Gentry 019C, Storrs, CT 06269, USA
* Corresponding author. Division of Child and Adolescent Psychiatry, Center for School Mental Health, University of Maryland School of Medicine, 737 West Lombard Street, 426, Baltimore, MD 21201.
E-mail address: sstephan@psych.umaryland.edu

Child Adolesc Psychiatric Clin N Am 24 (2015) 211–231
http://dx.doi.org/10.1016/j.chc.2014.12.002   childpsych.theclinics.com
1056-4993/15/$ – see front matter © 2015 Elsevier Inc. All rights reserved.

Abbreviations	
ADHD	Attention deficit hyperactivity disorder
CBITS	Cognitive Behavioral Intervention for Trauma In Schools
EBP	Evidence-based practice
IEPs	Individualized education programs
MOU	Memoranda of Understanding
PBIS	Positive Behavioral Interventions and Supports
RtI	Response to intervention

In the wake of No Child Left Behind and subsequent high-stakes testing, Common Core Standards, and teacher evaluation, schools are increasingly focused on instructional content and its effective delivery as a way to promote achievement and success for all students. Although focus on academics is important to advance student success, so too is attention to the social, emotional, and behavioral factors that are critical to student functioning. All students can benefit academically and socially when their classroom and school environments are positive, preventive, and responsive.[1–3] Furthermore, there are likely to be several students in each classroom that have impairments that impede their own and other students' learning, necessitating more targeted intervention or supports. Integrating mental health interventions into a multitiered system of educational, social, emotional, and behavioral supports has the potential to contribute to positive learning environments for all students, especially those who display significant risk for mental health difficulties.

Despite a growing evidence base for school mental health interventions, strategic integration of mental health supports into the education infrastructure has proved challenging. Efforts to implement are often incomplete, short in sustainability, limited in outcome durability, and narrow in spread.[4,5] Explanations for these shortfalls include limited funding, competing initiatives, inadequate training and professional development, insufficient school-community partnerships, low priority, lack of leadership.[6–8] To fully realize the potential of mental health supports in academic settings, it is essential to consider how to effectively integrate the mental health and education systems and their respective resources, staffing, and structures. The purpose within this article is to review best practices and strategies for school and community partners to systematically integrate mental health interventions within a school's multitiered system of student support. It is also suggested that schools may represent one of the best opportunities to facilitate an integrated implementation of mental health practices and systems. In addition, by improving the capacity of educators (ie, general and special education teachers, paraprofessionals, principals), and school and community mental health professionals (ie, psychiatrists, psychologists, counselors, occupational therapists, nurses, social workers) to work together to leverage their respective knowledge, skills, and resources to implement evidence-based mental health practices, improvements in student academic achievement and social and behavioral competence may be realized.[4,9,10]

HISTORICAL CONTEXT AND CHALLENGES

Historically, school mental health services have not effectively spanned a full continuum of care, from mental health promotion to treatment, and several implementation and service challenges have evolved. First, school mental health service provision has largely been characterized by tertiary clinical care models, serving students with identified mental health challenges that interfere with school functioning. These services have been offered by school-employed and community-employed mental health professionals, including counselors, social workers, psychologists, and psychiatrists and often involve pulling students away from their regular course work to receive targeted mental health interventions and then returning them to class. Such services are sometimes conducted in isolation of the larger school team, with limited consideration for the educational plan and related school supports already in place. When treatment occurs in isolation, opportunities are lost to complement tertiary care with existing universal and selected intervention efforts and to build on the many school personnel who could be part of a more comprehensive and informed treatment strategy. Similarly, students receiving special education services for emotional and behavioral problems may be receiving health and mental health care from community providers that, if coordinated, could help avoid duplication, address a broader array of needs, and have key strategies and skills reinforced across adults working with the student.

Second, even when school personnel have tried to implement services to support student mental health along a continuum of care, they often focus primarily on one component of support versus the full-tiered prevention approach. For example, a district or school may focus predominantly on universal systems of positive behavioral support, with limited attention to mental health supports for students at-risk for or already displaying mental health concerns. Conversely, the focus may be exclusively on serving only those youth with significant mental health problems, with limited to no attention to universal or whole-school approaches to supporting student behavior and mental health. When schools attempt to deliver comprehensive behavioral supports to students, lack of universal screening or consistent identification and referral processes may result in missing students with serious mental health problems; particularly, those with internalizing disorders often go undetected with current systems of behavior monitoring (eg, office discipline referrals, suspensions).[11]

Third, and related to the challenge noted above, when a tiered continuum of support is adopted, implementation is often not integrated. Practices are associated with tiers and not implemented in a manner that considers their interconnected purpose and impact. For example, students who are receiving intensive and individualized assistance from a specialist may not experience extensions of that treatment from personnel in other settings (eg, classrooms, lunchtime, after school), may not participate in activities (eg, social skills groups, lessons, or assemblies) that are provided to the larger student body, or may receive contraindicated supports being provided by another provider. Individual providers, specific interventions, and particular organizational routines and structures are implemented independently rather than in an interconnected and integrated manner across the tiered continuum logic.

Fourth, in some respects, special education structures and processes have also perpetuated delayed intervention for mental health problems by requiring symptoms to be severely impacting educational performance before services are mandated. Only in recent years has attention shifted more toward early identification and preventive intervention, in part related to greater understanding of onset and trajectories of mental illness. What has been a paradigmatic shift for the mental health field is the more recent understanding that child and adolescent mental illness cannot and should not be separated from adult mental illness. Financing systems and traditional training programs bifurcate adult and child mental illness in ways that are artificial and have undermined progress in the area of prevention and early identification. Most mental health problems begin before age 18 as is indicated in the World Health Organization's World Mental Health Surveys.[12]

Fifth, educators often have not been adequately prepared to address student mental health, and school-employed student support staff may have little experience in effectively partnering with community providers to provide a full continuum of mental health care for students. School-employed mental health professionals have often resisted partnering by community mental health professionals for a variety of reasons. For instance, school administrators may have concerns about their responsibility to fund mental health needs identified by the school, and school-employed mental health professionals may view "outside" providers as a threat to their job security and/or think that community partners do not understand schools, integrate educational components effectively, or have priorities that are consistent with schools. Also, some would argue that everything impacting educational success, including mental health concerns, should be identified and addressed exclusively by the school system; therefore, bringing in outside providers may be seen as a "failure" by the education system versus the recognition that the mental health of students is a shared responsibility of multiple child-serving systems.

Finally, efforts to integrate education and mental health have not produced effective and sustainable implementation systems. For example, since the mid 1980s, Systems of Care efforts[13] and related federal investments (eg, Safe Schools/Healthy Students) have recognized the importance of coordinated, cross-system care. Among traditional mental health services, however, education has not been effectively and durably included as partners in care. In addition, isolated silos of preservice and professional training (for both educators and mental health professionals) have further contributed to the disconnect between the mental health and education systems. A report by the Annapolis Coalition on the Behavioral Health Workforce[14(p233)] stated "mental health services in schools, and the associated workforce, often have been marginalized and viewed as 'add ons' that are not central to the academic interests of schools." The Coalition further argued that most of the US mental health workforce is lacking competency in some of the areas that are most relevant to school mental health; that is, prevention and promotion, evidence-based practice (EBP), and collaborative partnerships with recipients of services.

To conclude, several historical challenges and needs have affected the delivery of school mental health supports, in particular, implementation of effective approaches to mental health promotion and early identification and intervention, such as school-wide universal screening for mental health challenges or social emotional learning curricula. Although some factors have been identified as impediments (eg, cost, stigma, privacy), what appears to be fundamentally missing is an organizational framework that would enable effective, efficient, equitable, and relevant integration of the array of professionals, services, and practices that are available in independently functioning disciplines (eg, mental health, child welfare, social work, public health, justice). The authors suggest that schools are more than a partner in an integrated school mental health approach, in large part because of their important position in the American democratic culture.

SCHOOLS AS AN IMPLEMENTATION OPPORTUNITY

Schools offer an ideal and ready-made opportunity to improve the efforts to support the academic, social, emotional, and behavioral development of students. All children in the United States have a right to a free and public K-12 education, and if a child has a disability, special education supports are available from birth. In many communities, preschool opportunities are also available. As such, all children are in school about 6 hours a day, 180 days a year, and at least 12 years of their lives. In this context, adults have daily opportunities to observe and assess student strengths and needs, monitor learning progress and potential, and deliver academic, emotional, and social support.

More specifically, schools are increasingly recognized as an optimal setting for providing a full continuum of mental health supports and services to students.[15,16] With approximately 50 million children and adolescents served by the US public education system,[17] and with increased attention to the connection between mental health and academic success,[18,19] schools are widely considered a natural venue for promoting wellness and preventing the onset or worsening of students' emotional and behavioral difficulties.[20] In fact, the 2009 Institute of Medicine report, *Preventing Mental, Emotional, and Behavioral Disorders Among Young People: Progress and Possibilities*, emphasized the importance of schools as a site for mental health promotion and prevention and identified several promising and evidence-based mental health prevention practices designed for school-based delivery.[20] Support is growing for promoting students' mental health via the implementation of social emotional learning curricula in schools,[21] which focus on developing social and emotional skills and the impact of one's emotions on other aspects of life. Schools are also well-positioned to provide targeted mental health intervention and treatment to students, often in partnership with community mental health systems and providers. In fact, data are mounting that it is in the best interest of schools and districts to provide such interventions to effectively promote students' academic success.[3,9]

From a mental health perspective, one could not ask for a better opportunity to support the healthy social, emotional, and behavioral development of young children, and to identify and address mental health issues before or early after their onset. All mental health and school personnel could work together to support the healthy development of all students by strengthening protective factors, reduce the exacerbation of existing risk factors, and screen for conditions that might indicate development of later emotional, social, and mental health difficulties. In particular, early identification and intervention of mental illness have been linked to an array of positive outcomes, including higher academic achievement, less intensive services, higher social and occupational functioning, less psychological distress, and fewer costs/burdens to the larger system of care. Increasing amounts of research results support the positive impact of early universal interventions, including mental health literacy for teachers and students,[22] social emotional learning,[21] and classroom behavior management strategies.[20]

MULTITIERED SYSTEMS OF SUPPORT

Response to Intervention (RtI) is a multitiered approach to the early identification and support of students with learning and/or behavioral needs. Within an RtI framework, all students receive high-quality instruction in the general education classroom, and struggling learners are identified and provided with additional interventions to accelerate their rate of learning. Similarly, all students should be supported with universal behavioral and emotional supports (such as positive behavior support strategies and social emotional competencies), and those with emotional or behavioral challenges would then be offered additional support services. Services are often delivered within a 3-tiered framework of intensive, targeted, and universal supports (**Fig. 1**). These services may be provided by a variety of school staff, including educators (regular and special) and other support staff (eg, psychologists, occupational therapists).

In 1996, the reauthorization of the Education of Individuals with Disabilities Act legislated an increase in technical assistance to state and local education agencies

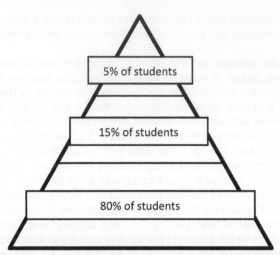

5% of students

15% of students

80% of students

Fig. 1. Multitiered system of support. Level 3: intensive supports that are individualized to meet the unique needs of each student who is already displaying a particular concern or problem. Level 2: targeted supports that are provided for groups of students who have been identified as being at risk for a given concern or problem. When problems are identified early and supports put in place, positive youth development is promoted and problems can be eliminated or reduced. Level 1: universal supports that all students receive. When there is a strong *foundation in promoting wellness and positive life skills,* concerns or problems can be prevented or significantly reduced.

to enhance educational supports for students with emotional or behavioral problems. The National Center on Positive Behavioral Interventions and Supports (PBIS) was established and has since refined and validated a behavior support and technical assistance framework developed around the RtI approach to enhance implementation of empirically supported behavioral interventions for students. As an example of a multitiered system of behavioral support, PBIS has several core features that can be applied to systematic integration of mental health supports into education: universal screening, continuous progress monitoring, team-driven data-based coordination and problem-solving, evidence-based behavioral interventions that are integrated into a continuum of support, sustained and scalable implementation fidelity, and cultural and contextual responsiveness[23,24] (www.pbis.org, Center on Positive Behavioral Interventions and Supports). Using the classroom and school opportunity, 4 specific strategies to improve integration of mental health into the education system are discussed: Workforce training, Family-School-Community Teaming, Resource Mapping, and EBP Implementation.

STRATEGIES TO INTEGRATE MENTAL HEALTH INTO EDUCATION
Workforce Training

In general, the mental health system in the United States is plagued with serious workforce issues, including challenges with recruitment and retention of staff, low wages and benefits, poor supervision, and lack of relevant and effective training, with perhaps the largest concern being quality of care.[25,26] As a concentrated effort to improve the quality of care, child and adolescent mental health is increasingly emphasizing EBPs in the provision of care. However, even when in-depth training is provided, child and adolescent mental health providers often fail to adopt and implement empirically supported interventions because of a lack of implementation support once the training is completed.[27–29] These workforce issues certainly exist in school mental health and may even be compounded by the marginalization of mental health in schools and the unique complexities of working in the school environment (eg, space, time constraints, educational pressures). Simultaneously, educators and school-employed support staff report inadequate training and limited support with respect to promoting student mental health and addressing student mental health problems.[30,31] It is essential that the community mental health workforce is prepared to engage with and work in schools, and educators and other school professionals are similarly prepared to address student mental health and to integrate community professionals into their systems of care for students.

There is limited research addressing the type of preservice and/or in-service professional training needed for a successful school mental health workforce. Ball and colleagues[32] identified professional competencies related to school mental health, including school social work, special education, general education, and school health. Results of their exploratory study yielded 7 core competencies areas in (1) key policies and laws; (2) interprofessional collaboration; (3) cross-systems collaboration; (4) provision of academic, social-emotional, and behavioral learning supports; (5) data-driven decision-making; (6) personal and professional growth and well-being; and (7) cultural competence. These 7 theme areas comprise 51 competencies, of which Brandt and colleagues[33] identified 17 as being unique to mental health practice in schools (**Box 1**). As the child and adolescent mental health workforce is being

---

Box 1
Competencies for mental health providers in schools

Building positive relationships

Representing mental health to school staff

Providing effective consultation

Promoting and supporting mental health

Knowledge of evidence-based learning supports

Identify, describe, and explain the differing roles and responsibilities

Provide classroom evidence-based strategies for students with behavioral and/or emotional difficulties

Identify and know the protocols for accessing various resources

Identify, describe, and explain risk and protective factors

Effectively navigate school-based services through appropriate prereferral and referral processes

Demonstrate an ability to prioritize mental health promotion, prevention, and early intervention

Collect, analyze, and synthesize data for evidence-based decision-making

Demonstrate knowledge of the three-tiered model of intervention

Provide classroom evidence-based strategies for students with learning difficulties or disabilities

Identify, describe, and explains key policies

Build the capacity of others by providing professional development

Understands typical school improvement planning processes

prepared, ways to improve their skills in these school-specific competencies may be considered, particularly given the increased attention to schools as a natural and important venue for mental health promotion and treatment.

In addition to the mental health workforce, it is critical to engage all school personnel in addressing student mental health. Given the prevalence of children's mental health concerns and the reality that mental health issues impact functioning in school, the modern job description for teachers includes aspects of mental health promotion, prevention, and intervention.[34] Of all the adults in the school building, teachers have the most access to students, are often the first to identify problems (eg, academic, social, emotional, behavioral), and are needed to help address the mental health issues that are barriers to learning for their students. In the United States, the Surgeon General has identified teachers as "frontline" mental health workers, who should be trained to recognize and manage childhood and adolescent mental health difficulties.[35] This sentiment was echoed by the President's New Freedom Commission on Mental Health,[16(p58)] which concluded that, "while schools are primarily concerned with education, mental health is essential to learning as well as to social and emotional development. Because of this important interplay between emotional health and school success, schools must be partners in the mental health of our children."

Although teachers generally accept that they have a duty to care for the mental health of their students, they feel unprepared to do so effectively.[34] Both new and experienced teachers report feeling unprepared to recognize and intervene with students facing mental health challenges.[36] As Burke and Paternite[37(p21-22)] poignantly describe, "Although teachers typically receive extensive pre-service and in-service preparation in curriculum and instruction, they receive little or no education concerning the intra- and interpersonal dimensions of teaching and learning in classrooms. Teachers, ill-equipped to deal with mental health needs—either their students' or their own—are left to their own devices to cope." Three areas of psychology are particularly relevant to teaching: (1) child and adolescent development, (2) mental health problem identification and early intervention, and (3) behavior management techniques. Currently, teacher training includes some instruction on child and adolescent development, but very little attention is given to topics on mental health or behavior management. Despite the recognition of a need for teachers to have mental health–related knowledge and skills to identify students in need and to help address the barriers to learning, currently no national mandates require teachers to receive training related to mental health.

Family-School-Community Teaming

To promote student mental health, schools and community partners, including families, must be committed to working together to build or enhance a multitiered, systemic approach that addresses the interconnected academic, social, emotional, and behavioral needs of *all* students. It is critical to integrate mental health and education teams into unified teams that consider the "whole child," addressing academic as well as social-emotional-behavioral considerations. To be successful, this integration requires that school partners are open to having community partners (eg, community mental health providers, child-serving agency workers, advocates, health care providers) and families engage in all aspects of the interconnected system.

Readiness requires a willingness to move beyond a "walled" model in which only school-based staff is part of a child's support team to one that embraces true cross-stakeholder and cross-system partnership. In forming such partnerships, it is necessary for school, family, and community partners to be willing to have a discussion about overlapping priorities and needs and to consider how a partnership could be beneficial to meeting the goals of each partner group. For instance, it may be important for school-employed and community-employed staff to discuss how their roles and responsibilities are distinct, how they will collaborate to facilitate seamless referral pathways and comprehensive care, and how they will avoid "turf battles." Ideally, these discussions will reflect a recognition of the unique requirements and mandates and strengths and limitations of each discipline or stakeholder group. Some questions to consider during the teaming process are included in **Box 2**.

A multitiered system of support at the school level often has 3 teams with one team focusing on the planning, implementation, and evaluation of universal interventions and the other teams focusing on second and third tier interventions (some schools, depending on size and number of team members, prefer to have only a universal team and a combined tier 2 and tier 3 team, and smaller schools may only be able to have one team to address all 3 tiers). It is helpful to have a regularly scheduled time and frequency for meeting and a process for holding meetings that includes clear rules, expectations, and action planning that are informed by and uses data throughout to track progress toward action items and to monitor success of interventions. Data can be used in many different ways, including helping to identify students who could most benefit from services and/or interventions and can help demonstrate the impact of services. For example, some teams are using measures, such as the Child and Adolescent Needs and Strengths Screening[38] and the Global Appraisal of Individual Needs[39] scale, to screen for or identify children who may be in need of mental health supports. Data are also used to track the progress of students who have received services to determine if the services are impacting outcomes important to the team (eg, academic, social, emotional, and behavioral indicators).

A challenge for coordination of efforts can result when data are not shared across school and community providers. Identifying issues related to data sharing (HIPAA, FERPA) should be done up front and consideration should be given to securing

---

Box 2
Questions to consider during family-school-community teaming

- What are the *outcomes valued* by all team members (families, schools, community partners), and how are these outcomes measured to document impact of interventions?

- How will all team members (including community mental health professionals) *support implementation* of interventions across all 3 tiers (universal, selected, targeted)?

- Can school-employed and community-employed mental health professionals provide care to the same student simultaneously? If so, how will they *ensure services are complementary*?

- *Who is authorized to provide services* mandated within students' IEPs?

- What factors determine whether a student with identified mental health problems is *referred to a school-versus-community*-employed mental health professional?

- Who is responsible for conducting *mental health screening and assessment*, and how are findings conveyed to all team members?

- How do school personnel (administrators, teachers, student support staff) *receive feedback* about referrals, intervention implementation, and outcomes from school-based community professionals?

- How is feedback about referrals, intervention implementation, and outcomes integrated into a *continuous quality improvement process*?

- What strategies will be used to engage and *meaningfully involve families* in the teaming process?

consents and release of information to allow sharing of data across system partners in an effort to have a more comprehensive picture of student progress across educational and social-emotional-behavioral domains. Consideration should also be given to how data will best be collected, analyzed, and shared from the inception of the partnership and should be clearly outlined in any Memoranda of Understanding (MOU).

Resource Mapping

Most schools and school districts have developed at least some partnerships with and regularly make referrals to an array of organizations and programs that can complement educational supports. Nevertheless, schools and school districts do not strategically map and identify the comprehensive array of school-based and community supports available for several reasons:

- The decision to implement a support was made because of a particular funding stream or mandate or as a reaction to a particular incident.
- Supports are often developed in isolation rather than as part of an integrated system.
- Awareness of a given program may be limited to a school or a small subset of individuals within a school—even when services may be available to the larger community.

Over time, tracking of available supports and resources, services provided, and eligibility requirements no longer occurs and significant gaps in care, as well as to an unintended duplication of services, are experienced.

Resource mapping offers a strategy to help schools and school districts to consider the array of supports and resources available to students and families and provides a visual picture of how services and programs are related and information on who can and how to access the supports and resources. Ideally, availability of resources is mapped across a multitiered system of support reflecting a more comprehensive system of care. Family-school-community teams can use mapping tools to identify student and family resources that promote student mental health across the continuum of support, from promotion and prevention to tertiary intervention. Identification of resources across both the school and the community can minimize duplication of services and support coordinated care. Mapping may also promote opportunities for cross-system and interdisciplinary training and facilitate streamlined referral and transition processes across systems and programs. An example of a school-community resource map, across 3 tiers of student support, is provided in **Fig. 2.**

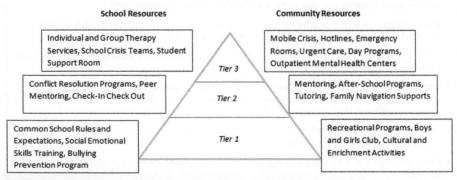

Fig. 2. School-community resource map, across 3 tiers of student support.

As part of the mapping process, it is important that school-community teams document not only the *existence* of programs and resources but also the *impact* of such programs and resources on expected and actual outcomes. By restricting mental health resources to only those with demonstrated impact on desired outcomes, schools and districts can be more prudent in their selection process, thereby increasing efficiency and likelihood of student success.

Resource mapping must be considered an on-going and data-informed process.[40] District and building teams should work together with community partners to develop MOU that specify partnership roles and responsibilities, referral processes, feedback loops, data systems and decision-making rules, and regular scheduled meetings. **Box 3** highlights the objectives of school and district mental health resource mapping.

Implementation of Evidence-Based Practices

As important as specifying EBPs are, so are the systems that are associated with the accurate, sustainable, and adapted implementation of those practices. Implementation science suggests that high-quality effective interventions will fail if specific drivers that promote implementation success are not addressed.[28,41,42] Unfortunately, mental health interventions are often poorly implemented in schools because of insufficient funding, initiative overload and overlap, poorly trained implementers, ineffective data-based decisions-making systems, and misalignment with intended and actual outcomes.[43,44] Poor implementation has resulted in iatrogenic effects, including reactive disciplinary practices, multiple changes in programs implemented, inequitable outcomes for disadvantaged students, and consumer dissatisfaction and lack of confidence.[9,45]

Given these consequences, education and mental health systems should consider using implementation science to more effectively integrate a full continuum of evidence-based mental health practices into schools. Sugai and Stephan[46] review key questions to consider when determining if and how to implement evidence-based mental health practices in schools: (1) Are need and intended outcome specified? (2) Is the most appropriate EBP selected? (3) Is practice adaptable to local context and culture? (4) Is support for local implementation developed? and (5) Is system level continuous progress monitoring and planning in place? These questions have been integrated into an EBP Implementation Framework Self-Assessment tool for schools (**Table 1**) and are considered in the school case example provided.

Box 3
Objectives of multitiered resource mapping

School and district resource mapping offers a systematic process to:

- Identify all available resources/programs in the school and surrounding community
- Recognize gaps in services/resources that can inform strategic planning and outreach
- Better understand program requirements to access services (eg, insurance, hours of operation, eligibility)
- Avoid duplication of services and valuable resources
- Better match service needs with available resources/programs
- Increase awareness of underused partnerships/resources
- Cultivate relationships with new programs/resources that can address gaps in care

Table 1		
Evidence-based practice implementation framework self-assessment		
Main Question	**Subquestions**	**Decision**
1. Are need and intended outcomes specified?	• Is need described in measurable terms? • Is importance for addressing need high? • Is intended outcome described in measurable terms?	Yes/No?
2. Is most appropriate evidenced-based practice selected?	• Does evidence exist to support effectiveness of practice? • Does outcome associated with practice align with stated need and intended outcome? • Is practice consistent with other practices and initiatives currently in place?	Yes/No?
3. Is practice adaptable to local context or culture?	• Are data for decision-making culturally valid? • Is practice culturally relevant? • Is intended outcome culturally equitable and representative? • Is implementer system culturally knowledgeable?	Yes/No?
4. Is support for local implementation developed?	• Is leadership support multileveled and distributed? • Is institutional or organizational support available? • Is implementation driver-based? • Is implementation action planning phase-based? • Are implementation exemplars documented? • Is continuous progress monitoring system available?	Yes/No?
5. Is system level continuous progress monitoring in place for implementation enhancements?	• Is practice being implemented with fidelity? • Are students benefiting from implementation? • Is interrelatedness of implementation fidelity and student progress/benefit examined concurrently?	Yes/No?

CASE EXAMPLE

In a suburban middle school, teachers in the seventh grade level meeting have been discussing concerns about many of their students this school year being out of their seat often, easily distracted, poorly organized, disruptive, and inattentive in class. Some teachers referred students for attention deficit hyperactivity disorder (ADHD) and executive functioning evaluations to their school mental health team and tried to share ideas about classroom management. Some of these same students are receiving special education services. In addition, after training provided as part of the workforce development efforts of their school district on trauma-informed schools, the teachers became concerned about whether their students' concentration problems could be due to trauma. Several teachers agreed, and they requested that the administration and student support team address the issue. Fortunately, the school had established a multitiered teaming process in which school and community mental health and student support providers regularly met to strategically discuss data and interventions for students across 3 tiers of student support (universal, selected, targeted).

Based on resource mapping conducted by their school administration and the current school mental health team, specific community resources for referral had been identified as well as a local community psychiatrist who partnered with the school to provide regular consultation. However, several gaps still remained for school resources, particularly at tiers 2 and 3, to address ADHD and trauma among students, and coordination of mental health and special education services was needed. Therefore, the Tier 2/Tier 3 team members agreed to review student data about hyperactivity and inattention (such as observing student behavior in the second grade classrooms and reviewing school mental health and 504 Plan referrals for these concerns), make intervention decisions according to the data findings, and report back to the teaching staff within 2 weeks. To reduce overlap, competing resources, and communication confusions, all staff also agreed to focus on student needs and strengths (rather than label or diagnosis), match of effective interventions and treatments to those needs and strengths (rather than provider), implementation fidelity and capacity (rather than unsupported use), and continuous progress monitoring and adaptation (rather than non-data-based decision-making).

Implementation Question 1: Are Need and Intended Outcome Specified?

Based on the Implementation Framework Self-Assessment, the team answered 3 important questions: (1) What is the need? (2) How important is addressing this need? and (3) What would the intended outcomes look like to have successfully addressed this need? An examination of the referral forms to the 504 team and school mental health staff over the past school year revealed that 70% of the referrals indicated some concern about hyperactivity such as out of seat behavior, inattention/poor concentration, and specific concern about ADHD or history of a traumatic event. However, classroom observations conducted by the Tier 2/Tier 3 team revealed that only 2 of the 6 second grade classrooms had student disruptive behaviors so severe that classroom-wide missed instruction resulted, although all of the classrooms had at least one student with disruptive behavior, inattention, and/or hyperactivity that required attention. Classroom observation indicated that 12% of teachers' instructional time across all classrooms in the second grade was missed having to attend to disruptive behaviors, and 7 students were missing more than 20% of instructional time related to disruptive/inattentive behavior.

In addition, the Tier 2/Tier 3 team, in consultation with the community psychiatrist and school mental health program, selected and collected brief universal screeners for trauma and ADHD. The results of these screeners were consistent with observational data; some classroom needs were identified and relatively few individual students would benefit from targeted support to reduce missed instruction. Team members agreed that the need to address classroom behaviors and to support the few students with identified problems was very important to the school.

They defined success as increases in uninterrupted instructional time, academic engagement, student compliance to academic-task requests by teachers, and quarterly grades. The criterion for success was specified as only 5% of teachers' instructional time devoted to correcting disruptive behaviors, and less than 10% of instructional time being lost for students with identified inattention and disruptive behaviors. Given that the need was clearly defined, the need for improvement was high, and the outcome important and achievable, the school was ready to look for possible solutions.

Implementation Question 2: Is Most Appropriate Evidenced-Based Practice Selected?

The team focused on practices supported by evidence to address the specified behavior issue. In particular, EBPs for all 3 tiers of support were desired, given the needs for supporting students with varying levels of need for behavior and executive functioning supports. Several online databases (examples include SAMHSA's National Registry of Evidence-based Programs and Practices, Blueprints for Healthy Youth Development, and Institute of Education Sciences What Works Clearinghouse) were reviewed to find evidence-based programs, with preference for programs that used experimental studies (eg, randomized control trials, quasi-experimental designs, single subject designs), and had been conducted in school settings.

For Tier 1, the team determined that current universal classroom and school-wide practices (Positive Behavior Implementation and Support; www.pbis.org) were sufficiently evidence-based, but implementation was haphazard across the school. Thus, effective implementation supports such as teacher retraining and ongoing support and coaching were targeted.[47]

For Tier 2, the team selected 2 programs to serve students with positive trauma or ADHD screenings, respectively, Cognitive Behavioral Intervention for Trauma in Schools (CBITS)[48] and Challenging Horizons Program.[49] These programs would be provided by school mental health teams as a pull-out group intervention for selected students on the basis of universal screening scores. In addition, school personnel, including general and special educators and special student support personnel, was involved to enable behavior and intervention support across settings, peers, and adults.

For Tier 3, the mental health team and community-partnered psychiatrist worked together to provide individual level evidence-based cognitive behavioral psychotherapies and executive functioning skill coaching to serve children with the most significant impairment. As for Tier 2, the activities and implementation efforts of the Tier 3 team were communicated and coordinated with all school personnel to ensure an integrated and comprehensive understanding and implementation.

To support efforts across all tiers, all professionals in the school building, including both community-partnered and school-employed mental health personnel, were trained in the basic logic, principles, and practices of a tiered continuum of support. For example, general education personnel learned about the importance of their Tier 1 efforts to maximize the impact of Tier 2/3 practices and of their active involvement and participation in Tier 2/3 plans for students in their classrooms. Similarly, Tier 2/3 team members learned the importance of their participation in Tier 1 activities with respect to prevention and supporting the academic goals of the school. Also, community mental health providers were invited to student 504 Plan and Individualized Education Programs (IEP) team meetings to exchange information with school staff about how to support individual students' educational goals. Before this collaboration, MOUs about data-sharing permissions, within the bounds of HIPPA and FERPA, were established collaboratively with family input and consent. The overall goal was to establish a common expectation about supporting the needs of all students, a common language and vocabulary about implementing behavior support, and a common routine or implementation process by which decisions were made and implementation was conducted.

Implementation Question 3: Is Practice Adaptable to Local Context or Culture?

Given the complexity of the school context, the team had to consider how implementation of the selected practice would be influenced by local contextual and cultural factors, such as language, social behavior variations in meaning, normative behaviors and expectations, individual or group cultural learning histories, and so on.[50,51] The team understood that selection, implementation, and impact of any practice would be affected by what students, their families, school personnel, community members, and mental health providers brought to the many opportunities to interact, communicate, and collaborate.

Thus, based on the Implementation Framework Self-Assessment, the team considered 4 main questions: (1) Are data for decision-making culturally valid? (2) Are practices culturally relevant? (3) Are intended outcomes culturally equitable and representative? and (4) Are implementer systems culturally knowledgeable?[52] For example, CBITS was selected by the Tier 2/3 team because it was developed specifically for a school-based group format to enhance coping for students exposed to traumatic life events. In addition, CBITS has been tested in grades 3 through 8, which matched the grade levels of the middle school and includes features that promote parent, teacher, and mental health personnel collaboration (eg, parent and teacher educational sessions). However, the team was also aware that the language systems of the families, the learning histories of the students, and the prior expectations and experiences of the implementers would need to be considered to ensure that communications were clear and understandable, implementation opportunities were engaging and participatory, implementation and outcome expectations were valued, and so on. By considering these contextual and cultural factors, the team could increase the likelihood that CBITS could have maximum impact on student outcomes and benefit.

Implementation Question 4: Is Support for Local Implementation Developed?

The school team understood that traditional professional development approaches (eg, 1-time in-services, passive video-training and Webinars, discussion-oriented communities of practices) alone have been insufficient in producing accurate, system-wide, and sustained implementation of an EBP.[53,54] Therefore, the team was careful to consider factors that support local implementation, such as leadership support and participation, comprehensive and continuous professional development, on-going coaching and implementation feedback, data based decision-making, team-driven implementation, and sustainable funding (PBIS Center, Implementation Blueprint, www.pbis.org, 2010). These implementation drivers or factors are important to support capacity for local implementation for practices and systems across all 3 tiers and represent the organizational structures or enablers of the implementation process and serve as the means for building expert implementation capacity.[28,55]

The school counselor was the chairperson of the Tier 2/Tier 3 team that also included the special educator, school psychologist, community psychiatrist, and the school-based community mental health clinician and was given authority to lead the development, adaptation, implementation, and evaluation of the 2 EBPs, CBITS and CHR. The school principal fully supported the EBP effort by attending team meetings, scheduling and protecting meeting times, supporting behavior policy recommendations, and communicating EBP support at school faculty meetings. The district superintendent acknowledged the school's EBP implementation efforts by reducing emphasis on district mandates that were not directly relevant to the school's improvement plan and permitting use of professional development days for preparing staff for the EBP implementation. The district student special support unit was made available to the school team.

The Tier 2/Tier 3 team in the example school was given authority by its principal to make scheduling adjustments and resource reallocations to enable professional development activities, material development, and data analyses. In addition, funds were combined from the school district budget and community-partnered mental health agencies to fund the training and material costs of the EBPs and to enable on-going district level coaching to maximize implementation fidelity and sustainability. Equally as important, the teams established a data system (see Implementation Question 5) that enabled (1) easy data input, (2) immediate data outputs, (3) decision-making on the most important evaluation questions for each tier, and (4) both summative and formative implementation fidelity and student progress monitoring.

The school understood that sustained and meaningful support for their EBP implementation was directly linked to institutional supports and engaged in a variety of activities to bolster support. The EBP team provided weekly data-based progress updates to faculty, parents, and district support units, and the principal included EBP progress reports in his monthly school board status presentations, which included student progress and staff implementation fidelity. The school-based community mental health clinician provided monthly updates to the community program's Clinical Director to ensure organizational support for continued involvement in the EBP efforts. The EBP team met 3 hours every other week in the first year with the district behavior support specialist who had expertise in the EBP practices and systems to develop an action plan for development and implementation of EBP. The team leader assumed coaching responsibilities and worked closely with the district behavior support specialist to increase adherence commitments and agreements included in the action plan.

The school-based community mental health clinician was actively involved with the development of the EBP team and helped administer a quarterly EBP self-assessment to evaluate establishment and operation of the EBP practices and systems. In year 2, the team's professional development schedule was reduced to 2-hour monthly meetings, and coaching and evaluation functions continued. The community mental health clinician role also shifted during the second year to include coleading training and coaching activities and conducting skill-based sessions for students who needed additional cognitive behavior techniques, such as coping skills and trauma-informed problem-solving techniques.

The assistant principal and team leader were given decision-making authority by the principal for the establishment and operation of the EBP practices and systems and provided monthly progress updates to the school faculty and semiannual progress reports to the district behavior support team and school board. At the end of the first school year, with all these efforts in place, the team was on their way to achieve full implementation in approximately 3 years.

Implementation Question 5: Is System Level Continuous Progress Monitoring in Place for Implementation Enhancements?

The final element in the development of support for local implementation of a practice is the continuous collection of data or information to guide enhancements and modifications that would improve implementation outcomes.[28,56,57] The EBP team completed a procedural self-assessment to examine the extent to which all EBP steps were being completed accurately and on schedule. The team also examined the progress being made by the EBP group as a whole and by individual students. If implementation inadequacies were noted, the EBP coach and team leader would provide a booster to improve accuracy of implementation. At weekly team meetings, individual student progress was reviewed. If progress was on track, discussions focused on enhancing outcomes further, changing outcome criterion, and/or modifying target behavior outcomes. If progress was not on track, the team discussed implementation fidelity, intervention adjustments or replacement, and setting of new outcome target behaviors and/or criterion.

DISCUSSION

Schools have an important responsibility to develop the academic competence of their citizenry; however, schools are also learning 2 important messages. First, academic achievement is linked to the social, emotional, and behavioral characteristics of their students, and second, classrooms and schools offer an important place for assessing and supporting the mental health needs of students. These 2 messages create an ideal opportunity for schools and mental health to join forces. In this article, the context and 4 strategies that might be considered in moving the mental health and education fields toward effective integration are described.

Three considerations are emphasized. First, research support that connects student mental health to academic success is rapidly accumulating.[9,58,59] Therefore, to support their academic mission, schools have a vested interest in improving and supporting student well-being and addressing mental health problems among students.

Second, recognition is growing that schools have an ethical imperative to attend not just to the "academic" success of students but also to the social, emotional, and behavioral development of students.[60] The total school experience influences student success in family, community, career, postsecondary education, and personal domains.

Finally, unlike any other social agency, schools offer a societal opportunity that is consistent, predictable, and available. Schools are open 8 hours a day, 180 days a year, every year for 12 years. Schools represent a place where kids can access the supports that will enable them to learn and grow emotionally, socially, and behaviorally. Therefore, the mental health field must strategically consider the structures and processes that will facilitate effective integration, including efforts to improve workforce development, family-school-community teaming, resource mapping, and application of implementation science to school-based mental health intervention delivery.

Child and adolescent psychiatrists are critical partners in the development of multi-tiered systems of student mental health support. As we move toward systematic implementation of such systems, schools and their mental health teams will be better able to identify and support those children with mental illness early, and hence, be better positioned to efficiently use the expertise of child and adolescent psychiatrists to support those students. Furthermore, child and adolescent psychiatrists can work with schools to consider how to support students across all tiers of the continuum. For example, their expertise in child development and brain science can be used to understand the complex interplay between academic development and social-emotional development and to develop school-based curricula and interventions that promote both personal well-being and academic success.

DISCLOSURE

The preparation of this article was supported in part by the Center for School Mental Health and a grant from the Office of Adolescent Health, Maternal, and Child Health Bureau, Health Resources and Services Administration, Department of Health and Human Services (U45MC00174), and by the Technical Assistance Center on Positive Behavioral Interventions and Supports and a grant from the Office of Special Education Programs, US Department of Education (H326S980003). Opinions expressed herein do not necessarily reflect the position of the US Department of Health and Human Services or the Department of Education, and such endorsements should not be inferred. For information about the Centers, go to https://csmh.umaryland.edu or www.pbis.org, or for information related to this article, contact the authors.

REFERENCES

1. Guerra NG, Williams KR. Implementation of school-based wellness centers. Psychol Sch 2003;40(5):473–87.
2. Horner RH, Sugai G, Anderson CM. Examining the evidence base for school-wide positive behavior support. Focus Except Child 2010;42(8):1–14.
3. Zins JE, Weissberg RP, Wang MC, et al. Building academic success on social and emotional learning: What does the research say? New York: Teachers College Press; 2004.
4. Domitrovich CE, Greenberg MT. The study of implementation: current findings from effective programs that prevent mental disorders in school-aged children. J Educ Psychol Consult 2000;11(2):193–221.
5. Durlak JA, DuPre EP. Implementation matters: a review of research on the influence of implementation on program outcomes and the factors affecting implementation. Am J Community Psychol 2008;41(3–4):327–50.
6. Aarons GA, Sommerfeld DH, Walrath-Greene CM. Evidence-based practice implementation: the impact of public versus private sector organization type on organizational support, provider attitudes, and adoption of evidence-based practice. Implement Sci 2009;4(1):83.
7. Forman SG, Olin SS, Hoagwood KE, et al. Evidence-based interventions in schools: developers' views of implementation barriers and facilitators. School Ment Health 2009;1(1):26–36.
8. Stephan S, Brandt N, Lever N, et al. Key priorities, challenges and opportunities to advance an integrated mental health and education research agenda. Adv Sch Ment Health Promot 2012;5(2):125–38.
9. Dix KL, Slee PT, Lawson MJ, et al. Implementation quality of whole-school mental health promotion and students' academic performance. Child Adolesc Ment Health 2011;17(1):45–51.
10. Elias MJ, Zins JE, Graczyk PA, et al. Implementation, sustainability, and scaling up of social-emotional and academic innovations in public schools. School Psych Rev 2003;32(3):303–19.
11. Mcintosh K, Mercer SH, Hume AE, et al. Factors related to sustained implementation of schoolwide positive behavior support. Except Child 2013;79(3):293–311.
12. Kessler RC, Angermeyer M, Anthony JC, et al. Lifetime prevalence and age-of-onset distributions of mental disorders in the World Health Organization's World Mental Health Survey Initiative. World Psychiatry 2007;6(3):168.
13. Stroul B, Goldman S, Pires S, et al. Expanding systems of care: Improving the lives of children, youth, and families. Washington, DC: Georgetown University Center for Child and Human Development, National Technical Assistance Center for Children's Mental Health; 2012.
14. Hoge MA, Morris JA, Daniels AS, et al. An action plan for behavioral health workforce development. Cincinnati (OH): Annapolis Coalition on the Behavioral Health Workforce; 2007.
15. Farmer E, Burns B, Phillips S, et al. Pathways into and through mental health services for children and adolescents. Psychiatr Serv 2003;54:60–6.
16. Hogan MF. New Freedom Commission report: the President's New Freedom Commission: recommendations to transform mental health care in America. Psychiatr Serv 2003;54(11):1467–74.
17. Chen C, Sable J, Mitchell L, et al. Documentation to the NCES common core of data public elementary/secondary school universe survey: school year 2009–10 (NCES 2011-348). U.S. Department of Education. Washington, DC: National

Center for Education Statistics; 2011. Available at: http://nces.ed.gov/pubsearch/pubs.info.asp?pubid=2011348.
18. Atkins MS, Hoagwood KE, Kutash K, et al. Toward the integration of education and mental health in schools. Adm Policy Ment Health 2010;37(1–2):40–7.
19. Hoagwood KE, Olin SS, Kerker BD, et al. Empirically based school interventions targeted at academic and mental health functioning. J Emot Behav Disord 2007; 15:66–92.
20. National Research Council and Institute of Medicine Committee on Prevention of Mental Disorders and Substance Abuse Children, Youth, and Young Adults: Research Advances and Promising Interventions. Preventing mental, emotional, and behavioral disorders among young people: progress and possibilities. In: O'Connell ME, Boat T, Warner KE, editors. Board of children youth, and families, division of behavioral and social sciences and education. Washington, DC: The National Academies Press; 2009.
21. Durlak JA, Weissberg RP, Dymnicki AB, et al. The impact of enhancing students' social and emotional learning: a meta-analysis of school-based universal interventions. Child Dev 2011;82(1):405–32.
22. Wei Y, Kutcher S, Szumilas M. Comprehensive school mental health: an integrated "school-based pathway to care" model for Canadian secondary schools. McGill J Educ 2011;46(2):213–29.
23. Sugai G, Horner RH, Dunlap G, et al. Applying positive behavior support and functional behavioral assessment in schools. J Posit Behav Interv 2000;2:131–43.
24. Walker HM, Horner RH, Sugai G, et al. Integrated approaches to preventing antisocial behavior patterns among school-age children and youth. J Emot Behav Disord 1996;4(4):194–209.
25. Paternite CF, Johnston TC. Rationale and strategies for central involvement of educators in effective school-based mental health programs. J Youth Adolesc 2005; 34(1):41–9.
26. Stemler SE, Elliott JG, Grigorenko EL, et al. There's more to teaching than instruction: seven strategies for dealing with the practical side of teaching 1. Educ Stud 2006;32(1):101–18.
27. Chorpita BF, Yim LM, Donkervoet JC, et al. Toward large-scale implementation of empirically supported treatments for children: a review and observations by the Hawaii Empirical Basis to Services Task Force. Clin Psychol Sci Pract 2002; 9(2):165–90.
28. Fixsen DL, Naoom SF, Blase KA, et al. Implementation research: a synthesis of the literature (Louis de la Parte Florida Mental Health Institute Publication No. 231). Tampa (FL): University of South Florida, Louis de la Parte Florida Mental Health Institute, National Implementation Research Network; 2005.
29. Kazdin AE. Evidence-based treatment and practice: new opportunities to bridge clinical research and practice, enhance the knowledge base, and improve patient care. Am Psychol 2008;63(3):146.
30. Brownell MT, Pajares F. Teacher efficacy and perceived success in mainstreaming students with learning and behavior problems. Teacher Education and Special Education 1999;22(3):154–64.
31. Walter HJ, Gouze K, Lim KG. Teachers' beliefs about mental health needs in inner city elementary schools. J Am Acad Child Adolesc Psychiatry 2006;45(1): 61–8.
32. Ball A, Anderson-Butcher D, Mellin EA, et al. A cross-walk of professional competencies involved in expanded school mental health: an exploratory study. School Ment Health 2010;2(3):114–24.

33. Brandt N, Gibson J, Lever N, et al. School mental health workforce competencies. Baltimore (MD): Center for School Mental Health; 2013.

34. Rothì DM, Leavey G, Best R. On the front-line: teachers as active observers of pupils' mental health. Teach Teach Educ 2008;24(5):1217–31.

35. US Public Health Service. Report of the Surgeon General's Conference on Children's Mental Health: A National Action Agenda. Washington, DC: Department of Health and Human Services; 2000.

36. Koller JR, Osterlind SJ, Paris K, et al. Differences between novice and expert teachers' undergraduate preparation and ratings of importance in the area of children's mental health. Int J Ment Health Promot 2004;6(2):40–5.

37. Burke RW, Paternite CE. Teacher engagement in expanded school mental health. In: Evans SW, Weist MD, Serpell ZN, editors. Advances in school-based mental health, vol. 2. Kingston (NJ): Civic Research Institute; 2007. p. 1–15.

38. Anderson RL, Lyons JS, Giles DM, et al. Reliability of the child and adolescent needs and strengths-mental health (CANS-MH) scale. J Child Fam Stud 2003; 12(3):279–89.

39. Dennis ML. Global appraisal of individual needs (GAIN) manual: administration, scoring, and interpretation. Bloomington (IL): Lighthouse Publications; 1998.

40. Lever N, Castle M, Cammack N, et al. Resource mapping in schools and school districts: a resource guide. Baltimore (MD): Center for School Mental Health; 2014.

41. Blase KA, Fixsen DL, Naoom SF, et al. Operationalizing implementation: strategies and methods. Tampa (FL): University of South Florida, Louis de la Parte Florida Mental Health Institute; 2005.

42. Blase K, Fixsen D. Core intervention components: identifying and operationalizing what makes programs work. ASPE research brief. Washington, DC: US Department of Health and Human Services; 2013.

43. Harn B, Parisi D, Stoolmiller M. Balancing fidelity with flexibility and fit: what do we really know about fidelity of implementation in schools? Except Child 2013;79(2): 181–93.

44. Forman SG, Fagley NS, Chu BC, et al. Factors influencing school psychologists' "Willingness to Implement" evidence-based interventions. School Ment Health 2012;4(4):207–18.

45. Marty D, Rapp C, McHugo G, et al. Factors influencing consumer outcome monitoring in implementation of evidence-based practices: results from the National EBP Implementation Project. Adm Policy Ment Health 2008;35(3):204–11.

46. Sugai G, Stephan S. Considerations for a school mental health implementation framework. In: Barrett S, Eber L, Weist M, editors. Advancing education effectiveness: interconnecting school mental health and school-wide positive behavioral support. 2013. p. 18–33. Available at: www.pbis.org/common/cms/files/pbisresources/Final-Monograph.pdf.

47. Hershfeldt PA, Pell K, Sechrest R, et al. Lessons learned coaching teachers in behavior management: the PBIS plus coaching model. J Educ Psychol Consult 2012;22(4):280–99.

48. Jaycox LH. Cognitive Behavioral Intervention for Trauma in Schools (CBITS). Sopris West; 2003.

49. Evans SW, Serpell ZN, Schultz BK, et al. Cumulative benefits of secondary school-based treatment of students with ADHD. School Psych Rev 2007;36(2): 256–73.

50. Burke RW, Stephan SH. Contextual features of public schools in the United States as settings for mental health promotion. Adv Sch Ment Health Promot 2008;1(1): 52–60.

51. Sugai G, O'Keeffe BV, Fallon LM. A contextual consideration of culture and school-wide positive behavior support. J Posit Behav Interv 2012;14:197–208.
52. Vincent CG, Randall C, Cartledge G, et al. Toward a conceptual integration of cultural responsiveness and schoolwide positive behavior support. J Posit Behav Interv 2011;13(4):219–29.
53. Beidas RS, Kendall PC. Training therapists in evidence-based practice: a critical review of studies from a systems-contextual perspective. Clin Psychol Sci Pract 2010;17(1):1–30.
54. Herschell AD, Kolko DJ, Baumann BL, et al. The role of therapist training in the implementation of psychosocial treatments: a review and critique with recommendations. Clin Psychol Rev 2010;30(4):448–66.
55. OSEP Technical Assistance Center on Positive Behavioral Interventions and Supports. Technical assistance and implementation blueprint for positive behavioral interventions and supports (PBIS). Eugene, OR: University of Oregon; 2014. Available at: www.pbis.org.
56. Aarons GA, Hurlburt M, Horwitz SM. Advancing a conceptual model of evidence-based practice implementation in public service sectors. Adm Policy Ment Health 2011;38(1):4–23.
57. Glasgow RE, Klesges LM, Dzewaltowski DA, et al. Evaluating the impact of health promotion programs: using the RE-AIM framework to form summary measures for decision making involving complex issues. Health Educ Res 2006;21(5):688–94.
58. Massey O, Armstrong K, Boroughs M, et al. Mental health services in schools: a qualitative analysis of challenges to implementation, operation and sustainability. Psychol Sch 2005;42(4):361–72.
59. Rimm-Kaufman SE, Fan X, Chiu Y, et al. The contribution of the responsive classroom approach on children's academic achievement: results from a three-year longitudinal study. J Sch Psychol 2007;45:401–21.
60. Fazel M, Hoagwood K, Stephan S, et al. Mental health interventions in schools in high-income countries. Lancet Psychiatry 2014;1(5):377–87.

Mental Health Literacy in Secondary Schools
A Canadian Approach

Stan Kutcher, MD, FRCPC, FCAHS[a],*, Alexa Bagnell, MD, FRCPC[b],
Yifeng Wei, MEd[c]

KEYWORDS

- Mental health literacy • School programs • Youth • Knowledge translation
- Mental health promotion

KEY POINTS

- Youth mental health literacy is a key factor in mental health awareness, reducing stigma and improving health-related decision making.
- Schools are an ideal environment within which to embed mental health and health literacy programs.
- Programs for youths need to incorporate information in a twenty-first century learning context, with media and electronic accessibility to material and tools, to develop lifelong health literacy skills and improve mental health outcomes.
- Sustainable and effective mental health literacy knowledge translation programs can be developed for educators using train-the-trainer models with evidence-based materials and tools for use within and beyond the classrooms.
- In Canada, 2 complementary mental health literacy approaches in secondary schools have been advanced to accomplish this goal and have been widely adopted across the country.

INTRODUCTION: HEALTH LITERACY

The long-term health and well-being of all individuals is inextricably linked with the level of education and literacy that individuals attain over the course of their lifetime, including education around health and mental health.[1] The World Health Organization

The authors have nothing to disclose.
[a] Department of Psychiatry, Sun Life Financial Chair in Adolescent Mental Health, IWK Health Centre, Dalhousie University, 5850 University Avenue, PO Box 9700, Halifax, Nova Scotia B3K 6R8, Canada; [b] Child and Adolescent Psychiatry, Department of Psychiatry, IWK Health Centre, 5850 University Avenue, PO Box 9700, Halifax, Nova Scotia B3K 6R8, Canada; [c] Sun Life Financial Chair, IWK Health Centre, 5850 University Avenue, PO Box 9700, Halifax, Nova Scotia B3K 6R8, Canada
* Corresponding author.
E-mail address: Stanley.Kutcher@iwk.nshealth.ca

Child Adolesc Psychiatric Clin N Am 24 (2015) 233–244
http://dx.doi.org/10.1016/j.chc.2014.11.007
1056-4993/15/$ – see front matter © 2015 Elsevier Inc. All rights reserved.

childpsych.theclinics.com

Abbreviations	
CDC	Centers for Disease Control and Prevention
DRSB	Durham Regional School Boards
TDSB	Toronto District School Board
WHO	World Health Organization

(WHO)[2] and national governments, such as Canada, the United States, and Australia, have recognized the importance of enhancing health literacy to improve population health outcomes.[3–5] Health literacy has been both narrowly and more broadly defined. The Centers for Disease Control and Prevention (CDC), for example, defines health literacy as "the capacity to obtain, process and understand basic health information and services to make appropriate health decisions"[6]; other organizations, such as the WHO, have identified health literacy as the knowledge and competencies needed to enhance health care, disease prevention, and health promotion at both individual and population levels.[2] Further extension of this construct has recently been suggested by the WHO as comprising 3 components: functional health literacy, conceptual health literacy, and health literacy as empowerment.[7] Understood in this framework, health literacy goes beyond the individual competencies that the CDC describes to recognize the need for creating the capacity of individuals to be actively applying evidence-based and contextually informed knowledge so that they can act effectively on their own behalf and also on behalf of their families and communities. Mental health literacy is an integral component of general health literacy and has been gaining increasing attention as an important focus globally for mental health interventions. With about one-fifth of the population being affected by mental illness in their lifetime and the high cost of these illnesses to individuals and society,[8] mental health literacy is a critical area for public health intervention. In Canada, youth mental health is increasingly recognized as a key national health concern and has received more focused attention than ever before within our health system.[9] Several unique homegrown national initiatives have addressed youth mental health literacy within Canadian schools.

MENTAL HEALTH LITERACY

Our understanding of mental health literacy has developed from relatively circumscribed definitions in which mental health literacy was primarily understood as the knowledge needed to be able to identify mental disorders[10] to a more nuanced and complex understanding of the requirements for improving mental health outcomes. For example, Jorm,[11] expanding on his early pioneering work in mental health literacy, has identified the following components: recognition of developing mental disorders to facilitate early help seeking, knowledge of professional help and effective treatments available, knowledge of effective self-help strategies, knowledge and skills to give mental health first aid and support to others, and knowledge of how to prevent mental disorders.

Such direction recognizes that mental health literacy is the foundation for mental health care, prevention of mental disorders, and promotion of good mental health. This perspective is consistent with the wider definition of health literacy as described by the WHO.[2] According to Kutcher and colleagues,[12] who have further refined this concept, mental health literacy comprises 4 distinct but related components: (1) understanding how to optimize and maintain good mental health, (2) understanding mental disorders and their treatment, (3) decreasing stigma, and (4) enhancing help seeking efficacy. Although consistent with Jorm's definition of focusing on the recognition of mental disorders and help sources/strategies for oneself and others, this construct of mental health literacy by Kutcher and colleagues[12] extends to emphasize the importance of fighting stigma, maintaining good mental health, and empowering a person to improve their help-seeking efficacy (knowing when to seek help, where to seek help, what to expect when seeking help, and being empowered to receive the best available help). This more complex construct also provides the basis for mental health decision making and can be applied at the individual and population levels, thus, addressing key factors in determining mental health outcomes.

As approximately 1 in 5 young people show signs of emotional/behavioral impairment,[8,13] the development of mental health literacy (**Box 1**) could possibly become the foundation for a lifetime of improved mental health and better outcomes for mental disorders. Given that young people begin making decisions about their health during their early adolescent years, there is a credible argument that health decision-making skills should be an integral part of the school curriculum from an early age.[14] Accordingly, youths should be a primary audience for whom mental health literacy is provided, ideally as a matter of course and not as add-on or unique events that occur infrequently (such as mental health parades, student assembly for mental health, and so forth). These one-off events may raise initial awareness of mental health concerns but often have little if any lasting or positive value in enhancing mental health literacy in young people.[12,15,16]

MENTAL HEALTH LITERACY AND SCHOOL

Given the importance of supporting the development of mental health literacy in young people, the reality that most youths attend school, and that schools are the preferred social structures through which literacy (for example, language literacy, mathematic literacy, scientific literacy, and so forth) is taught, it is both reasonable and rational to focus on developing and delivering evidence-based mental health literacy interventions in schools. School-based mental health literacy interventions can be provided through curriculum and through other school-based initiatives. These interventions may be particularly important for junior high and secondary school students who are demographically situated near the beginning of the rapidly ascending curve that marks the onset of diagnosable mental disorders (between 12–25 years of age).[8,13] For young people, the development of good mental health literacy during this period of the life cycle may be instrumental in achieving improvements in mental health, mental health care, and the decrease of stigma associated with mental disorders.

Globally, however, school-based mental health literacy interventions for this age group have been few and far between. Although there has been substantial interest in mental health promotion in schools[17] and whole-school approaches to student well-being, much of this work has been focused on primary grades, and the evidence

---

Box 1
Mental health literacy is defined as

1. Understanding how to optimize and maintain good mental health
2. Understanding mental disorders and their treatments
3. Decreasing stigma
4. Enhancing help-seeking efficacy

for a substantive and lasting positive impact is not as robust as early expectations.[18-20] Other approaches have addressed various models for meeting mental health care needs in schools, either through site-based services or through integration of schools with health care services, either by providing services within schools or linking schools to off-site services.[21-25] However, most of these interventions applied an approach in which external resources are brought into school settings. Such approaches require substantial additional investment and may not be sustainable over time. Further, evidence that they are substantially better than mental health literacy activities applied using existing school resources is not available. Indeed, such externally applied approaches may actually not be as effective as those embedded within usual school ecologies, such as curriculum presented by usual classroom teachers.[18]

Regarding mental health literacy specifically, a recent systematic review[26] on the effectiveness of school-based mental health literacy programs identified 27 studies addressing knowledge, attitudes/stigma, and help-seeking behaviors. However, most of these interventions were delivered by noneducators, and programs were not sustained once the intervention was completed. Although some studies demonstrated preliminary positive results in the 3 outcomes, the results are difficult to interpret as most studies lacked scientific rigor in study designs. As general health promotion initiatives, the interventions did not all fully address the 4 domains of mental health literacy as defined earlier and, thus, may not have included the components required improving mental health awareness and decision making. Stigma does not seem to be impacted by one-off interventions,[27,28] and teacher beliefs and perceptions regarding mental health problems and mental disorders need to be considered within any training program.[29] Mental health literacy needs to be embedded in schools, integrated and led by educators, to facilitate the creation of a school-wide environment of acceptance and normalization of mental illnesses and to facilitate recognition and help seeking in young people.

Furthermore, many of the mental health literacy resources described in the literature may not be designed to meet the evolving needs of students. For example, resources such as textbooks or classroom handouts may not be as acceptable to students today. The core concepts of twenty-first century learning are moving from static information to discovery of information and developing skills in managing new and changing information relevant to the individual. In particular, youths today are highly focused on interactive media as a primary resource and generator of information. Initiatives in mental health literacy must prepare youths to cope with an ever-changing and progressing health care landscape and to be able to apply these skills to the decisions they are making.[30] Thus, classroom resources that use interactive media opportunities and online resources while concurrently maintaining a high level of evidence-based content may be an appropriate vehicle to help address teaching mental health literacy to young people.[31-33]

These considerations raise both a challenge and a solution. A natural approach to addressing mental health literacy in schools, building on existing social ecologies of schools and using existing school structures and the professional capacities of educators, could be realized by developing 2 separate but mutually dependent streams. These streams are (1) a mental health literacy curriculum resource designed to be taught in classrooms by usual teachers who are trained in its use and (2) interactive Web-based mental health literacy resources that can be used by both teachers and students in the classroom setting. The authors here describe 2 separate but mutually supportive approaches that address these streams in Canadian schools: the Mental Health and High School Curriculum Guide (the Guide) (http://teenmentalhealth.org/curriculum/) and MyHealth Magazine (http://www.myhealthmagazine.net).

The Guide: Development, Application, and Evaluation with Teachers

The Guide was developed in collaboration between one of the authors (Stan Kutcher) and the Canadian Mental Health Association, the largest national organization addressing mental health in Canada. It was created using input from educators and mental health experts nationally in conjunction with national curriculum development organizations and designed to be a resource that could be used to meet curriculum guidelines and outcomes, as they exist in all Canadian provinces. The Guide is a comprehensive and best evidence–created resource available to support curricula across Canada and is available in both hard copy and Web-based formats (www.teenmentalhealth.org). The resources include a teacher's self-study guide, teacher's knowledge self-assessment, student evaluation materials, and 6 core modules in which teachers are trained: the stigma of mental illness, understanding mental health and wellness, information about specific mental illnesses, experiences of mental illness, seeking help and finding support, and the importance of positive mental health (**Box 2**).[12]

Supplemental resources accompany each module and include animated videos, first voice videos, digital story-telling videos, PowerPoint (Microsoft Corporation, Redmond, WA) slides, in-class handouts, and Web-linked resources. All materials have been vetted and approved by mental health clinicians, educators, parents, and young people who contributed to the development of the Guide. Total duration of in-class time for teaching the modules is between 8 and 12 hours.

Because initial pilot studies found that teachers were not comfortable with and did not have comprehensive enough knowledge to teach many components of the Guide, 2 authors developed a 1-day training program, designed to introduce teachers to the Guide, model the teaching of various components of the core curriculum, and provide more detailed information about the material addressed in the curriculum. The developers of the program initially provided this teacher's training. More recently, the direct training model has changed to a train-the-trainer model whereby the program developers train trainers (usually a combination of teachers, student services providers, and health care providers) within school boards who become a local resource for new-teacher training and support of current educators delivering the program.

Program evaluations of mental health literacy outcomes for teachers directly trained by developers of the Guide demonstrate significant improvements in teachers' knowledge and attitudes with effect sizes (Cohen's d) ranging from 1.4 to 1.8 for knowledge

---

Box 2
The Guide (www.teenmentalhealth.org)

- Teacher's self-study guide
- Teacher's knowledge self-assessment
- Student evaluation materials
- 6 core modules
  - The stigma of mental illness
  - Understanding mental health and wellness
  - Information about specific mental illnesses
  - Experiences of mental illness
  - Seeking help and finding support
  - Importance of positive mental health

and 0.5 to 1.2 for attitudes.[12,34] Recent evaluation of the train-the-trainer model has been conducted in different Canadian sites to ensure the knowledge transfer to teachers remains consistent. In the Province of Nova Scotia, each of the 9 school boards across the province has developed a training team that was trained by the program developers. Each training team consisted of classroom teachers, student services providers, and health/mental health professionals. Results from each train-the-trainer session demonstrated similar highly positive and substantial results with no significant differences between groups noted. Each of the teams applied their training by teaching teachers in the use of the Guide. Results demonstrated highly significant ($P<.0001$) and substantial improvements in 3 components of mental health literacy: understanding how to optimize and maintain good mental health, understanding mental disorders and their treatments (knowledge: Cohen's d = 1.85), and decreasing stigma (attitudes: Cohen's d = 0.51)[35]; In Alberta and Ontario, trainer teams were developed within the school districts to receive the training from the program developers and thereafter apply the Guide training to teachers in their school districts. Results were similar to those obtained in Nova Scotia (Cohen's d = 1.48–2.03 [knowledge]; Cohen's d = 0.21–1.26 [attitudes]),[36,37] suggesting that this train-the trainer modification may be a more effective and sustainable approach for widespread program dissemination while building local capacity and skills to maintain the program. Other provinces are now adopting this approach, and the results have been replicated in diverse (geographically, socioeconomically, culturally) locations across Canada, with more than 1000 teachers in 5 different provinces having received the training to date. Outcomes obtained from each training application have been similar, suggesting that this approach is not site dependent but rather has general applicability across all types, backgrounds, and previous academic exposure.

Taken as a whole, these data strongly suggest that providing teachers with a best evidence–based mental health resource, designed for ease of application for classroom teaching in combination with readily accessible online resources and training them in the use of this program, has a significant and substantial impact on improving teachers' mental health literacy. This improvement is achieved as part of the usual manner in which teachers worldwide prepare for their classroom activities. They are provided with curriculum resources and use their professional expertise to educate youths in mental health using these modules in their classrooms. This approach is in contrast to commonly considered mental health literacy approaches that set out to improve teachers' mental health literacy by providing them with one-time courses in mental health. These courses are time consuming (a few days compared with 1 day of curriculum guide training), can be costly to obtain and apply, are not part of the usual social ecology of schools, and have not been demonstrated to provide greater positive impact on teachers' mental health literacy than the simple method of training teachers in the use of the Guide resource. Furthermore, when school boards develop and maintain their own training teams, they can provide sustainable and potentially cost-effective capacity to continue this intervention as part of usual and ongoing professional education for classroom teachers. Research on the potential within school diffusion of mental health literacy from teachers trained on the use of the Guide to teachers not trained in its use is now underway.

The Guide: Application and Research with Students

To date, 3 studies have been independently conducted regarding the application of the Guide by teachers trained in its use in their usual classrooms. Two studies have been nonrandomized cohort designs (Toronto District School Board [TDSB]; Durham Regional School Boards [DRSB], Ontario, Canada) and one has been a randomized controlled trial (Ottawa Region, Ontario, Canada). In 2 (TDSB and DRSB) of the sites, a students' mental health literacy evaluation was conducted at baseline, following the application of the Guide in regular classroom teaching and at a 2-month follow-up. Results demonstrated significant and substantial improvements in students' mental health literacy (Cohen's d = 0.7–1.11 [knowledge]; Cohen's d = 0.18–0.66 [attitudes]) in both sites, immediately after the training and at a 2-month follow-up (McLuckie A, Kutcher S, Wei Y, et al: Sustained improvements in students' mental health literacy and attitudes toward mental illness with use of a mental health curriculum in Canadian schools. Submitted for publication).[38] In the Ottawa region, help-seeking efficacy was also evaluated along with mental health literacy. The results of improvements in mental health literacy were similar to the other sites (Cohen's d = 0.46 [knowledge]; Cohen's d = 0.30 [attitudes]); additionally, self-reported help-seeking efficacy improved significantly (Cohen's d = 0.2).[39] Although each site contained several schools that differed from each other in terms of geographic location, socioeconomic status, and cultural mix, no significant cross-site differences in outcomes were noted.

These results demonstrate that an approach using the application of classroom-ready mental health literacy materials that are easily Web-accessible paired with a 1-day training opportunity for teachers may be a relatively cost-effective and sustainable approach to improving mental health literacy for educators and students in junior high and high schools with several advantages. First, this model can be applied in schools in parallel with and in conjunction with any other school mental health interventions, be that specific mental health–promotion strategies, whole-school health and well-being strategies (such as health promoting schools) or health/mental health intervention strategies. Second, this approach builds on existing school ecologies with 3 common elements: teachers, students, and curriculum. Thus, it should be able to be universally applied within every school, as teachers teach curriculum based on their knowledge of the material using their professional skills. No two teachers teach any curriculum materials in exactly the same way, but all teachers can achieve results that can be verified by independent means. The fidelity is provided in the content of the Guide materials, and the training process that parallels the usual pedagogical processes used by teachers to familiarize themselves with new curriculum materials provides reasonable assurance that the teachers have appropriately engaged with the material. Thus, this model does not require potentially complicated and costly process fidelity of application evaluations, making it an ideal approach to widespread dissemination across many different educational constructs. Indeed, early results of the application of this approach, using the Guide materials that have been modified and adapted for context, have shown similarly highly significant and substantial results in the training of teachers in Malawi[40] and of trainers in Nicaragua. Third, this approach provides mental health literacy education to teachers and students within the context of their usual learning processes and environments. This approach does not require special stand-alone courses or programs, and it links classroom-ready materials to educator mental health literacy enhancement. As educators apply these materials over time, they reinforce and may even be able to improve their mental health literacy. Further research is currently underway addressing the impact of this approach in long-term gains in educator mental health literacy.

MYHEALTH MAGAZINE

MyHealth Magazine is a Canadian-developed resource that provides online interactive health and mental health programming and materials for students and educators developed around the core principles of mental health literacy and evidence-based understanding of effective learning and education delivery (www.myhealthmagazine. net).[30] It provides interactive online resources covering a variety of health and mental health topics and is composed of a series of online and classroom-based activities and workshops. The program was initiated approximately 10 years ago[32] and was designed to increase mental health literacy and foster help seeking in young people. The scientific integrity of the magazine content is overseen by the program codirectors working with experts in the field, whereas the format and layout of the magazine and all of its components are overseen by an independent creative director (**Box 3**).

The core elements of the program had been initially developed with research and institutional funds and had been validated in a series of studies for a local youth mental health literacy and help-seeking resource.[32,41,42] However, to implement the program on large scales, there was a need of further funding and a significant overhaul to both the program and dissemination strategy.[43] Expansion of the program included a site for teachers to address educators' reported need around more mental health literacy training and how to help young people struggling with mental health issues.[29] With support from foundations supporting youth mental health promotion, the program has grown and is now used in 5 provinces across Canada and has youth, educator/parent, and university/young adult versions. The core learning principles around which it is designed are (1) that learning be always accessible; (2) that learning be modular and brief allowing the learner to focus on specific topics; (3) that learning be interactive, providing immediate feedback; (4) that learning be very practical and skills based; and (5) that resources can be used with minimal training. Through this resource, educators, students, and parents have access to high-quality, relevant, engaging health and mental health information and tools that are updated every week.

To improve the appeal to youths and increase accessibility to the resource in keeping with modern media access tools, a phone application version of MyHealth Magazine using both smartphone and desktop/tablet versions was created. An additional innovation has been the creation of the Mental Health Minutes specifically designed for educators within the classroom to promote timely mental health education that does not depend on fixed curriculum and that can be delivered in conjunction with whatever mental health–related teaching opportunity is being delivered (**Box 4**).

Box 3
MyHealth Magazine (www.myhealthmagazine.net)

- Online mental health and wellness program for students and educators
- Goals: increase mental health literacy, improve coping strategies, and facilitate help seeking in young people
- Educator, youths, and college student versions
- Mobile application available
- Learning materials should be
  - Always accessible, daily presence
  - Modular and brief allowing the learner to focus on specific topics
  - Evidence based
  - Interactive, providing immediate feedback
  - Practical and skills based
  - Based on resources that can be used with minimal training
  - Useful for schools in supporting students

> **Box 4**
> **Mental Health Minutes**
>
> Brief, practical learning materials on health and mental health topics
> - Delivered by teacher in classroom
> - Easy to use, no prior training required
> - 5 minutes of classroom time
> - Stand-alone modules, but can be sequenced
> - Relevant and easily integrated in daily life of students
> - For example, impact of energy drinks, prevalence of mental illness in youths

User-friendly and immediate feedback tools have been created based on online feedback, including questions and answers (with topic search feature), pop-up quizzes (eg, stress quiz), and how-to sheets (eg, how to talk to your parent about a problem). Current research is under way in assessing outcomes with delivery of integrated brief classroom workshops using online materials by teachers on specific health topics (eg, "Bullying: Do the Right Thing"). The various components of the program have been formally evaluated in the past 10 years, and the program has continuously evolved to address the ongoing challenges faced in realizing these goals. Key findings from the evaluations are that a high percentage of students use these online resources for health information; students with more distress use more online resources and are more likely to access further help (eg, visit to school-based health center); and there is a high satisfaction rating of the Web site from youths and schools.[41–43]

SUMMARY

Mental health literacy is the foundation for mental health promotion, prevention, and health decision making. It is essential that young people become literate in mental health and that opportunities to do so be made widely available within the world they live. Ideally these opportunities would include related and complementary components to address the range of ways young people learn and integrate information. Through everyday classroom instruction by teachers literate in mental health, and integrating user-friendly online resources that can provide accurate and immediate mental health information, easily accessed and personalized to meet the needs of young people, mental health literacy becomes a daily presence in the lives of youths. In Canada, 2 complementary mental health literacy approaches in secondary schools have been advanced to accomplish this goal and have been widely adopted across the country.

The Guide has demonstrated a significant, substantial, and sustained impact on improving mental health literacy for both teachers and students and recently has shown promise when applied in low-income countries globally. This approach uses the Guide resource to integrate mental health into everyday learning and builds on existing school ecologies and well-established pedagogic interventions. Its further value is in its use of core best evidence–based materials created in accordance with best knowledge translation techniques presented to teachers using familiar pedagogical approaches that can be successfully applied in various situations without geographic, socioeconomic, or other common constraints. MyHealth Magazine is an interactive online mental health literacy resource for youths and educators with multiple formats and involves educators by providing information and resources they can use in and out of the classroom. It provides an ongoing daily presence that is youth oriented, with interactive and accessible mental health literacy opportunities unconstrained by classroom walls. These two programs incorporate principles of training the educators in mental health literacy by providing accurate and youth-relevant materials to promote mental health and reduce stigma around mental illness while improving mental health decision making and help seeking. The application of one or both of these resources can be expected to help address some of the many challenges of school mental health literacy, not only in Canada and the United States but also globally.

REFERENCES

1. Berkman ND, Sheridan SL, Donahue KE, et al. Low health literacy and health outcomes: an updated systematic review. Ann Intern Med 2011;155(2):97–107.
2. World Health Organization. Health literacy: the solid facts. 2013. Available at: http://www.euro.who.int/__data/assets/pdf_file/0008/190655/e96854.pdf. Accessed July 13, 2014.
3. Rootman & Gordon-El-Bihbety for the Canadian Public Health Association. A vision for a health literate Canada: report of the expert panel on health literacy. 2008. Available at: http://www.cpha.ca/uploads/portals/h-l/report_e.pdf. Accessed July 16, 2014.
4. U.S. Department of Health and Human Services, Office of Disease Prevention and Health Promotion. National action plan to improve health literacy. 2010. Available at: http://www.health.gov/communication/HLActionPlan/pdf/Health_Literacy_Action_Plan.pdf. Accessed July 16, 2014.
5. Australian Bureau of Statistics. Health literacy, Australia. 2006. Available at: http://www.ausstats.abs.gov.au/ausstats/subscriber.nsf/LookupAttach/4102.0Publication30.06.093/$File/41020_Healthliteracy.pdf. Accessed July 14, 2014.
6. Centers for Disease Control and Prevention. Learn about health literacy. Available at: http://www.cdc.gov/healthliteracy/Learn/. Accessed July 21, 2014.
7. Kanj M, Mitic W, World Health Organization. Promoting health and development: closing the implementation gap. 2009. Available at: http://www.who.int/healthpromotion/conferences/7gchp/Track1_Inner.pdf. Accessed July 16, 2014.
8. Kessler RC, Berglund P, Demler O, et al. Lifetime prevalence and age-of-onset distributions of DSM-IV disorders in the national comorbidity survey replication. Arch Gen Psychiatry 2005;62(6):593–602.
9. Waddell C, McEwan K, Shepherd CA, et al. A public health strategy to improve the mental health of Canadian children. Can J Psychiatry 2005;50:226–33.
10. Jorm AF. Mental health literacy: public knowledge and beliefs about mental disorders. Br J Psychiatry 2000;177:396–401.
11. Jorm A. Mental health literacy: empowering the community to take action for better mental health. Am Psychol 2012;67(3):231–43.
12. Kutcher S, Wei Y, McLuckie A, et al. Educator mental health literacy: a program evaluation of the teacher training education on the mental health & high school curriculum guide. Adv Sch Ment Health Promot 2013;6(2):83–93.
13. Strang NM, Pruessner J, Pollak SD. Developmental changes in adolescents' neural response to challenge. Dev Cogn Neurosci 2011;1(4):560–9.
14. Gray NJ, Klein JD, Noyce PR, et al. Health information-seeking behaviour in adolescents. Soc Sci Med 2005;60(7):1467–78.
15. Wei Y, Kutcher S. International school mental health: global approaches, global challenges, and global opportunities. Child Adolesc Psychiatr Clin N Am 2012; 21(1):11–27.

16. Canadian Alliance on Mental Illness and Mental Health. Mental health literacy: a review of the literature, 2007. Available at: http://www.camimh.ca/files/literacy/LIT_REVIEW_MAY_6_07.pdf. Accessed July 14, 2014.
17. Joint consortium for school health. Schools as a setting for promoting positive mental health: better practices and perspectives, 2010. Available at: http://www.jcsh-cces.ca/upload/PMH%20July10%202011%20WebReady.pdf.   Accessed July 16, 2014.
18. Weare K, Nind M. Mental health promotion and problem prevention in schools: what does the evidence say? Health Promot Internation 2011;26(S1):i29–69.
19. Mukoma W, Flisher A. Evaluations of health promoting schools: a review of nine studies. Health Promot Internation 2004;19:357–68.
20. UK Department of Education. Me and my school: findings from the national evaluation of targeted mental health in schools 2008-2011. 2011. Available at: http://www.gov.uk/government/uploads/system/uploads/attachment_data/file/184060/DFE-RR177.pdf. Accessed September 1, 2014.
21. Kornblum C, Vandermorris A, Thompson G, et al. It is time to make the grade: reaching Canadian youth through school-based health centers. Paediatr Child Health 2013;18:235–6.
22. Council on School Health. School-based health centers and pediatric practice. Pediatrics 2012;129:387–93.
23. Weist M, Evans S, Lever N, editors. Handbook of school mental health: advancing practice and research. New York: Springer; 2003.
24. Robinson K, editor. Advances in school-based mental health interventions. Kingston (NJ): Civic Research Institute; 2004.
25. Evans SW, Weist MD, Serpell Z. Advances in school-based mental health interventions: best practices and program models, vol. II. New York: Civic Research Institute; 2007.
26. Wei Y, Hayden JA, Kutcher S, et al. The effectiveness of school mental health literacy programs to address knowledge, attitudes and help seeking among youth. Early Interv Psychiatry 2013;7(2):109–21.
27. Skre I, Friborg O, Breivik C, et al. A school intervention for mental health literacy in adolescents: effects of a non-randomized cluster controlled trial. BMC Public Health 2013;13(1):1–15.
28. Wang J, Lai D. The relationship between mental health literacy, personal contacts and personal stigma against depression. J Affect Disord 2008;110(1–2): 191–6.
29. Whitley J, Smith JD, Vaillancourt T. Promoting mental health literacy among educators: critical in school-based prevention and intervention. Can J Sch Psychol 2013;28(1):56.
30. Bagnell A, Santor D. Building mental health literacy: opportunities and resources for clinicians. Child Adolesc Psychiatr Clin N Am 2012;21:1–9 In: Bostic JQ, Bagnell A, editors. Evidence-Based School Psychiatry.
31. Bergsma L. Media literacy and health promotion for adolescents. J Media Lit Educ 2011;3(1):25–8.
32. Santor D, Bagnell A. Enhancing the effectiveness and sustainability of school-based mental health programs: maximizing program participation, knowledge uptake and ongoing evaluation using internet-based resources. Adv Sch Ment Health Promot 2008;1(2):17–28.
33. Sitzmann T, Kraiger K, Stewart D, et al. The comparative effectiveness of web-based and classroom instruction: a meta-analysis. Person Psychol 2006; 59(3):623–64.

34. Kutcher S, Wei Y. Challenges and solutions in the implementation of the school-based pathway to care model: the lessons from Nova Scotia and beyond. Can J Sch Psychol 2013;28(1):90–102.
35. Wei Y, Kutcher S, Hines H, et al. Successfully embedding mental health literacy into Canadian classroom curriculum by building on existing educator competencies and school structures: the mental health & high school curriculum guide for secondary schools in Nova Scotia. Lit Inf Comput Educ J, in press.
36. Kutcher S, Wei Y, Hines H. Training of educators on the mental health & high school curriculum guide. 2013. Available at: http://teenmentalhealth.org/new/toolbox/mental-health-high-school-curriculum-guide-training-report-calgary-area/. Accessed July 16, 2014.
37. Kutcher S, Wei Y, Shea M, et al. Training of educators on the mental health & high school curriculum guide. 2013. Available at: http://teenmentalhealth.org/new/toolbox/mental-health-high-school-curriculum-guide-training-report-ontario/. Accessed July 16, 2014.
38. Kutcher S, Wei Y, McLuckie A, et al. Successful application of the mental health & high school curriculum guide in the Toronto District School Board. 2014. Available at: http://teenmentalhealth.org/new/toolbox/successful-application-mental-health-high-school-curriculum-guide-tdsb/. Accessed July 16, 2014.
39. Milin R, Kutcher S, Lewis S, et al. Randomized controlled trial of a school-based mental health literacy intervention for youth: impact on knowledge, attitudes, and help-seeking efficacy. Poster presentation at the 60th AACAP Annual Meeting. Orlando (FL), October 22–27, 2013.
40. Kutcher S, Gilberds H, Morgan C, et al. Improving Malawian teachers' mental health knowledge and attitudes: an integrated school mental health literacy approach. Global Mental Health, in press.
41. Santor D, Poulin C, LeBlanc J, et al. Facilitating help seeking behavior and referrals for mental health difficulties in school aged boys and girls: a school-based intervention. J Youth Adolesc 2007;36(6):741–52.
42. Santor DA, Poulin C, Leblanc J, et al. Adolescent help seeking behavior on the Internet: opportunities for health promotion and early identification of difficulties. J Am Acad Child Adolesc Psychiatry 2007;46:50–9.
43. Santor DA, Bagnell AL. Maximizing the uptake and sustainability of school-based mental health programs: commercializing knowledge. Child Adolesc Psychiatr Clin N Am 2012;21(1):81–92.

Being Present at School

Implementing Mindfulness in Schools

Jeff Q. Bostic, MD, EdD[a],*, Michael D. Nevarez, MD[a], Mona P. Potter, MD[b],
Jefferson B. Prince, MD[a], Margaret M. Benningfield, MD, MSCI[c],
Blaise A. Aguirre, MD[a]

KEYWORDS

- Mindfulness • Schools • Students • Meditation

KEY POINTS

- Mindfulness training helps students and staff learn to accept and tolerate distress, and to work through distress to resume effective functioning.
- Practicing mindfulness frequently, even for short intervals, results in positive health benefits and neurobiologic changes in reactivity to stress.
- Mindfulness programs in schools have shown benefits in cognitive performance and resilience to stress.
- Several mindfulness/yoga programs have been developed for elementary, middle, and high school students, and can be adapted to new settings.
- Mindfulness and yoga can be implemented into schools most effectively by being sensitive to the developmental stages and needs of students.

MINDFULNESS

Mindfulness is often defined as the awareness that arises through intentionally attending to one's moment-to-moment experience in a nonjudgmental and accepting way.[1] Mindfulness seeks to bring into awareness, in a specific way, a person's relationship to their experiences (thoughts, emotions, and behaviors). Bishop and colleagues[2] emphasized that mindfulness is characterized by an attentional awareness to fluctuating experiences of the individual, and an attitude of curiosity or thoughtfulness to the various reactions to these experiences. Different than psychotherapy, mindfulness is not about changing one's thoughts or experiences, but instead about being aware of thoughts and feelings as they flow without being reactive. Mindfulness

The authors have nothing to disclose.
[a] Massachusetts General Hospital, Child Psychiatry, Yawkey 6, 55 Parkman Street, Boston, MA 02114-3139, USA; [b] McLean Psychiatric Hospital, Boston, MA, USA; [c] Vanderbilt University, Department of Psychiatry, 1601 23rd Avenue South, #3068C, Nashville, TN 37212, USA
* Corresponding author.
E-mail address: jbostic@partners.org

Abbreviation	
AOB	Awareness of breathing

is not relaxation, even if relaxation ensues. It is noticing sensations, thoughts, and emotions with the eventual intention of having a better understanding of the brains habitual patterns. Expanding on the work of Linehan,[3] the developer of dialectical behavioral therapy, Aguirre and Galen[4] described the skills of mindfulness, which are provided in **Table 1**.

As an example, the differences in responding to anxiety are provided in **Table 2**. In this example, the unmindful reaction rapidly judges anxiety as bad, and cultivates fear responses and expectations that create new, dysfunctional neuronal pathways that only sensitize the brain to, and intensify, anxiety reactions. Alternatively, mindfulness allows the person to practice recognizing factual reactions, rather than to draw conclusions or make judgments, while also allowing the person to label rather than evade distressing reactions. This allows the brain to catalog reactions associated with anxiety, but simultaneously to allow the brain to integrate these sensations, yet in a more calm reaction, to not form stronger fear-based and evasive reactions to distress; rather, the brain practices accepting time-limited distressing sensations without pairing these intense fear.

Fears, such as attachment or clinging, usually increase suffering; yet, trying to avoid these fears only increases fear (and suffering). Efforts to accept the body's signals, and to remain present with those experiences, provide clues to what underlies distress. Sitting with this distress, even briefly, allows the body to recognize it will not be harmed or destroyed by these sensations or thoughts, and diminishes the need for people to make reactive or poorly considered responses. Moreover, this sitting with distress prevents the formation of inappropriate tactics to evade distress, which then become additional obstacles (reactive efforts that evade distress) to being calm and mindful.

Relevant Mindfulness Impacts in Adults

Interest in mindfulness-based approaches with adults has grown rapidly, and an expanding research base suggests that these are efficacious interventions with meta-analytic reviews showing a medium-sized effect on a variety of mental health

Table 1
Mindfulness components

Mindfulness	Skill	Defined
WHAT skills	Observe	Notice without labeling; attend with all senses
	Describe	Describe facts, not conclusions or opinions
	Participate	Fully enter the experience as if it is the only moment that matters
HOW skills	Intentional	Know and act mindful in this moment
	Nonjudgmental	Avoid quick assessments of an experience; stay with facts
	Focus on one thing	Do only one thing; avoid multitasking or thinking of other things
	Nonreactive	Embrace the experience, listen to all your body: open, curious, accepting
	Effective	Do what the situation calls for, rather than being "right"

From Aguirre B, Galen G. Mindfulness for borderline personality disorder: relieve your suffering using the core skill of dialectical behavior therapy. Oakland (CA): New Harbinger; 2013.

Table 2	
Mindful versus unmindful responses to anxiety: describe anxiety	
Unmindfully and Judgmentally	**Mindfully**
1. I am getting anxious	1. I am getting anxious
2. This is BAD	2. My heart is racing
3. I will always get anxious	3. My palms are sweating
4. This is awful	4. I am breathing faster
5. This will never end	5. My thoughts are racing
6. What is wrong with me?	6. I feel hot

outcomes.[5,6] Specifically, mindfulness has been shown to decrease, anxiety/panic, depression (including relapse), binge eating, numbness/avoidance in posttraumatic stress disorder, chronic pain, stress levels, and even blood pressure.[4] At the same time, mindfulness has improved self-regulation, attention/concentration, interpersonal functioning, immune response in HIV patients, and response to medication treatments.[4] Accordingly, interest has spread regarding the effectiveness of mindfulness-based approaches with younger populations.

Mindfulness Impacts on the Brain

Mindfulness has been associated with specific brain changes. Patients with depression or bipolar disorder treated for 8 weeks of mindfulness showed increased left-sided prefrontal lobe activity. Monks who meditate have enlarged left prefrontal cortical activity. People who meditate also show decreased hyperreactivity in emotional regions of the brain. Similarly, mindfulness training has shown significant reductions in stress hormone levels, such as cortisol.[1] Although still being elucidated, multiple brain structures are now being implicated and are described, as are proposed relationships to the "mechanisms of mindfulness," such as attention, automatic thoughts, and self-referential thinking, and emotional regulation.[7]

MINDFULNESS MODELS IN PSYCHIATRY

The primary mindfulness-based approaches include mindfulness-based stress reduction, mindfulness-based cognitive therapy, dialectical-behavior therapy, and acceptance and commitment therapy. Mindfulness-based stress reduction and mindfulness-based cognitive therapy use traditional mindfulness meditation practices to develop mindfulness skills, whereas dialectical-behavior therapy and acceptance and commitment therapy use mindfulness techniques and/or nonmeditative component skills of mindfulness.[8] Interventions based on mindfulness-based stress reduction/mindfulness-based cognitive therapy typically involve experiential learning programs that include weekly group practice, a core curriculum of mindfulness practices (body scan, sitting, movement, and walking meditations), and emphasis on intentional mindful awareness of activities of daily living. A common focus is to use the sensation of the breath and the body as "anchors" for attention, when attention wanders or becomes scattered. Through these practices, participants develop skills and attitudes that include focusing, sustaining, and switching attention and accepting their present moment experience without judgment or elaboration.[8]

MINDFULNESS INTERVENTIONS IN CHILD PSYCHIATRIC DISORDERS

Mindfulness interventions in adolescents have shown significant benefit in clinical and nonclinical populations. In individuals with autism spectrum disorder, studies showed improvements in social interactions and impulsive behavior,[9] and decreases in aggression.[10,11] Studies in those with substance abuse found that mindfulness practice frequency correlated with increased sleep duration and improvement in self-efficacy about substance use.[12,13] Patients with attention-deficit/hyperactivity disorder have shown improvement in self-reported attention-deficit/hyperactivity disorder symptoms and some significant changes in neurocognitive measures.[14] A study of mindfulness in adolescents with learning disabilities and anxiety showed significant differences in self-rated anxiety and social skills, teacher-rated social skills, and academic achievement.[15] A 4-week intervention in adolescents with conduct disorder found a 52% decrease in number of aggressive and noncompliant acts.[16] A randomized controlled trial with 102 adolescents from a clinical sample showed significantly decreased stress and anxiety.[17] In addition, more time spent in sitting meditation practice led to improved clinician-rated functioning, and declines in self-reported depressive and anxiety symptoms at 3-month follow-up ($P<.05$). In an intriguing study with a nonclinical sample, Hilt and Pollak[18] found adolescents were better able to disengage from negative ruminative states with a mindfulness intervention rather than distraction or problem solving. Given the short duration of the intervention (8-minute audio recording), the authors concluded that mindfulness might not need to be intensively practiced to be beneficial.

MINDFULNESS IN SCHOOLS

Mindfulness-based interventions in schools have become increasingly popular, and the first systemic review and meta-analysis specific to school settings was recently published.[19] Zenner and colleagues[19] examined 24 studies that included a mindfulness intervention; in total 1348 students were instructed in mindfulness and 876 served as the comparison group. Grades ranged from grade 1 through grade 12, and ages from 6 to 19 years old, with studies differing in how they described the setting, intervention, and sample. The authors of this meta-analysis grouped various study outcomes into different domains and found significant overall effect sizes for cognitive performance (0.80), stress (0.39), and resilience (0.36). The overall effect sizes between groups was 0.40 ($P<.0001$), which is in the same range as results of other meta-analyses of school-based prevention programs. For example, a meta-analysis of school-based social and emotional learning programs revealed an overall effect size of 0.30.[20] The authors concluded that mindfulness-based interventions in school settings hold promise, particularly in relation to improving cognitive performance and resilience to stress.[20]

Mindfulness Benefits in Schools

Emerging research indicates that mindfulness yields diverse benefits across school settings. A recent issue of *Advances in School Mental Health Promotion*[21] described recent findings, and cautioned that methodologic limitations in the existing studies preclude yoga currently reaching "evidence-based practice" status. Emerging evidence suggests mindfulness programs benefit school performance, and is summarized in **Table 3**.

The components of mindfulness programs most pertinent and impactful remain unclear. However, findings from teacher and staff reports provide some clarity. The Learning to BREATHE program was adjusted to be provided weekly for 15 to

Table 3
Mindfulness benefits for school success

Study	Population	Intervention	Duration	Findings
Berger et al,[22] 2009	71 fourth and fifth graders	Yoga, breathing, meditation	60 min/wk for 12 wk	Fewer self-report negative behaviors to stress
Broderick & Metz,[23] 2009	120 12th grade girls	Body awareness, working with thoughts, working with feelings, integrating awareness of thoughts, feelings and bodily sensations, reducing harmful self-judgments, and integrating mindful awareness into daily life	35 min twice weekly for six sessions (3 wk)	Decreased negative affect, increased calmness, relaxation, self-acceptance; improved emotional regulation; decreased tiredness
Mendelson et al,[24] 2010	Fourth and fifth graders	Yoga	45 min for 4 d/wk for 12 wk	Decreased ruminations, intrusive thoughts, and emotional arousal
Powell et al,[25] 2008	8–11 years old	Yoga postures, breathing, positive touching	45 min/wk for 12 wk	Better scores on Strengths/Difficulties Questionnaire
Napoli et al,[26] 2008	191 first through third graders	Yoga, body scanning, sensory awareness	45 min every other wk for 24 wk	Self-reported improvements in attention, social skills, anxiety
Parker et al,[27] 2014	111 fourth and fifth graders	Yoga, awareness, application to real-world	15 min daily for 20 sessions	Improved performance on executive functioning skills; fewer teacher-rated social problems and aggressive behaviors; decreased anxiety in girls; no difference from control subjects in teacher-rated attention, or intentions regarding substance use
Peck et al,[28] 2005	10 attention issue elementary students	Yoga	30 min twice per wk for 3 wk	Improved attention and compliance
Schonert-Reichl & Lawlor,[29] 2010	246 fourth through seventh graders	Quieting the mind; mindful attention, managing negative emotions/thinking; acknowledge self/others	Ten 45 min lessons over 10 wk AND 3 min three times daily practice	Improved optimism; teachers perceived greater student social competence
Sibinga et al,[30] 2013	41 seventh and eighth grade urban boys	Mindfulness-based stress reduction	12 sessions	Decreased anxiety, less rumination; stable cortisol levels (control group increased cortisol as academic demands increased)

Data from Smith BH, Connington A, McQullin S, et al. Applying the deployment focused treatment development model to school-based yoga for elementary school students: steps one and two. Adv Sch Ment Health Promot 2014;7(3):140–55; and Smith BH, Mendelson T. Special issue on yoga and mindfulness in schools. Adv Sch Ment Health Promot 2014;7(3):137–39.

Table 4
Mindfulness and yoga programs designed for school use

Program Name	Grade Level	Description	Web Site/Reference
Mindfulness			
Mindful Life School Program	K–12	Curriculum of 1- to 5-min mindfulness lessons to be incorporated into classroom education. Letters to parents included for reinforcement of skills at home. Training includes a 1-d intensive program for educators, online training.	http://www.mindfullifetoday.com/
Mindful Schools	K–12	Online or in-person course on mindfulness fundamentals and mindfulness curriculum for educators.	www.mindfulschools.org
Wellness Works	K–12	Trained consultants implement curriculum in schools. Professional development for teachers also offered.	http://www.wellnessworksinschools.com/
Attention Academy Program	1–3	45-min sessions during physical education classes. Implemented by trained mindfulness instructors. Twelve bimonthly sessions, which included breathing exercise, body scan, body movement task, and postsession debriefing.	Napoli et al,[26] 2008
Learning to BREATHE	5–12	Mindfulness curriculum for adolescents, 6- or 18-session versions available 45-min sessions, intended to be integrated into classroom instruction; sessions can be broken into smaller pieces for implementation. Six core themes: (1) body awareness; (2) understanding and working with thoughts; (3) understanding and working with feelings; (4) integrating awareness of thoughts, feelings, and body sensations; (5) reducing harmful self-judgments; (6) integrating mindful awareness into everyday life. Teachers complete 8-wk MBSR and 2 d in-service on Learning to Breathe curriculum	http://learning2breathe.org/
Mindfulness in Schools Program	9–12	Mindfulness curriculum implemented in classroom. Nine scripted lessons on mindfulness delivered by trained classroom teachers "learning to direct attention to immediate experience, moment by moment, with open-minded curiosity and acceptance."	Kuyken et al,[37] 2013
Meditation Fluir	9–12	90-min sessions once a week for 10 wk. Mindfulness meditation; body scan.	Franco et al,[38] 2011

Yoga

Program	Grades	Description	Reference
The School Yoga Project	PreK–12	30-wk curriculum for students delivered by trained yoga instructors. 1-d teacher workshops offer training on how to integrate mindfulness in the classroom.	http://littlefloweryoga.com/programs/the-school-yoga-project
PowerMoves Kids	PreK–8	Focus is on building character traits with physical training.	http://www.crossculturefitness.com/powermoves-kids-.html
Yoga 4 the Classroom	K–8	Classroom-based practice; brief exercises delivered by classroom teachers. Program implementation supported by staff development, classroom residency, parent education, and adult classes for school staff.	http://www.yoga4classrooms.com
YogaKidz	1–5	Implemented in high poverty, minority population; emphasis on respect, hope, gratitude.	www.gogrounded.com
Here and Now: Yoga in School	3–6	13 yoga sessions over 4 mo delivered by trained yoga instructors, integrated into the school day; based on Iyengar yoga for school children.	Ehud et al,[39] 2010
Bent on Learning	4–5	Afterschool program for inner city youth. 1-h session per week for 12 wk. Delivered by certified yoga instructors from nonprofit group Bent on Learning. Groups of about 20 children. Written curriculum based on school physical education standards.	http://bentonlearning.org/
Training of Relaxation with Elements of Yoga for Children (TorweY-C)	5	German program focused on stress reduction and response to "high psychological demands and pressure in everyday life." Fifteen 60-min sessions in three parts: (1) relaxation, (2) yoga exercises (based on Shivananda-Yoga, Rishikesh/India); (3) social interaction/integration of skills.	Stueck & Gloeckner,[40] 2005. http://dx.doi.org/10.1080/03004430420000230537
Mindful Awareness for Girls through Yoga	4–5	8-wk curriculum based on MBSR delivered afterschool by trained instructor. Daily homework assignments.	White,[41] 2012
Yoga in My School	PreK–grade 12	Offers on-line training and in-person workshops for teachers; based in Alberta, Canada. World Wide Web-based resources available with subscription.	https://yogainmyschool.com/

Abbreviation: MBSR, Mindfulness Based Stress Reduction.

Data from Lawlor MS. Mindfulness in practice: considerations for implementation of mindfulness-based programming for adolescents in school contexts. New Dir Youth Dev 2014;2014(142):83–95.

25 minutes over 18 weeks, to accommodate schedule needs (provided during choir class).[31] Smith and colleagues[32] identified specific tactics that seem to improve implementation of mindfulness programs into school:

- Teacher-identified prompting was often required for students to use techniques.
- Breathing seemed the most useful technique for elementary students.
- Techniques were most needed during transitional times, or to calm down, more so than to focus.
- Most teachers did not perceive that weekly instruction was sufficient for students to use mindfulness techniques when they needed them. Fifteen minutes per day was preferable to a longer session less frequently.[27]
- Students who practiced mindfulness outside of school derived greater benefits from these programs.[33]
- Students were reluctant to remove socks, and struggled with reacting to tight-fitting clothes (on others), such that programs should allow socks and encourage loose-fitting clothing for body positioning (eg, yoga, breathing) mindfulness components.
- Identifying preferred or "favorite" poses increased student effort and applications outside of class.[32]

Measuring Mindfulness in Schools

Measuring the impact of mindfulness continues to evolve. A summary of common measures is available at http://www.mindfulexperience.org/measurement.php. One measure of mindfulness specifically designed for children and adolescents is the Child and Adolescent Mindfulness Measure,[34] which has been used internationally.[35]

Mindfulness Programs Designed to Be Implemented in Schools

The growth of mindfulness-based approaches is spreading rapidly. Educators seeking mindfulness-based or contemplative educational programs can look to the Garrison Institute's Contemplative Education Database (www.garrisoninstitute.org). The database has specific inclusion criteria, and was created in part to aid educators in finding contemplative education programs within their geographic area in the United States and Canada.[36] A sample of some of these programs is provided in **Table 4**.

A PROPOSED MINDFULNESS PARADIGM FOR ELEMENTARY, MIDDLE, AND HIGH SCHOOL

Implementation of any additional program into contemporary schools requires addressing likely barriers. Smith and colleagues[32] and Miller and colleagues[42] have identified barriers with yoga and mindfulness programs being adapted in the United States. A list of likely barriers and potential tactics to address is provided in **Table 5**.

As children mature, they usually can perform more complex physical moves, and also more complex and multistep cognitive tasks.[43] Frequent (daily) practice, including outside school, outward looking or separation among students to decrease self-consciousness, emphasis on breathing and preferred poses, and use in preparation for potentially stressful situations enhance student benefits to mindfulness training at school. A developmentally sensitive mindfulness program is proposed to match the needs of children at various ages with mindfulness practices likely to be acceptable and effective with these students.[42] A proposed program across school levels is

Table 5
Potential obstacles to implementation of mindfulness in schools

Potential Obstacle	Tactics to Address This Obstacle
Perceptions by staff/parents the program competes with religious/cultural principles	1. Provision of the actual events/curriculum proposed so that adults can view 2. Clarification of how mindfulness components "fit" (not compete) with diverse religious/cultural practices
Competition with other academic priorities	1. Staff/teacher information on benefits of mindfulness for academic achievement 2. Inclusion as part of health/physical education
Feasibility (how mindfulness will be implemented and delivered)	1. Identification of staff or local providers willing to train staff and/or conduct student sessions 2. Creation of a motivated school committee to develop an implementation plan attentive to specific needs/concerns of that school 3. Piloting of the proposed program to identify benefits and potential other obstacles
Safety (risks associated with the program)	1. Identification of staff to respond to/address any injuries or complaints 2. Comparison of students receiving mindfulness with students not receiving
Age-appropriateness (eg, physical "positions" that could be embarrassing, or mental practices that could be seen as "weak" by peers)	1. Reviewing/eliminating particular physical postures that may be perceived as too vulnerable, provocative or potentially embarrassing for secondary school students 2. Providing context descriptions for practices that may be perceived initially negatively by students/staff
Attendance and retention	1. Provided at convenient times, make-up times available during week 2. Reinforcement/rewards for regular participation

Data from Smith BH, Mendelson T. Special issue on yoga and mindfulness in schools. Adv Sch Ment Health Promot 2014;7(3):137–39; and Miller S, Herman-Stahl M, Fishbein D, et al. Use of formative research to develop a yoga curriculum for high-risk youth: implementation considerations. Adv Sch Ment Health Promot 2014;7(3):171–83.

described in **Table 6**, and pictures of yoga poses are available at http://www. namastekid.com/learn/kids-yoga-poses/.

SCHOOL STAFF APPLICATIONS

An additional component to consider in mindfulness programming for schools concerns applications for school staff. A mindfulness-based stress reduction program[44] has been adapted for teachers.[45] Ancona and Mendelson[46] piloted a six-session yoga/mindfulness program for 43 elementary and middle school teachers in low-income Baltimore schools who volunteered (21 receiving the intervention, and 22 into a control condition). Teachers received breathing and yoga poses around weekly themes of breath, stress, anger, thoughts, energy, and love, with reflection to conclude each session. A total of 83% of teachers completed the program, and 72% attended four or more of the six sessions. Findings from this pilot study indicated that teachers may need an introductory video to clarify what the intervention provides, and that the intervention after school too often competes with other demands and responsibilities, inhibiting participation. Providing skills that teachers use to reduce stress, but also that they perceive will be helpful for stress-reduction for their students,

Table 6
Suggested mindfulness program components for elementary, middle, and high schools

School Level	Component	Lesson
Elementary school		
Attentional	Breathing	AOB (or "belly breathing"): becoming familiar with directing attention to the breath moving in (as stomach expands outward) and with the breath moving out (as stomach returns toward middle)
		Useful to practice standing, sitting, and laying down (practice breathing with a buddy placing stuffed animal on the belly and move the animal up and down with movements of breathing)
		• Conductor breathing
		• Bumble bee breathing
		• Lion's breath
		• Power breath
		• Counting breathing
		In the nose and out the mouth slow breathing; noticing that they can observe how they feel about emotions amid breathing
		Focus on stomach coming in and out
		Other usual practices include
		• Stress body: where and what color is stress in the body?
		• Relaxed or joyful of grateful body: where and what "color" is this experience in the body?
		• Tasting meditation: usually students can focus on the tastes of fruit or chocolate completely from start to finish of eating
		• Listening meditation: listening to the bells, following the sound all the way until no longer hear it, or while listening to a story
		• Walking meditation: as students walk, having an image of themselves as a quiet cat/lion moving around the jungle
		• Songs: listening or singing to any appropriate to that group and that allow them to focus clearly on what they hear
		• Journaling: writing about what I love, what I am grateful for, what adults worry about, what is stressful for my friends, and so forth
	Yoga poses	Simple poses: child's pose, chair, mountain, picking grapes, ball, bee, boat, butterfly, bridge, cat/cow, dolphin, downward dog, tree, airplane
		Chaining together simple sequences of yoga
Attitudinal		Image of "planting seeds of kindness" toward self and those we care for (as tend to their "garden")
		Pairing AOB with the poses and working toward but not beyond limits, practice being gentle with self/others, evading self-judgments regarding ability to do poses

Middle school		
Attentional	Breathing	AOB: standing, sitting in chair, and if lying down in the astronaut pose; language built around noticing sensations of breathing, where does one feel the breath most easily (nostrils, chest, belly); feeling the breath inside; letting things (eg, stresses) go with each breath
		Other usual practices include
		• Stress body: where and what color is stress in the body?
		• Relaxed or joyful of grateful body: where and what color is this experience in the body?
		• Eating meditation: focusing on the entire experience of eating (eg, fruit pieces and chocolate that melts)
		• Listening meditation: listening to the bells, following the sound all the way until no longer hear it
		• Walking meditation: practicing AOB while noticing sensations on bottoms of feet
		• Journaling: example topics include what I love, what I am grateful for, what adults worry about, what is stressful for my friends in middle school, what is stressful about grades, social media, and so forth
	Yoga poses	Focus on diaphragmatic breathing; poses more appropriate for middle school children include monkey, mermaid, reverse warrior, giraffe, salutation, tree, mountain, kite, rainbow, crescent moon, lion, chair, plank, airplane
Attitudinal		Image of planting seeds of kindness; toward self and those we care for
		Gentle and patient with this body so may become gentle and patient with others
		Lessons of differences in perception; how I see the world is not usually exactly the way others see the same things; using perception exercises, such as magic eye book, to experience
		Sensitivity to "provocative poses" for each gender; configuring yoga events with students in a circle and legs going outward
High school		
Attentional	Breathing	AOB as foundation of cultivating a calm mind; calm mind helpful to see clearly (using example of glitter settling down within a "snow globe") and AOB as thread of attention through day-to-day activities; turning/focusing inward through breathing
	Yoga poses	Gradated breathing (slow to more quickly) to sustain a pleasant state; both middle school and elementary (and advanced) yoga poses can be used, based on the maturity (not seeing poses as sexually suggestive) and physical dexterity of the participants

(continued on next page)

Table 6
(continued)

School Level	Component	Lesson
Attitudinal		Learning and practicing being gentle with self (and therefore others)
		Impact of perception (using trump d'oeil [eye-tricking/deceiving] images); test of selective attention (eg, http://www. theinvisiblegorilla.com/videos.html)
		Conditioning (eg, ladder of inference: http://www.mindtools.com/pages/article/newTMC_91.htm)
		Other usual practices include
		• Stress body: where and what "color" is stress in the body?
		• Relaxed or joyful or grateful body: where and what color is this experience in the body?
		• Eating meditation: savor and fully notice fruit pieces or chocolate that melts
		• Listening meditation: listening to the bells, following the sound all the way until no longer hear it
		• Walking meditation: practicing AOB while noticing sensations on bottom of feet; usually not slow walking
		• Journaling: writing about what I love, what I am grateful for, what adults worry about, what is stressful for my friends in high school, what is stressful about grades, social media
		• Videos (eg, One Minute Meditation [http://www.wikihow.com/Meditate-in-One-Minute]; for older adolescents: This is Water [https://www.youtube.com/watch?v=DKYJVV7HuZwJ])

Abbreviation: AOB, awareness of breathing.

may also encourage teacher participation and "link" teachers and students in use of mindfulness techniques.[47]

REFERENCES

1. Kabat-Zinn J. Mindfulness-based interventions in context: past, present, and future. Clin Psychol Sci Pract 2003;10:144–56.
2. Bishop SR, Lau M, Shapiro S, et al. Mindfulness: a proposed operational definition. Clin Psychol Sci Pract 2004;11(3):230–41.
3. Linehan M. Cognitive-Behavioral Treatment of Borderline Personality Disorder. New York: Guilford Press; 1993.
4. Aguirre B, Galen G. Mindfulness for borderline personality disorder: relieve your suffering using the core skill of dialectical behavior therapy. Oakland (CA): New Harbinger; 2013.
5. Goyal M, Singh S, Sibinga EM, et al. Meditation programs for psychological stress and well-being: a systematic review and meta-analysis. JAMA Intern Med 2014;174(3):357–68.
6. Grossman P, Neimann L, Schmidt S, et al. Mindfulness-based stress reduction and health benefits: a meta-analysis. J Psychosom Res 2004;57:35–43.
7. Marchand WR. Neural mechanisms of mindfulness and meditation: evidence from neuroimaging studies. World J Radiol 2014;6:471–9. http://dx.doi.org/10.4329/wjr. v6.i7.471. Available at: http://www.wjgnet.com/1949-8470/full/v6/i7/471.htm.
8. Burke C. Mindfulness-based approaches with children and adolescents: a preliminary review of current research in an emergent field. J Child Fam Stud 2010;19:133–44.
9. Bogels S, Hoogstad B, van Dun L, et al. Mindfulness training for adolescents with externalizing disorders and their parents. Behav Cognit Psychother 2008;36: 193–209.
10. Singh N, Lancioni G, Manikam R, et al. A mindfulness-based strategy for self-management of aggressive behavior in adolescents with autism. Res Autism Spectr Disord 2011;5:1153–8.
11. Singh N, Lancioni G, Singh A, et al. Adolescents with Asperger syndrome can use a mindfulness-based strategy to control their aggressive behavior. Res Autism Spectr Disord 2011;5:1103–9.
12. Bootzin R, Stevens S. Adolescents, substance abuse, and the treatment of insomnia and daytime sleepiness. Clin Psychol Rev 2005;25:629–44.
13. Britton W, Bootzin R, Cousins J, et al. The contribution of mindfulness practice to a multicomponent behavioral sleep intervention following substance abuse treatment in adolescents: a treatment-development study. Subst Abus 2010;31:86–97.
14. Zylowska L, Ackerman D, Yang J, et al. Mindfulness meditation training in adults and adolescents with ADHD: a feasibility study. J Atten Disord 2008;11(6): 737–46.
15. Beauchemin J, Hutchins T, Patterson F. Mindfulness meditation may lessen anxiety, promote social skills, and improve academic performance among adolescents with learning disabilities. Compl Health Pract Rev 2008;13(1):34–45.
16. Singh N, Lancioni G, Subhashni D, et al. Adolescents with conduct disorder can be mindful of their aggressive behavior. J Emot Behav Disord 2007;15(1): 56–63.
17. Biegel G, Brown K, Shapiro S, et al. Mindfulness-based stress reduction for the treatment of adolescent psychiatric outpatients: a randomized clinical trial. J Consult Clin Psychol 2009;77(5):855–66.

18. Hilt L, Pollak S. Getting out of rumination: comparison of three brief interventions in a sample of youth. J Abnorm Psychol 2012;40:1157–65.
19. Zenner C, Herrnleben-Kurz S, Walach H. Mindfulness-based interventions in schools: a systematic review and meta-analysis. Front Psychol 2014;5:603.
20. Durlak JA, Weissberg RP, Dymnicki AB, et al. The impact of enhancing students' social and emotional learning: a meta-analysis of school-based universal interventions. Child Dev 2011;82:405–32.
21. Smith BH, Mendelson T. Special issue on yoga and mindfulness in schools. Adv Sch Ment Health Promot 2014;7(3):137–9.
22. Berger D, Silver E, Stein R. Effects of yoga on inner-city children's well-being: A pilot study. Alternative Therapies in Health and Medicine 2009;15:36–42.
23. Broderick PC, Metz S. Learning to BREATHE: a pilot trial of a mindfulness curriculum for adolescents. Adv Sch Ment Health Promot 2009;2:35–46.
24. Mendelson T, Greenberg MT, Dariotis JK, et al. Feasibility and preliminary outcomes of a school-based mindfulness intervention for urban youth. Journal of Abnormal Child Psychology 2010;38(7):985–94.
25. Powell L, Gilchrist M, Stapley J. A journey of self-discovery: An intervention involving massage, yoga and relaxation for children with emotional and behavioural difficulties attending primary schools. European Journal of Special Needs Education 2008;23(4):403–12.
26. Napoli M, Krech PR, Holley LC. Mindfulness training for elementary school students: the attention academy, (November 2014). J Appl Sch Psychol 2008;37–41. http://dx.doi.org/10.1300/J370v21n01.
27. Parker AE, Kupersmidt JB, Mathis ET, et al. The impact of mindfulness education on elementary school students: evaluation of the master mind program. Adv Sch Ment Health Promot 2014;7(3):184–204.
28. Peck HL, Kehle TJ, Bray MA, et al. Yoga as an intervention for children with attention problems. School Psychology Review 2005;34(3):415–24.
29. Schonert-Reichl KA, Lawlor MS. The effects of a mindfulness-based education program on pre- and early adolescents wellbeing and social and emotional competence. Mindfulness 2010;1(3):137–51.
30. Sibinga EM, Perry-Parrish C, Chung SE, et al. School-based mindfulness instruction for urban male youth: a small randomized controlled trial. Prev Med 2013; 57(6):799–801. http://dx.doi.org/10.1016/j.ypmed.2013.08.027.
31. Metz SM, Frank JL, Reibel D, et al. The effectiveness of the learning to BREATHE program on adolescent emotion regulation. Res Hum Dev 2013;10(3):252–72. http://dx.doi.org/10.1080/15427609.2013.818488.
32. Smith BH, Connington A, McQullin S, et al. Applying the deployment focused treatment development model to school-based yoga for elementary school students: steps one and two. Adv Sch Ment Health Promot 2014;7(3):140–55.
33. Huppert FA, Johnson DM. A controlled trial of mindfulness training in schools: the importance of practice for an impact on well-being. J Posit Psychol 2010;5: 264–74.
34. Greco LA, Baer RA, Smith GT. Assessing mindfulness in children and adolescents: development and validation of the child and adolescent mindfulness measure (CAMM). Psychol Assess 2011;23(3):606–14.
35. de Bruin EI, Zijlstra BJ, Bögels SM. The meaning of mindfulness in children and adolescents: further validation of the child and adolescent mindfulness measure (CAMM) in two independent samples from The Netherlands. Mindfulness 2014; 5(4):422–30.

36. Lawlor MS. Mindfulness in practice: considerations for implementation of mindfulness-based programming for adolescents in school contexts. New Dir Youth Dev 2014;2014(142):83–95.
37. Kuyken W, Weare K, Ukoummunne OC, et al. Effectiveness of the mindfulness in schools programme: non-randomized controlled feasibility study. Br J Psychiatry 2013;203:126–31.
38. Franco C, Mañas I, Cangas AJ, et al. Exploring the effects of a mindfulness program for students of secondary school. Int J Knowl Soc Res 2011;2(1):14–28. http://dx.doi.org/10.4018/jksr.2011010102.
39. Ehud M, An BD, Avshalom S. Here and now: yoga in Israeli schools. Int J Yoga 2010;3(2):42–7. http://dx.doi.org/10.4103/0973-6131.72629.
40. Stueck M, Gloeckner N. Yoga for children in the mirror of the science: working spectrum and practice fields of the training of relaxation with elements of yoga for children. Early Child Dev Care 2005;175(4):371–7. http://dx.doi.org/10.1080/0300443042000230537.
41. White LS. Reducing stress in school-age girls through mindful yoga. J Pediatr Health Care 2012;26(1):45–56. http://dx.doi.org/10.1016/j.pedhc.2011.01.002.
42. Miller S, Herman-Stahl M, Fishbein D, et al. Use of formative research to develop a yoga curriculum for high-risk youth: implementation considerations. Adv Sch Ment Health Promot 2014;7(3):171–83.
43. Weil LG, Fleming SM, Dumontheil I, et al. The development of metacognitive ability in adolescence. Conscious Cogn 2013;22:264–71.
44. Kabat-Zinn J. Full catastrophe living: using the wisdom of your body and mind to face stress, pain, and illness. New York: Delta; 1990.
45. Flook L, Goldberg SB, Pinger L, et al. Mindfulness for teachers: a pilot study to assess effects on stress, burnout, and teaching efficacy. Mind Brain Educ 2013;7:182–95.
46. Ancona MR, Mendelson T. Feasibility and preliminary outcomes of a yoga and mindfulness intervention for school teachers. Adv Sch Ment Health Promot 2014;7(3):156–70.
47. Roeser RW, Schonert-Reichl KA, Jha A, et al. Mindfulness Training and Reductions in Teacher Stress and Burnout: Results From Two Randomized, Waitlist-Control Field Trials. Journal of Educational Psychology 2013;105(3):787–804.

Educational Impacts of the Social and Emotional Brain

Margaret M. Benningfield, MD, MSCI[a],*, Mona P. Potter, MD[b], Jeff Q. Bostic, MD, EdD[c]

KEYWORDS

- Neuroscience • Cognitive • Emotional • Education • Students

KEY POINTS

- The way the brain is "wired" links cognitive and emotional processes so that one cannot function without the other.
- Emotion regulation skills develop as the prefrontal cortex matures, and can be promoted through direct instruction, behavior modeling, and provision of a stable, predictable environment.
- Adolescence is marked by a shift in the brain's emotion/cognition balance; emotion has greater influence during this developmental phase.
- These insights about brain development suggest educational strategies that can promote greater academic achievement.

INTRODUCTION

Recent developments in neuroscience related to social and emotional development have significant Implications for educational practice. Social and emotional development are closely linked with cognitive processes, thus significantly influencing overall student development and academic progress. Emotions affect how humans interpret experiences and adapt to changes in internal and external environments. This article asserts that integrating social-emotional learning (SEL) into classrooms is essential for academic achievement because of the way the brain is organized and the process through which brain development occurs. The understanding of these aspects of brain development suggests several strategies for the classroom setting that can influence student achievement (**Table 1**).

The authors have nothing to disclose.
[a] Vanderbilt University, Department of Psychiatry, 1601 23rd Avenue South, #3068C, Nashville, TN 37212, USA; [b] McLean Psychiatric Hospital, Boston, MA, USA; [c] Massachusetts General Hospital, Child Psychiatry, Yawkey 6, 55 Parkman Street, Boston, MA 02114-3139, USA
* Corresponding author.
E-mail address: meg.benningfield@Vanderbilt.Edu

Child Adolesc Psychiatric Clin N Am 24 (2015) 261–275
http://dx.doi.org/10.1016/j.chc.2014.12.001
1056-4993/15/$ – see front matter © 2015 Elsevier Inc. All rights reserved.

Abbreviations	
CBT	Cognitive behavioral therapy
SEL	Social-emotional learning

The importance of SEL is even greater for students affected by psychiatric illness. Up to 20% of students[1] will experience symptoms of anxiety, depression, poor attention, and impulsivity that frequently manifest as difficulties in learning. For students with these symptoms, incorporating SEL may be even more crucial to achieving academic targets. Understanding brain development related to social and emotional aspects of learning can serve as a bridge between the work of educators and that of child and adolescent psychiatrists and other mental health specialists engaged in school-based practice.[2]

OVERVIEW OF SOCIAL-EMOTIONAL LEARNING

SEL describes the features of education that attend to the social and emotional needs of youth that are necessary for supporting academic achievement. Meta-analytic reviews of SEL programming have demonstrated positive gains in academic achievement, improved behavior, and prevention of risk-taking.[3] Contemporary SEL programs promote these gains by mitigating the effects of negative emotion on learning through strengthening students' ability to regulate their responses, and by strengthening positive emotions that motivate students to set and achieve long-term goals. SEL programming accomplishes these goals through 2 related strategies: (1) direct instruction of skills in self-awareness, self-management, social awareness, relationship skills, and responsible decision making, and (2) cultivating a school environment that simultaneously encourages social, emotional, and academic development (http://www.casel.org/social-and-emotional-learning).

EMOTION AND COGNITION ARE ESSENTIALLY LINKED

The brain's wiring ensures that cognitions and emotions influence each other in the apperception of all experiences. Because emotion and cognition are so tightly linked, school classrooms that integrate the social and emotional aspects of learning enhance academic achievement. The appreciation of the tight link between emotion and cognition is relatively new. Until the mid-1990s, the field of neuroscience generally viewed emotion and cognition as distinct neurologic processes. Furthermore, "higher order" rational thought was often held as privileged over emotional processes, with a goal of supplanting emotional reactions with increasingly critical and analytical thinking.[4] What has become clear in the past 2 decades is that emotion and cognition markedly influence one another, and both must be addressed in the learning process.

This link is likely partly because emotions have evolved to help monitor and respond to the environment to promote survival.[5] Emotion serves the important function of coordinating diverse body functions in response to specific contextual demands through directing attention, limiting sensory input, attributing salience to stimuli, and directing the selection of behavioral output.[5] Through these processes, emotion influences what one sees, and as a result, how one behaves.[6,7] The environment holds far more information than humans can process. Therefore, the brain must prioritize sensory input and act on what is most important in the moment. In contexts of high emotional arousal, extraneous stimuli are ignored and attention is focused on information that is critical to survival.[8] When students feel threatened, their focus shifts from academic efforts, such as performing math calculations, toward seeking immediate safety, often through a fight-or-flight response. Social threats may generate similar responses and preoccupy the student's attention. Therefore, efforts to address perceived social-emotional threats could be essential to engaging a student in learning.

HUMANS TEND TO FOCUS MORE ON THE NEGATIVE

Perhaps because of the emotional system's role in maintaining safety, individuals tend to be primed to be alert for potential threats. Beginning in infancy, humans overvalue negative events compared with positive ones,[9] recognize negative events more quickly than positive ones, ascribe more value to negative experiences than positive ones, and remember negative events longer than positive ones.[10] Furthermore, greater emphasis is placed on adversity and loss compared with winning or positive experiences.[11]

This negativity bias is borne out in the anatomy of the amygdala, which is the brain structure most closely associated with responses to threat.[12] In addition, the right hemisphere of the brain more quickly processes and identifies negative experiences.[13] Negative experiences are recognized almost immediately in implicit memory, whereas positive experiences take 5 to 20 seconds to "register."[10] The tendency to focus selectively on the negative can be tempered by learning strategies for managing distress and through challenging negative interpretations of circumstances or events.

EMOTION REGULATION IS A SKILL THAT CAN BE LEARNED

Building emotion regulation skills begins with acquiring an awareness of emotional experience, then establishing a repertoire of responses to experience, and, finally, repetitive practice of these skills in a safe and supportive environment. The ability of adults in the environment to be aware of their own emotional experience and model effective regulation is one key to teaching youth how to regulate their emotions.[14] Children learn from an early age to use social referencing to assess the response of familiar caregivers.[15] Predictable routines and positive reactions from adults also serve as safe signals for children navigating the school environment. Learning to recognize these safe signals and calm emotional reactions can be challenging for youth who experience adversity outside the school environment.

Early experiences significantly influence the ability to regulate emotion, because development of emotion regulation skills begins during infancy.[16] Babies as young as 6 months look away from stimuli that cause distress.[17] By the time they have reached school age, most children have developed the rudimentary skills of identifying emotion in others and regulating their own emotional responses. However, lack of emotional readiness is one of the most consistent concerns reported by kindergarten teachers.[18] For children who have not developed emotion regulation skills, academic success is hard-won. These same children often disrupt learning for their peers because of their low frustration tolerance that often manifests in aggressive outbursts. Recognizing the individual differences in students' ability to regulate emotions and set realistic expectations for performance is key to promoting development in these skills. One avenue for improving emotion regulation skills is through the use of language.

The ability to use language to express a wide range of emotional experiences and to communicate needs and desires markedly increases the student's sense of control over feeling states.[19] Clinicians, teachers, and caregivers often recognize that

Table 1
Implications from recent advances in neuroscience

Neuroscience Finding	Significance	Brain Processes and Structures	Classroom Implications
Emotion and cognition cannot be completely separated	Emotion influences what is seen and the response. How one thinks about a situation influences what is felt about it	Prefrontal cortex, Limbic system, Amygdala, Sensory gating	Inclusion of social-emotional development is critical to academic success. Cannot exclusively focus on academic achievement without attending to social-emotional experience. Explicit positive self-talk (cognitive reframing) can shift emotional valence
Humans tend to overvalue negative emotional content. Negative stimuli are perceived more rapidly, more likely to be committed to memory	Negative events may receive greater attention because they are more critical for survival. Right hemisphere and amygdala focus on negative while left hemisphere responds more to positives	Amygdala	Although negatives, losses, and fears are selectively emphasized, a brain focusing on this becomes hypervigilant and "seeks trouble," vs learning how to adjust to negatives and feel comfortable
Executive function develops steadily through school-age years	Emotion regulation is a skill that can be learned	Prefrontal cortex	Modeling explicit attention to emotional content and effective regulation

Brain maturation during school-age years occurs through synaptic pruning or refining of connections between neurons Brain reaches 95% of adult size by age 6 y	Unnecessary connections are eliminated through synaptic pruning. Crucial connections are retained and strengthened Experience influences which connections are retained and which pathways become "superhighways" for rapid action	Gray matter: synaptic pruning; cortical thinning White matter: myelination (speeding up connections for greater efficiency) Myelin sheaths insulate the "wiring" between connections, increasing efficiency	Use it or possibly lose it Practice makes permanent Offer wide variety of experiences to stimulate connections
Student brain favors emotional over cognitive pathway	Students filter through emotional centers, whereas adults process similar stimuli through logical brain regions	Amygdala Frontal cortex	Engaging teens' passions may improve academic engagement Adults need reasonable expectations about how teens will engage Adults can "lend" frontal lobe function
Students are more sensitive than adults to social cues	Students take greater risks when they perceive their peers watching Appetitive cues are more distracting to teens Rewards are more enticing	Ventral striatum	Students may require direct instruction to recognize negative consequences of risks and to practice managing desire to impress peers Take advantage of sensitivity to reward: positive feedback for pleasing behaviors Reduce exposure to appetitive distractors (dress code)

frustration and disruptive outbursts sometimes emerge because of learning differences that escalate amid increased academic, social, or emotional demands.

The development of emotion regulation skills depends on the function of the prefrontal cortex (PFC), which shows steady increases in development throughout the school-age years and into early adulthood. In the elementary school years, with increasing PFC maturity, students are able to increase the number of strategies they can use for self-regulation and improve on the ability to flexibly select an optimal strategy.[14] Through the school-age years, children learn to respond to frustration with creative problem solving rather than by giving up.[20] Teachers play an important role in helping children to develop these problem-solving skills through modeling effective emotion regulation and offering multiple opportunities for students to practice emotion regulation skills frequently within daily classroom experiences. Frequent repetition of these skills is vital in development because the brain selectively eliminates neuronal connections that are not used.

TYPICAL DEVELOPMENT PROCEEDS BY PRUNING NEURAL CONNECTIONS

By the time most children enter first grade, the brain has already reached 93% of its adult size.[21] Beginning in late childhood and continuing through adolescence, development proceeds primarily through pruning of the neuronal connections or synapses that have been growing. Synapses that seem unnecessary are eliminated,[22] allowing space to enhance the connections that are deemed to be most critical.[23] The brain continues to develop in this manner into and throughout adulthood, pruning unnecessary branches to place more emphasis on generating more rapid and sophisticated responses to the environment's challenges. During this developmental process, patterns of behavior become codified into habits (ie, automated programs of response that can be generated reflexively in response to environmental cues).

These findings have clear implications for education. First, because underused synaptic connections will be eliminated, students exposed to broad and varied experiences during childhood seem to be better positioned for well-rounded development. Second, the "hard-wiring" of often-practiced cognitive and behavioral patterns suggests that habits learned early on can profoundly influence behavioral outcomes. Early development may represent a critical period for the development of social and emotional skills that are more difficult to master later in life.

EMOTION/COGNITION BALANCE SHIFTS IN ADOLESCENCE

Throughout the elementary school years, the PFC steadily increases in maturity and ability to provide top-down cognitive control of emotional responses. As youth enter adolescence, the development of subcortical emotion centers surges ahead of that of the PFC, shifting the balance of emotional and cognitive control.[24] The increased risk-taking frequently observed in students is likely a result of this imbalance in the development of emotional drive centers and cognitive control centers. Not until early adulthood does the maturity of the PFC catch up, bringing emotion and cognition back into balance.[24]

The cognitive/emotional imbalance during adolescence results in a greater influence of positive and negative emotions on behavior.[25] Teens are more drawn to novelty and thrill-seeking and are also more affected by distress. As parents of teenagers and middle- and high-school teachers have often observed, students tend to be more inclined to make rash decisions with little regard for thinking through consequences.[26] Brain imaging studies show that adolescents filter stimuli, such as facial emotions, through the amygdala, whereas adults process the same stimuli through frontal cortical regions.[27,28] These studies establish a neural basis for the passionate responses observed in adolescent students. The intensity of these responses can get in the way, but finding ways to engage student passion can significantly enhance the learning that occurs.

Peer influence is another important aspect of development that affects school performance in the teenage years. As students struggle with the necessary task of separating from parents/caregivers, peer appraisal becomes more important in their decision-making. Students take greater risks when they believe that their friends/peers are watching.[29] The brain seems to be programmed to reinforce students' tendency to remain attentive to the perceptions of their peers. A recent brain imaging study found that reward regions showed greater sensitization in students when they believed that peers were watching, and brain activation in these regions predicted risk-taking behavior.[30]

PSYCHIATRIC ILLNESS ADDS COMPLEXITY FOR 1 IN 5 STUDENTS

Optimizing education to meet the needs of the typically developing brain can be challenging. For nearly 1 in 5 students, psychopathology imposes additional vulnerabilities.[1] Students who are referred for mental health treatment in schools often face significant deficits in social-emotional domains that require additional support in the classroom (**Table 2**). Psychiatric illness often results in behaviors that impact academic performance not only for students with symptoms but also for classmates. Disruptive behaviors are among the most significant variables affecting classroom performance.[40] Strategies to address these difficulties can improve the learning environment for all students.

One effective clinical approach for treatment of anxiety and depression is cognitive behavioral therapy (CBT). CBT is grounded in the theory that thoughts, feelings, and behaviors influence one another. Treatment addresses problematic automatic thoughts by challenging assumptions and building arguments that promote a more positive self-view. Neuroimaging studies in adults with phobias have shown that CBT can produce changes in neural processes related to emotional responses.[41] Helping youth to understand the connections between their thoughts and their emotions has the potential to significantly shift the trajectory of illness. In addition to clinical efforts, school-wide efforts to address social and emotional development can have a significant impact on students with mental health challenges while promoting healthy development in typically developing youth.[3]

LIMITATIONS

The brain findings reviewed reveal an emerging, but far from complete, scientific understanding of normal brain development. Although these findings seem consonant with tasks of children in different developmental phases and seem to be consistent, they remain early pieces in a more comprehensive understanding of brain development. MRI and other technologies, such as neuropsychological screening and testing, which are likely more readily accessible to all students through advances in computer technology, will allow more thorough and sophisticated elucidation of brain findings regarding cognitive, emotional, and social development. As additional brain findings emerge, their implications for enhancing educational practices will remain a vital consideration.

Table 2
Psychopathology and the brain: school planning to optimize brain development

Psychiatric Disorder	Brain Development Considerations	Implications for School (to Create Compassion/Understanding)	Specific Strategies to Consider in the Classroom
ADHD	Maturation of the frontal cortex is delayed an average of 3 y compared with children without ADHD[31,32] Ability to delay gratification and make decisions may lag behind peers	Lag in ability to control thinking, attention, and planning compared with peers Might look like oppositional behavior when it is actually a deficit more appropriately viewed as a learning disability	Ensure that expectations are clear and reasonable, and skill deficits are being addressed to allow the student's brain to progress/catch up Provide instruction in shorter intervals Increase internalized speech/verbal mediation Assign staff to help with organization/planning and problem solving Change power arguments to reminding student of choices and consequences When behavior is inappropriate, first remind the student of what is expected, then reinforce efforts closer to classroom expectations Allow student to receive instructional content in multiple modalities Use rhyme, rhythm, or music to improve memory of academic content
	Altered reward processing[33]	Higher threshold for feeling rewarded by completion of a task Less likely to respond to delayed gratification	Expect that students with ADHD will be drawn to smaller, more immediate rewards vs larger delayed rewards Provide frequent, intermittent reinforcement of desired behaviors Present students with tasks that are not too frustrating to accomplish Praise effort rather than outcome Help with positive habit formation Use goal-setting and frequent reminders of long-term goals to increase motivation to persist in challenging tasks

Anxiety	Amygdala is activated in anticipation of anxiety-provoking situations much more in anxious than in nonanxious students[34] Perturbed engagement of amygdala and ventrolateral prefrontal cortex is seen in anxious students compared with healthy controls[35]	Anxious students are more likely to become emotionally revved up quicker and with more intensity than their peers Anxious students are less able to access the rational/"thinking" part of their brain during that arousal, making it difficult not only to accurately assess danger but also to engage meaningfully with cognitive tasks (eg, paying attention to teacher) and access skills to calm self down	Consider need for distress tolerance techniques, such as distraction or self-soothing, to help decrease the intensity so that the "thinking" part of the brain can engage Encourage the student to engage in a mindfulness exercise, such as mindful defusion, body scan, or "surf the wave" Help the student practice positive self-talk As much as possible (and when appropriate), do not avoid the triggering event (with the expectation that anxiety will eventually diminish on its own, so the student will have the experience of eventually winning over the anxiety): extinction/habituation training Focus on resilience (increase protective factors and decrease risk factors) and ability to take control back from the anxiety
Depression	Differences in brain volume and physiologic response to reward, inhibitory tasks, and emotional processing have been shown in multiple brain areas including amygdala, hippocampus, basal ganglia, and prefrontal cortex. Students with depression also show differences in activation in brain regions associated with rumination and self-referential thought. Rumination can interfere with performance on a task—especially when cognitive control is required. These abnormalities in brain function typically resolve with successful treatment[36]	The brains of students with depression seem to pass over the potential pleasure of winning a reward to focus on unpleasant emotions caused by the potential for failure. Engaging in tasks is more difficult for students during an episode of depression	Praise effort rather than outcome Encourage student to practice "opposite action to emotion" skills if the impulse is to give up because of sadness and fear of failure Help the student identify the gray areas vs seeing things as black and white (ie, either succeeding or failing) Help the student identify the evidence for and against failure Breakdown the task into smaller, easier-to-accomplish goals Encourage positive self-talk

(continued on next page)

Table 2
(continued)

Psychiatric Disorder	Brain Development Considerations	Implications for School (to Create Compassion/Understanding)	Specific Strategies to Consider in the Classroom
Bipolar disorder	Overactivation of amygdala with neutral and scary faces[37]	The student might misinterpret another person's facial expression, resulting in increased emotional response. This bias impacts behavior and the ability to appreciate the perspectives of others and the ability to establish relationships	If a student seems to become emotional during a conversation, stop and ask the student how the interaction is being interpreted
Substance use	Adolescents have greater risk for developing addiction than adults given similar amounts drug exposure[38] Neural circuits related to impulsivity, novelty seeking, and risk-taking are most influential in whether addiction develops[38] Neuroadaptive changes occur in response to exposure to drugs, and these changes may be permanent[39]	Experimentation with substance use is normative, and therefore identifying problematic consequences is key to engaging students in changing behavior	Programs that advocate a "Just say no" approach are not likely to make a significant impact Delaying onset of first use can significantly decrease risk for addiction Engagement in prosocial/safer risk-taking may be protective

Box 1
Classroom strategies that take advantage of neuroscience findings

1. Tendency to focus on the negative

   a. Practicing alternative self-talk throughout daily events becomes important to better discern which events require changes.

   b. Noticing what persists, viscerally, or haunts a student may reveal needs for additional or alternative self-talk or other accepting (eg, mindfulness) strategies to neutralize or tolerate negative attributions to events.

   c. Examining all of the evidence surrounding a student's conclusions of inadequacy, or negative self-attributions, may enhance the student's ability to integrate negative and positive experiences throughout each school day.

   d. Recognizing the cascade of negativity surrounding one event or a small number of events may alert the student to combating these negative perceptions.

2. Synaptic pruning eliminates connections that seem to be irrelevant to the individual

   a. Exploring students' lives outside of school clarifies what content may be most relevant. This understanding provides teachers with opportunities to encourage students to apply classroom teachings in their own real world. Becoming connected with life outside school can also offer an opportunity to encourage parents to reinforce classroom teachings in real-life circumstances.

   b. Providing predictable and stable experiences, both inside and outside of school, becomes relevant. If a student must use significantly different skills inside and outside of school (eg, gang-related events, domestic abuse/conflict, substance exposures), selection of the most important neuronal structures to retain versus prune may be compromised. Coordination with community outside of the school building has substantial importance for organized versus asynchronous brain development. Providing opportunities (eg, art, music, sports) and encouraging the skills a student needs to engage in these prosocial activities (eg, rehearsing refusal skills, staying engaged with long-term goals) may become priorities in a given school.

   c. Frequent return to previous learnings and connecting to subsequent learnings seems to be helpful in retaining desired neuronal structures and enhancing the student's connections with additional structures, perhaps useful for coordination with other skills. To be clear, preparing a student for functioning in a preferable, but realistic, environment may clarify what curriculum content should be emphasized.

3. Greater emotional than cognitive influence during adolescence

   a. Teacher acceptance of the passion surrounding student positions or perceptions may require teachers to acknowledge the student's intensity and support how important the topic or position is to a student. Caring about any topic is worthwhile and can increase investment in the educational activity. However, sometimes the student's position may be overly emotional and irrational; accordingly, helping students to recognize how their "good intention may go awry" (by alienating more neutral others) may be helpful so that students learn how rationales for positions may be more effective than impassioned pleas.

   b. Very direct, and often repetitive, evaluation of information from more logical schemas may need to be modeled by teachers, because these approaches may not be the natural preference of students. When teachers articulate the logical support for a student's emotionally driven position, the student may be able to integrate emotional amygdala reaction with rational cortical function. Similarly, students may relinquish some of their amygdalar propensities, and include more cortical involvement, if they champion a different, even countervailing opinion than their own perhaps emotionally charged initial reaction.

   c. Paradigms such as examination of a situation, including alternatives and consequences (both for the student and also for others), may shift amygdalar thinking to more rational structures.

4. Influence of peer approval in adolescence through early adulthood

   a. Teachers (and adults working with students) may benefit from recognizing this dynamic tension, which is always present (and making every choice somewhat unpredictable), wherein students balance following the adult-preferred learnings/practices against students' need to establish themselves within their peer group. Therefore, every situation warrants consideration of how the student will "look" to other students, and this can be elicited when problems are presented (eg, "how do you think your peers would perceive you if you chose to do _____?").

   b. Apprising students of this propensity may help them to sometimes recognize decision-making compromised by this circumstance, and potentially rethink choices.

   c. Information that students perceive will help them appear useful/vital to their peers may increase its attractiveness; consideration of the consequences of a decision for the student and the student's peers, and on how the peers will view this student, may help sophisticate the student's thinking.

   d. Consideration of risks and sudden impulses may help students pause during real-life circumstances. Accordingly, "practicing" likely situations students would encounter in real-life environments may help them cultivate a more viable routine when actually confronted with risky situations. This strategy has been used in drug abuse resistance and sexual behavior programs, yet, to the authors' knowledge, never with awareness of the "reward center" activation in the brain. Rather, the effort has been to provide competing responses ("just say no") or ascribe these risk-taking behaviors to "peer pressure," which is now recognized as indirect (peers are not actually pressuring the student) rather than "direct" pressure.

SUMMARY

Emerging brain research illuminates the significant role emotion plays in the developing brain. Social and emotional systems in the brain have evolved to promote survival. These neural systems allow an individual to adapt to the environment through monitoring internal and external signals and organizing advantageous responses. Selective attention to negative emotion, synaptic pruning, shifts in balance of emotional drive and cognitive control in adolescence, and the impact of psychopathology all have a marked influence on student development. Because cognitive processes cannot be fully disentangled from emotional ones, shaping learning environments to minimize negative emotion and enhance the intrinsic rewards of social engagement and mastery of new skills will enhance academic achievement. Child psychiatrists have a unique opportunity to engage with educators in promoting understanding of how these brain processes influence learning and behavior in the classroom across the course of school-age development. Brain findings in childhood psychopathology provide additional clarity about educational programming to address and minimize the impacts of psychiatric illness. Addressing the social and emotional aspects of development can ultimately improve academic achievement for all students (**Box 1**).

REFERENCES

1. Merikangas KR, He JP, Burstein M, et al. Lifetime prevalence of mental disorders in U.S. adolescents: results from the National Comorbidity Survey Replication–Adolescent Supplement (NCS-A). J Am Acad Child Adolesc Psychiatry 2010; 49(10):980–9. http://dx.doi.org/10.1016/j.jaac.2010.05.017.

2. Cohen J. Social, emotional, ethical, and academic education: creating a climate for learning, participation in democracy and well-being. Harv Educ Rev 2006; 76(2):201–37.

3. Durlak JA, Weissberg RP, Dymnicki AB, et al. The impact of enhancing students' social and emotional learning: a meta-analysis of school-based universal interventions. Child Dev 2011;82(1):405–32. http://dx.doi.org/10.1111/j.1467-8624.2010.01564.x.

4. Immordino-Yang MH, Damasio A. We feel, therefore we learn: the relevance of affective and social neuroscience to education. Mind Brain Educ 2007;1(1): 3–10. http://dx.doi.org/10.1111/j.1751-228X.2007.00004.x.

5. Damasio A, Carvalho GB. The nature of feelings: evolutionary and neurobiological origins. Nat Rev Neurosci 2013;14(2):143–52. http://dx.doi.org/10.1038/nrn3403.

6. Munakata Y, Casey BJ, Diamond A. Developmental cognitive neuroscience: progress and potential. Trends Cogn Sci 2004;8(3):122–8. http://dx.doi.org/10.1016/j.tics.2004.01.005.

7. Nelson EE, Lau JY, Jarcho JM. Growing pains and pleasures: how emotional learning guides development. Trends Cogn Sci 2014;18(2):99–108. http://dx.doi.org/10.1016/j.tics.2013.11.003.

8. Rozin P, Royzman EB. Negativity bias, negativity dominance, and contagion. Pers Soc Psychol Rev 2001;5(4):296–320. http://dx.doi.org/10.1207/S15327957PSPR0504_2.

9. Hamlin JK, Wynn K, Bloom P. Three-month-olds show a negativity bias in their social evaluations. Dev Sci 2010;13(6):923–9. http://dx.doi.org/10.1111/j.1467-7687.2010.00951.x.

10. Baumeister RF, Bratslavsky E, Finkenauer C, et al. Bad is stronger than good. Rev Gen Psychol 2001;5(4):323–70. http://dx.doi.org/10.1037//1089-2680.5.4.323.

11. Fiske ST. Attention and weight in person perception: the impact of negative and extreme behavior. J Pers Soc Psychol 1980;38(6):889–906. http://dx.doi.org/10.1037//0022-3514.38.6.889.

12. Zald DH. The human amygdala and the emotional evaluation of sensory stimuli. Brain Res Brain Res Rev 2003;41(1):88–123. Available at: http://www.ncbi.nlm.nih.gov/pubmed/12505650.

13. Alfano KM, Cimino CR. Alteration of expected hemispheric asymmetries: valence and arousal effects in neuropsychological models of emotion. Brain Cogn 2008; 66:213–20.

14. Siegler RS, DeLoache JS, Eisenberg N, et al. How children develop. 4th edition. New York: Worth; 2014.

15. Posner MI, Rothbart MK. Toward a physical basis of attention and self regulation. Phys Life Rev 2009;6(2):103–20. http://dx.doi.org/10.1016/j.plrev.2009.02.001.

16. Sheese BE, Voelker PM, Rothbart MK, et al. Parenting quality interacts with genetic variation in dopamine receptor D4 to influence temperament in early childhood. Dev Psychopathol 2007;19(4):1039–46. http://dx.doi.org/10.1017/S0954579407000521.

17. Mangelsdorf S, Shapiro J, Marzolf D. Developmental and temperamental differences in emotion regulation in infancy. Child Dev 1995;66(6):1817–28. Available at: http://www.ncbi.nlm.nih.gov/pubmed/8556901. Accessed August 19, 2014.

18. Blair C. School readiness. Integrating cognition and emotion in a neurobiological conceptualization of children's functioning at school entry. Am Psychol 2002; 57(2):111–27. http://dx.doi.org/10.1037//0003-066X.57.2.111.

19. Thompson R. Emotion regulation: a theme in search of definition. Monogr Soc Res Child Dev 1994;59(2–3):25–52. Available at: http://www.ncbi.nlm.nih.gov/pubmed/7984164.

20. Berg C. Knowledge of strategies for dealing with everyday problems from childhood through adolescence. Dev Psychol 1989;25(4):607–18. Available at: http://psycnet.apa.org/journals/dev/25/4/607/. Accessed August 19, 2014.

21. Giedd JN, Rapoport JL. Structural MRI of pediatric brain development: what have we learned and where are we going? Neuron 2010;67(5):728–34. http://dx.doi.org/10.1016/j.neuron.2010.08.040.

22. Craik FI, Bialystok E. Cognition through the lifespan: mechanisms of change. Trends Cogn Sci 2006;10(3):131–8. http://dx.doi.org/10.1016/j.tics.2006.01.007.

23. Chechik G, Meilijson I, Ruppin E. Neuronal regulation: a mechanism for synaptic pruning during brain maturation. Neural Comput 1999;11(8):2061–80. Available at: http://www.ncbi.nlm.nih.gov/pubmed/10578044.

24. Casey BJ. The teenage brain: an overview. Curr Dir Psychol Sci 2013;22(2):80–1. http://dx.doi.org/10.1177/0963721413486971.

25. Somerville LH, Jones RM, Casey BJ. A time of change: behavioral and neural correlates of adolescent sensitivity to appetitive and aversive environmental cues. Brain Cogn 2010;72(1):124–33. http://dx.doi.org/10.1016/j.bandc.2009.07.003.

26. Dreyfuss M, Caudle K, Drysdale AT, et al. Teens impulsively react rather than retreat from threat. Dev Neurosci 2014;36(3–4):220–7. http://dx.doi.org/10.1159/000357755.

27. Yurgelun-Todd D. Emotional and cognitive changes during adolescence. Curr Opin Neurobiol 2007;17(2):251–7. http://dx.doi.org/10.1016/j.conb.2007.03.009.

28. Giedd JN. The teen brain: insights from neuroimaging. J Adolesc Health 2008;42:335–43. http://dx.doi.org/10.1016/j.jadohealth.2008.01.007.

29. Gardner M, Steinberg L. Peer influence on risk taking, risk preference, and risky decision making in adolescence and adulthood: an experimental study. Dev Psychol 2005;41(4):625–35. http://dx.doi.org/10.1037/0012-1649.41.4.625.

30. Chein J, Albert D, O'Brien L, et al. Peers increase adolescent risk taking by enhancing activity in the brain's reward circuitry. Dev Sci 2011;14(2):F1–10. http://dx.doi.org/10.1111/j.1467-7687.2010.01035.x.

31. Shaw P, Eckstrand K, Sharp W, et al. Attention-deficit/hyperactivity disorder is characterized by a delay in cortical maturation. Proc Natl Acad Sci U S A 2007;104(49):19649–54. http://dx.doi.org/10.1073/pnas.0707741104.

32. Shaw P, Ph D, Gilliam M, et al. Cortical development in typically developing children with symptoms of hyperactivity and impulsivity: support for a dimensional view of attention deficit hyperactivity disorder. Am J Psychiatry 2011;168(2):143–51.

33. Castellanos FX, Tannock R. Neuroscience of attention-deficit/hyperactivity disorder: the search for endophenotypes. Nat Rev Neurosci 2002;3(8):617–28. http://dx.doi.org/10.1038/nrn896.

34. Guyer AE, Lau JY, Mcclure-tone EB, et al. Amygdala and ventrolateral prefrontal cortex function during anticipated peer evaluation in pediatric social anxiety. Arch Gen Psychiatry 2008;65(11):1303–12.

35. Tromp DP, Grupe DW, Oathes DJ, et al. Reduced structural connectivity of a major frontolimbic pathway in generalized anxiety disorder. Arch Gen Psychiatry 2012;69(9):925–34. http://dx.doi.org/10.1001/archgenpsychiatry.2011.2178.

36. Drevets WC, Price JL, Furey ML. Brain structural and functional abnormalities in mood disorders: implications for neurocircuitry models of depression. Brain Structure & Function 2008;213(1-2):93–118. http://dx.doi.org/10.1007/s00429-008-0189-x.

37. Perlman SB, Fournier JC, Bebko G, et al. Emotional face processing in pediatric bipolar disorder: evidence for functional impairments in the fusiform gyrus. J Am Acad Child Adolesc Psychiatry 2013;52(12):1314–25.e3. http://dx.doi.org/10.1016/j.jaac.2013.09.004.

38. Chambers RA, Taylor JR, Potenza MN. Developmental neurocircuitry of motivation in adolescence: a critical period of addiction vulnerability. Am J Psychiatry 2003; 160(6):1041–52. Available at: http://www.ncbi.nlm.nih.gov/pubmed/12777258. Accessed January 16, 2013.

39. Koob GF, Volkow ND. Neurocircuitry of addiction. Neuropsychopharmacology 2010;35(1):217–38. http://dx.doi.org/10.1038/npp.2009.110.

40. Hattie J. Visible learning: a synthesis of over 800 meta-analyses relating to achievement. New York: Routledge; 2009.

41. Paquette V, Lévesque J, Mensour B, et al. "Change the mind and you change the brain": effects of cognitive-behavioral therapy on the neural correlates of spider phobia. Neuroimage 2003;18(2):401–9. http://dx.doi.org/10.1016/S1053-8119(02)00030-7.

Safety Assessment in Schools: Beyond Risk

The Role of Child Psychiatrists and Other Mental Health Professionals

Nancy Rappaport, MD[a],*, William S. Pollack, PhD[b], Lois T. Flaherty, MD[c], Sarah E.O. Schwartz, PhD, MEd[a], Courtney McMickens, MD, MPH[a]

KEYWORDS

- School violence • School shootings • School safety • Threat assessment
- Risk assessment • Safety assessment

KEY POINTS

- It is critical to empower the family and student at a time when they may feel threatened while simultaneously upholding the school standards of safety for all students.
- When the consultant has the capacity to create a careful balance between family, student, and school standards, schools are better able to provide a more substantive assurance that they are taking the necessary steps to not only provide immediate safety but also make critical outreach to students and families.
- A truly positive safe school climate that nurtures students and families while also enhancing the educational mission of the school can be created.

INTRODUCTION

A spate of school shootings in the 1990s, culminating in the rampage at Columbine High School, led to heightened vigilance toward severe violence in schools and precipitated focused efforts to develop effective methods of detection and response.[1] More recent school shootings, such as the mass murders at Sandy Hook Elementary School, continue to fuel a sense of urgency and create increased pressure on schools to identify students at risk for violent behavior and to act decisively. Often educators

Disclosures: None.
[a] Cambridge Health Alliance, Harvard Medical School, 1493 Cambridge Street, Cambridge, MA 02139, USA; [b] Cambridge Health Alliance, Harvard Medical School, 47 Prentice Road, Newton Center, MA 02459, USA; [c] Cambridge Health Alliance, Harvard Medical School, 9 Saint Mary Road, Cambridge, MA 02139, USA
* Corresponding author.
E-mail address: nancy@nancyrappaport.com

Child Adolesc Psychiatric Clin N Am 24 (2015) 277–289
http://dx.doi.org/10.1016/j.chc.2014.11.001
1056-4993/15/$ – see front matter © 2015 Elsevier Inc. All rights reserved.

childpsych.theclinics.com

Abbreviations	
IEP	Individualized Education Program
SSI	Safe School Initiative

must decide if a student can return to school, needs a more restrictive school setting, or should be expelled immediately. In such cases, the school's primary priority is to ensure the safety of the students and staff.

Empirical data demonstrate that schools today are generally safe places and that multiple shootings, homicide, and suicide are relatively rare at school. In fact, the most recently published data from the Centers for Disease Control and Prevention showed that during the 2009 to 2010 school year, there was approximately one homicide or suicide of a school-aged youth at school per 2.7 million students enrolled.[2] However, both covert aggression and potential overt violence remain significant concerns. A nationally representative sample of students in grades 9 to 12 showed that 7.1% of all students did not go to school during the year at least once because they felt unsafe; 19.6% reported being bullied on school property; 8.1% reported being in a physical fight on school grounds during the year; 5.2% reported carrying a weapon; and 6.9% were threatened with a weapon on school property at least 1 day during the school year.[3]

When students and staff feel threatened, schools may turn to a child psychiatrist or other mental health consultant to evaluate imminent and long-term risk and to suggest an action plan. (As the article title suggests, in addition to child and adolescent psychiatrists, other highly trained mental health experts may serve as "consultants." School personnel who hold specialized expertise in risk assessment may play comparable roles. For convenience, the role of "consultant" is referred to throughout.) The consulting clinician will likely want to do more than just a rapid risk assessment (although rapid assessment may be necessary at times). He or she should also examine the context of the events or concerns, the potential underlying precipitants to the student's disruptive behavior, and the reasons for concern. This process ideally takes into account the perspectives of all involved, including student, family, teachers, and administrators. This approach evaluates whether the student's threatening behavior is a symptom of a mental illness, explores interactions between the staff and the student, examines how school climate may be contributing to the crisis, and addresses relevant family factors. This analysis can help educators generate a thoughtful treatment plan rather than resorting to immediate expulsion. The history of assessing threats of violence is briefly reviewed; the first author's (N.R.) model of assessment is introduced, and case vignettes are provided to illustrate the process.

FROM ASSESSMENT OF RISK TO THREAT ASSESSMENT

Numerous techniques have been developed to assess potential threats to school safety. Unfortunately, several of these techniques are not only invalid, but may cause additional harm by stigmatizing students who pose no danger and by overlooking students who need evaluation and support. In "What Can Be Done About School Shootings?," Randy Borum and colleagues[4] summarize the negative effects of zero-tolerance programs, excessive security measures, and so-called profiling and warning lists. They conclude that these measures are counterproductive in helping to detect high-risk students and actually create negative school climates wherein more harmful acts toward students may occur.[5,6]

Too many schools adopt a zero-tolerance stance for any kind of "violent" behavior—ranging from an immature boy who brags that he is making a bomb, to a second-grade child who accidentally brings a water gun to school, to an explosive girl who makes unsubstantiated threats. There is no research to demonstrate the efficacy of these policies. As a result, educators sometimes respond to trivial potential threats or minor transgressions of school rules with mandatory expulsion. Although zero-tolerance should, in theory, increase school safety by setting firm limits, in many cases, it may actually undermine school cohesion and true school safety by making no distinction between various types and levels of putative violence or social context and by treating all "offenders" the same.[7] In addition, minority students are disproportionately affected by such policies.[8]

Consider the story of Patrick, who is highlighted in the vignette provided. When he was in ninth grade, he found a Swiss Army knife on the way to school and unwittingly "played" with it during class. The school expelled him without conducting a thorough assessment, and his biracial family harbored animosity and distrust as a result. Patrick later presented a different kind of threat, and an outside consultant was called in to sort out the lingering resentment the family had for the school. The zero-tolerance policy, in this case, led to further issues that could have been avoided if a more comprehensive risk assessment had been done after the first incident.

According to Borum and colleagues,[4] the best school-based risk-assessment technique is to have thoughtful, well-trained personnel engage in investigative "threat assessment." When properly implemented, this technique will also address equally damaging nonphysical aggression acts, such as bullying and sexual harassment. This approach can result in an improved school climate, school connectedness, and genuine emotional security, which, in turn, can improve and enhance educational outcomes.[8]

The earliest evidence-based model of modern threat assessment for targeted violence in school shootings was developed by the Safe School Initiative (SSI), a collaborative effort of the US Department of Education and the US Secret Service.[9,10] The SSI studied 37 incidents of targeted school violence and 41 attackers. It used and modified key concepts of targeted violence by defining the target as "a specific individual, such as a particular classmate or teacher, or a group or category of individuals, such as 'jocks' or 'geeks'... or the school itself."[9] The study yielded 10 key findings (**Box 1**) to aid in future attempts to interrupt paths to violence; a model of investigative techniques; key questions that educators and mental health consultants can use to investigate students who actually pose threats; and suggestions that allow schools to respond to danger while diminishing unwarranted fears. The findings highlight the importance of a thorough evaluation that identifies resources to support students, because most attackers were known to have difficulty coping with significant losses or personal failures, had a sense of being persecuted or injured by others before the attack, and engaged in concerning behavior before the incident.

The SSI protocol emphasizes a questioning analytical and skeptical mind-set. This type of thinking is methodical, reasoned, and evaluative, leading to the development of a clinical formulation that deepens understanding about the student's concerning behavior.

The SSI argued that the best way to avoid a targeted school attack is to foster a student-friendly school climate in which students and adults are connected.[5,10] **Box 2** presents a series of 11 investigative questions that can help determine whether a student might *pose* a threat. In the 2004 final SSI report, Robert A. Fein and colleagues[11] emphasized, "Many persons who make threats do not pose threats... [and] some persons who pose threats never make threats."

Box 1
Ten key findings of the Safe School Initiative

1. Incidents of targeted violence at school are rarely sudden, impulsive acts.

2. Before most incidents, other people knew about the attacker's idea and/or plan to attack.

3. Most attackers did not threaten their targets directly before advancing the attack.

4. There is no accurate or useful "profile" of students who engage in targeted school violence.

5. Most attackers engaged in some behavior, before the incident, that caused concern or indicated a need for help.

6. Most attackers were known to have difficulty coping with significant losses or personal failures. Many had considered or attempted suicide.

7. Many attackers felt bullied, persecuted, or injured by others before the attack.

8. Most attackers had access to and had used weapons before the attack.

9. In many cases, other students were involved in some capacity.

10. Despite prompt law enforcement responses, most shooting incidents were stopped by means other than law enforcement intervention.

From Fein RA, Vossekuil B, Pollack W, et al. Threat assessment in schools: a guide to managing threatening situations and to creating safe school climates. United States Secret Service; United States Department of Education; 2002. Available at: http://www.secretservice.gov/ntac/ssi_guide.pdf.

Box 2
Eleven key questions to determine if a student poses a threat

1. What are the student's motive or motives and goals?

2. Have there been any communications suggesting ideas or intent to attack?

3. Has the student shown inappropriate interest in any of the following?
   - School attacks or attackers
   - Weapons (including recent acquisition of any relevant weapon)
   - Incidents of mass violence (terrorism, workplace violence, mass murders)

4. Has the student engaged in attack-related behaviors?

5. Does the student have the capacity to carry out an act of targeted violence?

6. Is the student experiencing hopelessness, desperation, and/or despair?

7. Does the student have a trusting relationship with at least one responsible adult?

8. Does the student see violence as acceptable—or desirable—or the only way to solve problems?

9. Is the student's conversation and "story" consistent with his or her actions?

10. Are other people concerned about the student's potential for violence?

11. What circumstances might affect the likelihood of an attack?

From Fein RA, Vossekuil B, Pollack W, et al. Threat assessment in schools: a guide to managing threatening situations and to creating safe school climates. United States Secret Service; United States Department of Education; 2002. Available at: http://www.secretservice.gov/ntac/ssi_guide.pdf.

Building on the SSI guidelines, Dewey G. Cornell and Peter L. Sheras have conducted several studies examining threat assessment in schools. Their research led to a manual, "Guidelines for Responding to Student Threats of Violence," which presents a field-tested model to assess school threats.[12] The goal was to develop a user-friendly model of threat assessment and to distinguish what they came to call "transient threats" (which can be handled with routine discipline) from "substantive threats," which require more immediate precautions, mental health consultation, and, in extreme cases, law enforcement involvement.

In their first study, over the course of one school year, 188 cases were identified for assessment with only 30% rising to the level of "substantive threats" that required protective plans and consultation.[13] Ultimately, no threats were ever carried out. There were a few expulsions, but the vast majority of students coming to the attention of the assessors were allowed to return to their original schools.

The researchers tested their model as part of the 2007 Virginia High School Safety Study and found that schools using this threat-assessment approach reported decreased bullying, greater willingness among students to seek help, and more positive school climates than schools that did not implement their threat-assessment approach.[14] Although only loosely related to the SSI model, the Virginia program drew on the same underlying principles: connecting threat assessment to an enhanced school climate; appropriate reaction to threats; and consultation with mental health professionals regarding substantive threats.[10] This approach thus provides a bridge from mere risk assessment to a more sophisticated threat assessment.

In this model, consultants work with school systems to foster an environment of genuine safety. An integral component of the school's educational mission is to provide interventions for potentially harmful students before they act out.

OUR MODEL: BEYOND THREAT ASSESSMENT TO SAFETY ASSESSMENT

Developing a program of school safety consultation involves a larger perspective than that of many threat-assessment approaches. It emphasizes an in-depth understanding of a student's and family's objective and subjective experience, and it is best undertaken by a professional who has experience in school consultation and a sophisticated level of mental health training. The consultant should have the clinical experience necessary to pull multiple perspectives together.

An important objective is to move from the phase of crisis evaluation and safety assessment to an effort to mobilize resources of resilience[15,16] and create a climate that strengthens the relationships between students and adults.[6] A sophisticated mental health consultant who uses empathic interviewing and the principles of threat assessment can ultimately enhance a student's capacity for mental health and emotional balance as well as "safety." Although many assessments are limited to only establishing whether the student is safe or not, these evaluations also offer recommendations—once safety is assessed and established—to increase the capacity for how schools can work with the identified student and family. The goal is to enhance the student's learning and to build a safe and civil school climate by fostering emotionally meaningful connections between staff and students alike.[1,5,17,18]

A comprehensive psychiatric safety-assessment approach developed by the lead author (N.R.) is illustrated. This approach was created as part of a school outreach program based within a Harvard Medical School teaching hospital's Department of Psychiatry, located in an urban setting. This 14-year collaboration between the school assessment program and the local school system, elementary through high school, has resulted in more than 140 safety assessments performed to date by N.R. as well as attending psychologists and supervised child psychiatry fellows.

SCHOOL REFERRALS FOR SAFETY ASSESSMENT

School psychologists, guidance counselors, and clinical social workers are often asked to conduct an assessment on a student who may make a threat. In some cases, when the situation is perceived as a high-level threat, the students will be referred to a multidisciplinary team, which often includes an administrator, a school resource officer, and a clinician. When a student is referred for a safety assessment, usually the school has made a decision that they need a more thorough psychiatric evaluation but there is not imminent risk of harm. The clinician conducting the safety assessment should be familiar with the SSI threat-assessment protocols[9,10] and the emphasis on a questioning analytical and skeptical mind-set.

Students are referred for psychiatric safety assessment when their behavior is concerning but not sufficiently serious to result in immediate referral to the police. Although the student may not seem to pose an immediate risk of serious harm, the school asks for consultation to understand the context of the student's behavior and to share the responsibility of making the weighty decision about whether the student is safe to return to school. The consultant can help allay staff anxiety and provide meaningful suggestions about how to effectively continue to intervene with the student.

Reasons for referrals have included threats made or posed (directly or indirectly) to an adult or peer and assaults without a weapon. Some of the referred students have also threatened or assaulted siblings or parents.[19] Behaviors have included escalating explosiveness; swearing at a teacher or threatening to harm a teacher, student, or parent; destroying property in the classroom; fighting with peers; assaulting staff; engaging in inappropriate sexualized behavior; and posting something potentially threatening, or perceived to be threatening, on the Internet.

SAFETY ASSESSMENT: A CASE-BASED EVALUATION MODEL

This assessment model involves review of school records including, but not limited to, the incident report, academic transcript, and, if applicable, any psychological testing or Individualized Education Program (IEP). It involves discussions with school personnel and other involved mental health professionals, a psychiatric interview with the referred student, and a separate interview with his or her family or guardians (**Box 3**).

The first step always is to focus on whether a student is safe and to assess the immediacy of the student's potential for harm (**Box 4**). The consultant must create a therapeutic alliance that allows for deeper psychological understanding and delves into the motivation and context of the student's threat. Therefore, the assessment includes a detailed review of the incident and context that led to the referral; the student's current mental status; questions about involvement in bullying; drug and alcohol and other substance use and abuse; current level of psychosocial stressors for the student and his or her family; questions of exposure to domestic violence; and assessment of school context and previous educational history.

This assessment is done objectively, as well as subjectively, through the eyes of the referred student and the family. Access to weapons is always ascertained. Factors of resilience are also assessed, identifying resources that can be mobilized to enhance the student's higher functioning by expediting access to treatment. The consultant also addresses, if appropriate, how to increase the "goodness of fit" between the

---

Box 3
Components of the assessment model

Record review
- Incident report
- Academic transcript
- Psychological and neuropsychological testing
- IEP

Interviews
- School personnel
- Student
- Parents or guardians

Components of the interview
- Rapport building
- Limits of confidentiality
- Safety assessment
- Exposure to violence/domestic violence
- Mental health assessment, family history, school history
- Questions about bullying
- Access to weapons
- Substance use/abuse

Potential recommendations
- Additional accommodations
- Mental health treatment
- Home-based services
- Functional behavioral analysis
- Academic accommodations
- Mediation
- Alternative educational/therapeutic setting

---

capacity of the student, the parents or legal guardians, and the expectation of the school.[7] The consultant then formulates all of the findings into a written consultation report, in addition to meeting with school personnel, the family, and, at times, the student to discuss findings and recommendations and to participate in treatment and educational planning for the student.

The goal is to work collaboratively with the school team, student, and family to identify interventions that can mobilize support. It is critical to have a clinician who is familiar with school resources and has the capacity to connect vulnerable families to therapeutic services, including those outside the school.

A clinician who is not part of the school staff has the potential to defuse tension if the school and family are in conflict. An outside clinician also may have the added benefit of helping to share responsibility with the school in making a judgment call about whether the student is safe to return to school. Although there are benefits to using

Box 4
Identifying concerning behavior

Behavior that is within typical developmental range

- Impulsivity
- Exploration of provocative topics
- Low frustration threshold and misdirected anger
- Struggles with authority

Concerning behavior (see Meloy and O'Toole[20] for more detail)

- Bizarre statements or behavior
- Obsession with themes of blame or desperation or increasingly concerning obsession with a person or cause, including stalking
- Threatening gestures
- Violent drawing or writing (outside of an assignment)
- Seeking information about weapons and their acquisition and/or a "warrior mentality" that identifies with previous attackers or as an agent of a cause or belief
- Communication of the intent to harm to a third party
- Escalating acts of violence
- Increasing desperation or distress
- Repetitive threats and past history of aggression
- Agitation

an outside clinician, some schools may not have the capacity to employ one. Whether the clinician is drawn from within the school or an outside agency, the clinician must be able to engage families and students, to conduct a thorough assessment that explores the strengths and vulnerabilities of the student and family, and to generate a clinical formulation and recommendations to most effectively support the student and the family.

The consultant is in a privileged position to both validate the school's concerns about safety and respond to the staff's fear that a student may harm others, while also recognizing the feelings and concerns of the family. The consultant mediates among school, student, and family so that the entire system can move forward productively. Although it must be clear that the written evaluation is provided for the school and that the information shared by the family is not confidential, the consultant can still offer a valuable empathic stance. He or she can assist the family to understand what initiated the school crisis and to create a narrative of their experience. The consultant can help the student and family to advocate for what they reasonably need to feel empowered at a time when they may otherwise feel vulnerable or stigmatized and, as a result, misunderstood. Ultimately, the family may come to experience this type of safety-assessment process as a therapeutic intervention, which may, in turn, make them more amenable to following through on suggestions for continued help without feeling criticized or judged, but rather encouraged to promote their own growth.

At the same time, the consultant needs to recognize that the school's duty is to provide safety for all students and to find the appropriate and delicate balance between the student's needs and the school's response. The consultant can help to appropriately diminish the level of tension with the hope of creating a more constructive dialog. However, even when the school is receptive to investing in these types of evaluations, a productive outcome is not guaranteed. The school staff's referral of a disruptive student for a psychologically oriented safety assessment demonstrates a willingness to address the student's needs. However, educators can, at times, be reluctant to follow through on the consultant's recommendations, such as adequately addressing or modifying the school climate, providing the student with the necessary therapeutic services, and remaining open to the needs of the family as well.

The school's resistance to change can occur for a variety of reasons: a lack of resources, external pressure for academic performance over emotional climate, or ambivalence because some school personnel may be exasperated or fearful by this point and therefore not as invested in understanding the depth or context of the student/family perspective. The consultant who remains open to understanding objections or resistance on the part of the school allows for the best chance for a continuing dialog and better receptivity to the consultant's recommendations over time.

SAFETY ASSESSMENT: CASE VIGNETTES

Patrick

Patrick, a biracial adolescent in his junior year of high school, was referred for a safety assessment after teachers learned that he was looking at, and suggesting others visit, a Web site that referred to killing teachers. One of Patrick's teachers viewed the Web site and expressed that she felt unsafe having Patrick in her class. Rather than wait for the administrator and school security to complete their assessment, she immediately contacted other teachers and Patrick's friends to sound the alarm and to share her concerns.

Patrick had a history of initially engaging his teachers with his keen intellect, but then, at some point, would "cross a line." Some teachers struggled with his somewhat rigid sense of self-righteousness when concerns were raised. In the interview with the consulting child psychiatrist, he described how he would argue a matter passionately when someone in power asserted or "forced their control."

Patrick and his parents described the Web page in question as a "stream of consciousness" that contained provocative ideas about the organization of the school and the state of education. Patrick's parents saw the school's response to the incident as overly emotional and excessively harsh. In ninth grade, Patrick had been suspended and subsequently expelled for "playing" with a Swiss Army knife in class after picking it up en route to school. His parents were still angry about what they saw as the school's rigid decision that led to that expulsion, even though the weapon was not used to threaten anyone. The family thought that teachers should know how to avoid getting into power struggles. Patrick suggested that a teacher "should be like a comedian who doesn't get derailed by the hecklers."

Patrick's exploration and curiosity were reframed by the consultant as provocative but not sinister, which allowed Patrick to reenter school and addressed the staff member's anxiety. After comprehensively assessing for threat and finding nothing imminent, but noting an ongoing disconnection between Patrick and some of his teachers, the child psychiatrist formed a plan. The assessment included interviewing the teacher; evaluating the threat; establishing that the student had no intent to hurt the teacher; and determining that he had no history of antisocial behavior, family violence, rage outbursts, aggression, impulsivity, agitation, restlessness, alcohol or drug use, or access to a weapon.

With this information, the focus shifted to understanding the student's sensitivity to humiliation and his struggle with authority, which could lead him to provocative behavior. The goal was to help the school staff contain their anxiety closer to the level of the reality of the problem and to help them see through the bravado of Patrick's normative adolescent curiosity and questioning, which might at times be viewed as menacing. In turn, the psychiatrist worked with Patrick and his parents to let down their guard enough to feel less outraged at the school and to be reflective about how Patrick communicated in a way that could feel threatening to his teachers. Consequently, any potential chance of risk of harm was assessed and alleviated, and the rift in the connection between the school and the student and his parents was repaired.

Problems still arose, such as Patrick negotiating disagreement with teachers, but they could now be resolved without resorting to another safety assessment. Teachers were encouraged to engage in strategies that measured expectations and balanced accountability with flexibility, rather than resorting to demands for apologies and control struggles, which only served to escalate the conflicts. These approaches were key factors to fostering an open dialog, which ultimately allowed Patrick to be more pro-social and less self-sabotaging. The incident at school had made Patrick initially decide not to apply to college, but after the assessment, he chose to pursue the application process and ended up being admitted to an elite college.

Robert

Robert was an eighth grader who lit a fire in a garbage can behind the school after hours. He had also brought a sharp metal object to school, which he threw against a tree during recess. He subsequently denied this, even though adults observed the behavior. He escalated to stealing a cell phone from the assistant principal's office. The school requested consultation to assess whether he was safe to be at school and to understand what was necessary for him to make progress.

During the psychiatric consultation, Robert's mother revealed that her son had problems with his anger, which had gotten significantly worse since both she and Robert's brother became ill. Robert had also been exposed to significant domestic violence aimed toward his mother in early childhood, including observing his mother being burned, hit, and stabbed by her ex-boyfriend. More recently, Robert had become increasingly aggressive at home. His mother also shared that he had recently pinned her up against a wall, kicked his brother without provocation, and held a hot metal rod to his sister's arm. His mother said she discovered him keeping knives under his bed. His mother agreed that he could be aggressively out of control at school.

Robert had also been arrested and charged for alleged sexual assaults in his neighborhood. During the individual interview, Robert was agitated and barely cooperated answering the questions. He seemed to show no remorse about harming his family members. He thought that the school was out to get him and took minimal responsibility for his aggression. He said that he would not participate in outpatient therapy because it was a waste of time. The information that the mother provided to the clinician warranted a report to the child protective services (which was already providing home-based treatment in which Robert was refusing to participate). Because he was so guarded and had prior history of acts of aggression, it was difficult to assess his access to a weapon. His sadism toward his brother and escalation of aggressive behavior and agitation also were extremely concerning. The school had not been aware of the extent of this behavior. His unwillingness to participate in any type of therapy precluded that option to address his anger. To return to a public school setting, Robert needed to be less aggressive and show that he was motivated to develop new skills to replace his reliance on intimidation as a source of power.

In this case, the consultant concluded that Robert could not safely return to his regular educational setting and required more intensive clinical monitoring within a structured residential/therapeutic school. The school was comforted to have shared the responsibility for this difficult placement, which required significant financial investment but seemed necessary. His mother was relieved to finally have the opportunity to speak to the consultant about these increasingly frightening experiences with her much-loved son.

DISCUSSION

In these examples, the school saw each of these students' behaviors as threatening, although neither of them met the threshold of threats of targeted violence. The school's apprehension was understandable: Patrick's obsession with the Web site that seemed to endorse violence against teachers was frightening, and Robert's rising aggression was becoming extremely ominous.

In the first case, the student and family experienced the consultant as a neutral third party who was able to objectively assess the information surrounding the incident. Based on the information gathered, the student was deemed safe to return to school, and recommendations around school climate allowed the student to engage more effectively with teachers. The second case illustrates the cumulative risk factors that led a consultant to determine that a student was at substantive risk to a school, to his family, and perhaps even to himself, and warranted placement in an alternative school setting.

Ongoing retrospective research study of a sample of these comprehensive psychiatric safety assessments performed over the last 5 years has yielded preliminary findings that suggest that some parents and students initially experience the school as overreacting and aligned against them. They react with anger and defensive behavior and may approach the psychiatric evaluation feeling attacked and vulnerable or helpless. Without this safety-assessment process, they might easily have waged an unproductive standoff against the school, which would have diminished the likelihood of the youth's returning to school, much less having a successful outcome. The assessment process shifted this dynamic.

It is critical for the consultant to recognize the asymmetrical nature of the relationship during the process of the evaluation and to act as a neutral, yet empathic, party who can help to realign the goals of the school and the family so that they can move forward. The first step is to understand the complexity and multiplicity of the factors involved in the student's behavior and to determine the context of the threat. The clinician can then leverage his or her role as a mediator among the student, the family, and the school and often address the underlying tensions that are creating an impasse. The process is often high stakes in terms of the decision about whether a child is safe to return to school, but the opportunity for reflection should occur after that decision has been made.

The evaluation can potentially be therapeutic for families and students and affect more wide-ranging life outcomes. The consultant can work with the school to alter the trajectory of the student by determining what course of action is helpful based on the understanding of the student's behavior from the safety assessment. The consultant can help students and families to understand the school rules regarding unsafe behavior and help facilitate access to resources and mental health professionals. Educators often struggle with the responsibility to be responsive to individual students' needs and to keep all students safe. The consultant can provide an opportunity to have a measured approach to evaluating situations in which students may act in alarming ways or make provocative comments. He or she can help tease out the meaning in the context of the student's development and decipher what the student may be communicating. This information may help the school to feel less threatened and to resume a more caring, connected stance, which can, in turn, create a safer environment for all.

SUMMARY

The safety-assessment model presented here expands beyond classic risk assessment. It not only shares the responsibility with educators in making informed decisions about the safety of students but also uses the consultant's expertise to discover the complexity and deep meaning of all the variables that created the crisis of safety and to understand the context. School consultants empathically interview school staff, the student, and the family and construct a narrative encompassing all 3 sides of the story while also attempting to balance and address (or diminish) underlying tension. In this way, the consultant can increase the family's receptiveness for additional scaffolding for the student; galvanize mental health resources; enhance communication among the school, the family, and student; and catapult the school system and family past an impasse. This process, in turn, can provide greater safety and, whenever possible, intensify support at a time when the student needs to shift his or her developmental trajectory in a more positive direction.

This is a delicate process that is not formulaic, but which requires an ability to successfully negotiate when conflict is high. It is critical to empower the family and student at a time when they may feel threatened while simultaneously upholding the school standards of safety for all students. When the consultant has the capacity to create this careful balance, schools are better able to provide a more substantive assurance that they are taking the necessary steps to not only provide immediate safety but to make critical outreach to students and families; this creates a truly positive safe school climate in a way that nurtures students and families while also enhancing the educational mission of the school.

TIPS FOR EDUCATORS

- Zero-tolerance policies are not supported by research and may actually undermine school safety.
- Differentiation of students who may pose a substantial threat from those who make threats is key.
- Comprehensive safety assessments are the best means to avoid a targeted school attack, allowing schools to enhance a positive school climate and to maintain safety while diminishing impasses between school, students, and families.

REFERENCES

1. Nader K, Pollack W. Early interventions: preventing aggression and enhancing connection among youth and adults. In: Nader K, editor. School rampage shootings and other youth disturbances: early preventative interventions. New York: Routledge/Taylor & Francis Group; 2012. p. 245–64.
2. Centers for Disease Control. Youth violence: facts at a glance. 2012. Available at: http://www.cdc.gov/violenceprevention/pdf/yv-datasheet-a.pdf. Accessed July 7, 2014.
3. Centers for Disease Control. Trends in the prevalence of behaviors that contribute to violence on school property: National YRBS 1991-2013. 2014. Available at: http://www.cdc.gov/healthyyouth/yrbs/pdf/trends/us_violenceschool_trend_yrbs.pdf. Accessed July 7, 2014.
4. Borum R, Cornell DG, Modzeleski W, et al. What can be done about school shootings?: a review of the evidence. Educ Res 2010;39:27–37.
5. Pollack W, Modzeleski W, Rooney G. Prior knowledge of potential school-based violence: information students learn may prevent a targeted attack. Washington, DC: United States Secret Service; United States Department of Education; 2008. Available at: http://www.secretservice.gov/ntac/bystander_study.pdf. Accessed July 7, 2014.

6. Resnick MD, Bearman PS, Blum RW, et al. Protecting adolescents from harm: findings from the National Longitudinal Study on Adolescent Health. JAMA 1997;278:823–32.
7. Rappaport N. Survival 101: assessing children and adolescents' dangerousness in school settings. Adolesc Psychiatry 2004;28:157–81.
8. Skiba RJ, Knesting K. Zero tolerance, zero evidence: an analysis of school disciplinary practice. In: Skiba RJ, Noam GG, editors. Zero tolerance: can suspension and expulsion keep school safe?. New directions for youth development, vol. 92 San Francisco (CA): Jossey-Bass; 2002. p. 17–43.
9. Vossekuil B, Fein RA, Reddy M, et al. The final report and findings of the safe school initiative: implications for the prevention of school attacks in the United States. Washington, DC: United States Secret Service; United States Department of Education; 2002. Available at: http://www.secretservice.gov/ntac/ssi_guide.pdf. Accessed July 7, 2014.
10. Fein RA, Vossekuil B, Pollack W, et al. Threat assessment in schools: a guide to managing threatening situations and to creating safe school climates. Washington, DC: United States Secret Service; United States Department of Education; 2002. Available at: http://www.secretservice.gov/ntac/ssi_guide.pdf. Accessed July 7, 2014.
11. Fein RA, Vossekuil B, Holden GA. Threat assessment: an approach to prevent targeted violence. Washington, DC: US Department of Justice, Office of Justice Programs, National Institute of Justice; 1995. p. 1–7.
12. Cornell D, Sheras P. Guidelines for responding to student threats of violence. Longmont (CO): Sopris West; 2006.
13. Cornell D, Sheras P, Cole J, et al. Guidelines for student threat assessment: field-test findings. School Psych Rev 2004;33:527–46.
14. Cornell D, Sheras P, Gregory A, et al. A retrospective study of school safety conditions in high schools using the Virginia threat assessment guidelines versus alternative approaches. Sch Psychol Q 2009;24:119–29.
15. Brooks R, Goldstein S. Raising resilient children: fostering strength, hope, and optimism in your child. New York: McGraw-Hill; 2001.
16. Goldstein S, Brooks R. Handbook of resilience in children. New York: Kluwer Academic/Plenum Publishers; 2005.
17. Cohen J. Social, emotional, ethical, and academic education: creating a climate for learning, participation in democracy, and well-being. Harv Educ Rev 2006;76:201–37.
18. Cohen J, McCabe E, Michelli N, et al. School climate: research, policy, practice, and teacher education. Teach Coll Rec 2009;111:180–213.
19. Rappaport N, Flaherty LT, Hauser ST. Beyond psychopathology: assessing seriously disruptive students in school settings. J Pediatr 2006;149:252–6.
20. Meloy J, O'Toole M. The concept of leakage in threat assessment. Behav Sci Law 2011;29:513–27.

The Role of Schools in Substance Use Prevention and Intervention

Margaret M. Benningfield, MD, MSCI[a],*, Paula Riggs, MD[b],
Sharon Hoover Stephan, PhD[c]

KEYWORDS

- Substance use disorder • Adolescent • School mental health

KEY POINTS

- Schools provide an ideal setting for screening, brief interventions, and outpatient treatment of substance use disorders (SUD).
- Individual treatment for SUD is effective at decreasing substance use as well as substance-related harm.
- In some contexts, rather than being helpful, group interventions can result in harm to participants; therefore, individual treatment may be preferred.
- Early interventions for adolescents using alcohol and other drugs (AOD) are generally effective in decreasing frequency and quantity of AOD use and decreasing risky behaviors.

INTRODUCTION

Most youth who have mental health problems do not receive appropriate services. This treatment gap is especially pronounced for problems related to or co-occurring with substance use.[1] In the United States, about 5% of youth aged 12 to 17 will develop a substance use disorder (SUD) each year, but fewer than 10% of the 1.3 million youth who meet diagnostic criteria for a SUD receive treatment.[2] Many schools implement evidence-based drug/alcohol prevention programs; however, the vast majority of these programs target youth who have not yet initiated substance use. In the community, the vast majority of adolescents who receive treatment are mandated to receive care by juvenile justice. Treatment resources are extremely limited for the estimated 10% to 15% of high school students who regularly use or

[a] Division of Child and Adolescent Psychiatry, Vanderbilt University School of Medicine, Nashville, TN, USA; [b] Division of Substance Dependence, School of Medicine, Mail Stop F478, 12469 East 17th Place, Building 400, Aurora, CO 80045, USA; [c] Center for School Mental Health, Division of Child and Adolescent Psychiatry, University of Maryland School of Medicine, 737 West Lombard Street, 426, Baltimore, MD 21201, USA
* Corresponding author.
E-mail address: meg.benningfield@Vanderbilt.Edu

Child Adolesc Psychiatric Clin N Am 24 (2015) 291–303
http://dx.doi.org/10.1016/j.chc.2014.12.004
1056-4993/15/$ – see front matter © 2015 Elsevier Inc. All rights reserved.

Abbreviations

ACRA	Adolescent Community Reinforcement Approach
AOD	Alcohol and other drugs
CBT	Cognitive–behavioral therapy
CM	Contingency management
CYT	Cannabis Youth Treatment
MDFT	Multidimensional family therapy
MET	Motivational enhancement therapy
SUD	Substance use disorder

---

meet diagnostic criteria for a SUD, but who are not (yet) involved with the juvenile justice system. Co-locating high-quality substance/behavioral health treatment in schools, including in school-based health centers, has the potential to improve screening, treatment access and availability, continuing care, and coordination of medical/behavioral health care.[3] Compared with community-based treatment settings, youth who have access to school-based health centers are 10 times more likely to make a mental health or substance use visit and participate in screening for other high-risk behaviors.[4] Implementing evidenced-based substance treatment interventions in schools also has the potential to reach youth at earlier stages of substance severity and to reduce the risk of progression to more chronic addiction with considerable cost savings to society.[5]

PREVALENCE OF SUBSTANCE USE IN ADOLESCENTS

The National Survey on Drug Use and Health found that 2.2 million youth ages 12 to 17 years reported using illicit drugs in the past month and 1.6 million youth reported binge drinking (consuming 4 or more drinks in 1 sitting for females or 5 or more drinks in 1 sitting for males) in the past month.[2] Most youth who engage in substance use do not meet diagnostic criteria for clinical disorders; however, any substance use during adolescence is concerning because the risk for developing a SUD increases significantly with earlier age of initiation of use.[6] For each year beyond age 14 that first alcohol use is delayed, the odds of subsequent alcohol use disorder drop by 14%. Lifetime prevalence of alcohol dependence was nearly 40% in those who reported first drinking alcohol before age 14 compared with about 10% in those who started drinking at age 20 or older.[6] Thus, efforts to delay the initiation of substance use may significantly impact public health and dramatically decrease the cost to society of SUD.

SCHOOL BASED PREVENTION OF SUBSTANCE USE DISORDERS
School Climate and Connectedness

Connection with school has a bidirectional relationship with adolescent substance use. Youth who drop out of school have a significantly increased risk for cigarette, marijuana, and alcohol use and those who use alcohol and other drugs (AOD) are more likely to leave school.[7] School connectedness is characterized by students having positive relationships with teachers, administrators, and peers at school and expressing a sense of commitment to the school. Connectedness is facilitated by provision of a safe learning environment where students feel they are treated fairly. Even in ideal circumstances, school connectedness often declines as youth enter middle school[8]—a time when rates of AOD use are on the rise. In a study of more than 2000 students, low school connectedness was associated with a 2-fold increase in regular alcohol drinking, cigarette smoking, and marijuana use.[9] It follows that efforts to increase school connectedness by engaging students and families in the school community can impact AOD use.[10] A report from the Centers from Disease Control and Prevention provides a list of guidelines for increasing school connectedness that includes both curricular and logistical actions. These recommendations fall under 4 general categories: adult support, belonging to a positive peer network, commitment to education, and school environment (**Box 1**).[7] Another element of school climate that affects initiation of AOD use is access to drugs on school grounds. In the 2009 Youth Risk Behavior Study, 23% of high school students reported that they had been offered drugs on school property. More robust efforts to define and enforce policies that establish school as a drug-free environment are associated with lower rates of use.[11] In addition to these global strategies targeting the school environment, schools are ideal settings to implement universal, selective, and indicated prevention as well as SUD treatment.

Universal Prevention of Substance Use and Other Risky Behaviors

Schools have been identified as an ideal setting for substance use prevention programs because they can be incorporated into the usual curriculum to reach large populations of youth before beliefs and expectations about AOD use have been firmly established. Beginning in elementary school, some programs targeting aggression and disruptive behaviors are effective in preventing multiple risky behaviors including initiation of substance use and prevention of SUD.[12] A recent Cochrane (2011) review, however, concluded that only a small number of drug/alcohol prevention programs had sufficient empirical support for their efficacy.[13] One example of such a program is the Good Behavior Game, a method of classroom behavior management used by teachers in first and second grade classrooms.[14] The specific target of this intervention was to improve classroom socialization of children who displayed aggressive, disruptive behavior. Longitudinal follow-up of students in classrooms where teachers were randomized to receive Good Behavior Game training found significant decreases in SUD when the students were aged 19 to 21 years.[15] The rate of lifetime SUD in

---

Box 1
Factors that can increase school connectedness

Adult Support

School staff can dedicate their time, interest, attention, and emotional support to students.

Belonging to a Positive Peer Group

A stable network of peers can improve student perceptions of school.

Commitment to Education

Believing that school is important to their future, and perceiving that the adults in school are invested in their education, can get students engaged in their own learning and involved in school activities.

School Environment

The physical environment and psychosocial climate can set the stage for positive student perceptions of school.

From Centers for Disease Control and Prevention. School connectedness: Strategies for increasing protective factors among youth. Atlanta (GA): U.S. Department of Health and Human Services; 2009.

males was significantly lower in those who were in Good Behavior Game classrooms (19%) compared with control classrooms (38%) and the decrease in risk was most pronounced for youth at greatest risk.

Other interventions have been developed for middle school students to delay the onset of first substance use and prevent progression to SUD. These programs typically target sixth or seventh grade students who have not yet begun using AOD and focused on increasing knowledge about potential risks of AOD use, drug refusal skills, resistance to peer pressure, and improved decision making skills.[16] Notably, even the best prevention interventions have only modest effect sizes that attenuate over time. Programs that engage students in active processes have been found to be more effective than didactic lecture-based programs.

Indicated Prevention and Early Intervention for Mild to Moderate Substance Use

As noted, most adolescents who use substances do not meet criteria for clinical disorders; however, early interventions to reduce quantity and frequency of AOD use may prevent or delay progression to SUD. Several systematic reviews have examined brief interventions to address subclinical AOD use in adolescents.[17,18] In general, early intervention can be effective in decreasing AOD-related harm, but the benefits may be short lived and the study design has a significant impact on results. For example, in a recent review of brief interventions delivered in schools, brief interventions were more effective than assessment only, but no more effective than a control condition that provided teens with information about substance use.[17]

Although brief interventions can be effective in decreasing harm in youth who do not meet diagnostic criteria for SUD, more intensive school-based motivational enhancement therapy (MET)/cognitive–behavioral therapy (CBT) interventions are needed for the estimated 10% to 15% of adolescents who have clinically significant patterns of AOD use.

SCHOOL BASED SCREENING AND REFERRAL TO TREATMENT

Most youth who have SUD problems will not seek treatment, and youth who receive treatment in schools are even less likely than peers in clinic settings to recognize substance use as a problem or understand the need for treatment.[19–21] Therefore, effective screening is essential to providing services that may prevent long-term consequences of disease. Screening Brief Intervention and Referral to Treatment (SBIRT) refers to a model for intervention that applies universal screening for all students and offers brief motivational enhancement to address mild to moderate problems. When more severe problems are identified, referral to more intensive treatment is indicated.[22]

Use of a formal screening instrument increases dramatically the likelihood of positive reports in multiple settings. In 1 study of pediatricians who screened for substance use in routine clinical care, a standard screening identified 100 youth with problem substance use and 86 who met full diagnostic criteria for SUD, whereas a clinical examination without a formal screening tool identified only 16 with problem use and 10 with a SUD.[23] Many screening tools have been validated for use in adolescents and may be administered in school settings (**Table 1**). One convenient screening tool is the CRAFFT questionnaire that asks 6 yes or no questions regarding experience with AOD (**Box 2**).[27] These questions screen for problematic AOD use and can be administered by any concerned adult. Adolescents who answer yes to any of these questions should undergo additional assessment of the frequency and quantity of use as well as negative consequences of AOD use. The additional information gathered in a clinical interview can guide decisions about referral for treatment to the

Table 1
Evidence-based assessment for SUD

Screening Instrument	Primary Focus	No. of Items	Estimated Time to Complete (min)	Cost	Reference
Adolescent Diagnostic Interview (ADI)	Comprehensive review of symptoms related to SUD	213	50	$75 per kit (includes 5 assessment booklets)	24
Adolescent Drug Involvement Scale (ADIS)	Developed as a research tool to distinguish heavy, problematic users from lower risk users	13	5	Free	25
Alcohol Use Disorders Identification Test (AUDIT)	Screening for problem alcohol use across health care settings	10	10	Free	26
CRAFFT	Screener to identify youth who require further assessment	6	<5	Free	27
Drug Use Screening Inventory (DUSI)	Measures severity of problems in 10 domains, including substance use and psychiatric symptoms	159	20	$3 per assessment; $495 for computer scoring	28
Fagerstrom Test for Nicotine Dependence	Assessment for tobacco dependence	6	<5	Free	29
Global Assessment of Individual Needs (GAIN)	Recency, breadth, and frequency of problems and service use related to substance use	1606	60–120	$1 per use	30
Marijuana Problem Inventory (MPI)	Adapted from RAPI; assesses problem behaviors associated with cannabis use	23	10	Free	31

(continued on next page)

Table 1
(continued)

Screening Instrument	Primary Focus	No. of Items	Estimated Time to Complete (min)	Cost	Reference
Personal Experience Screening Questionnaire (PESQ)	Screener to identify youth who require further assessment	40	10	$70 per 25	[32]
Rutgers Alcohol Problem Index (RAPI)	Developed to assess problems related to alcohol use in adolescents and young adults (ages 12–20)	23	10	Free	[33]
Rutgers Alcohol Problem Index–brief version	Adapted from RAPI to address concern regarding biases	18	10	Free	[34]
Severity of Dependence Scale (SDS)	Developed for adults to measure severity of different drugs in the context of SUD	5	<5	Free	[35]
Substance Abuse Subtle Screening Inventory-Adolescent Version (SASSI)	Identifies low or high probability of SUD and provides clinical insight into family and social risk factors, level of defensive responding, and consequences of substance misuse teens endorsed.	100	15	$135 for starter kit including 25 assessments	[36]

Abbreviation: SUD, substance use disorder.

recommended level of care. Assessment should include evaluation for other co-occurring psychiatric illness as well as SUD.

Notably, even if schools effectively screened for substance abuse and SUD, it is highly unlikely that students who screen positive for SUD and who are referred to

---

Box 2
The CRAFFT questions

C   Have you ever ridden in a **CAR** driven by someone (including yourself) who was "high" or
     had been using alcohol or drugs?

R   Do you ever use alcohol or drugs to **RELAX**, feel better about yourself, or fit in?

A   Do you ever use alcohol or drugs while you are by yourself, **ALONE**?

F   Do you ever **FORGET** things you did while using alcohol or drugs?

F   Do your family or **FRIENDS** ever tell you that you should cut down on your drinking or
     drug use?

T   Have you ever gotten into **TROUBLE** while you were using alcohol or drugs?

© John R. Knight, MD, Boston Children's Hospital, 2015. All rights reserved. Reproduced with
permission. For more information, contact ceasar@childrens.harvard.edu.

---

substance treatment would enter treatment in non-school community settings. Even if they are wiling to go, the lack of third- party payers and distance from community-based substance treatment settings typically prohibit follow-through with referrals to community-based substance use treatment. Ideally, treatment should be located at the screening site; however, to sustain this model in schools, existing third-party payers and reimbursement systems will have to evolve (or align incentives) with this progressive health care reform.

School-Based Treatment for Substance Use Disorders

When outpatient SUD treatment is the appropriate level of care, it may be most convenient to provide these services on site at the school. School-based treatment can increase access to care, reduce barriers (including transportation), and can promote ongoing connectedness with the school community, which may be protective. Effective treatments for adolescent SUD have been conducted in clinic settings, but are only more recently being implemented and evaluated in schools. Results from a recently completed pilot study provide empirical support for this conjecture.[37,38] The study adapted an existing 16-week evidence-based MET/CBT plus contingency management (CM)/motivational incentives intervention (Encompass) as a briefer (8-week) school-based intervention. Fifteen students who committed drug- or alcohol-related school offences were consecutively referred for clinical evaluation. All met DSM-5 diagnostic criteria for cannabis use disorder and 13 of the 15 enrolled in the 8-session intervention after adolescent assent and parental consent. Nine (69%) completed treatment with 95% compliance (CBT session attendance) and more than one-half (56%) achieved at least 1 month of sustained abstinence during treatment based on weekly urine drug screens.[37]

WHICH TREATMENTS WORK BEST FOR ADOLESCENT SUBSTANCE USE?

According to recent published reviews, the following psychosocial interventions are considered to have "well-established efficacy": (1) individual CBT with or without a component of MET, (2) multidimensional family therapy (MDFT), (3) functional family therapy, and (3) group CBT.[39–44] Interventions deemed to be "probably efficacious" include (1) brief strategic family therapy, (2) behavioral family therapy, and (3) multisystem therapy.[41] Taken together, these interventions have comparable and moderate acute treatment effect sizes on reductions in substance and more modest effects on sustained abstinence.[39,41,45–47] Of the treatment strategies listed, interventions that utilize individual MET or CBT have consistently shown greater sustained or emerging post-treatment effect size compared with family-based interventions.[39,41,45] Other studies have shown that CM using motivational incentives (ie, voucher payments or prize drawings) increase significantly rates of sustained abstinence when added to individual MET/CBT compared with MET/CBT alone.[48,49] In a randomized controlled trial of CM in 69 adolescents (ages 14–18) with cannabis use disorders, 50% of the participants who receive CM plus MET/CBT achieved at least 10 weeks of abstinence compared with 18% who received MET/CBT alone. In this study, between group differences were maintained at 6 months, but not the 9-month post-treatment follow-up.[50]

Treatment Format: Group, Family, or Individual Based

Selecting the best format for treatment requires careful balance of the needs of the population and available resources. The primary question must be whether the selected format is effective in treating the problem; arguably as important is the efficiency and cost effectiveness of the program to be delivered. Group interventions may be particularly appealing because a greater number of youth can be treated in a short amount of time with fewer therapist resources. Considerable evidence has shown group treatments to be effective for treatment of adolescent mental health problems, including SUD.[41] A good example is the group-based MET and CBT tested in the Cannabis Youth Treatment (CYT) study. This study compared a 5-session group-based treatment condition (MET/CBT5) with a 12-session condition (MET/CBT12) and a third condition that added a family education component to MET/CBT12. Participants in each of the conditions reduced the quantity and frequency of drug use with no significant difference between group assignments.[51] This study suggests that a group format can be effective in treatment for youth with cannabis use disorders and that as few as 5 sessions may be needed to produce meaningful benefit. Group treatments are not always appropriate, however, for adolescents with SUD.

Individuals with co-occurring conduct problems were excluded from the CYT study. This is critical, because high-risk youth may be sensitive to the influence of "deviant friendships" that can worsen outcomes.[52] Group treatment settings can provide a format for youth to receive positive feedback from peers regarding discussion of deviant behavior. In 1 longitudinal study, involvement in group-based treatment resulted in poorer outcomes and counselor report of strong rapport and youth engagement in treatment was not associated with more favorable outcome.[52] Potential negative effects of group treatment may be mitigated by strong leadership from a skilled therapist and inclusion of nondeviant participants.[53,54]

Family treatments for adolescent SUD are appealing because of the potential roles of family discord, parental substance use, and parental monitoring in the developmental processes that contribute to adolescent SUD. Family treatments have been shown to be effective in decreasing substance use, but these treatments are typically more challenging and more expensive to implement than individual or group-based treatment.[51] The CYT provides additional relevant data regarding the question of cost effectiveness of family-based treatment. A second trial in the CYT compared group-based MET/CBT5 with Adolescent Community Reinforcement Approach (ACRA) and MDFT. Both ACRA and MDFT combine individual, parent, and family session with case management and were delivered over 12 to 14 weeks. In this trial, as in the previous one described, youth improved in all 3 conditions without significant between-group differences. A cost-effectiveness analysis found MET/CBT5 and ACRA to be superior to MDFT.

Given the potential risks of group-based treatment and the challenges inherent in providing family treatment in school settings (related to limited school hours and some families' poor past experiences with the school system),[55] individual treatment may be the most appropriate format for delivery in schools. Further support for this conclusion comes form a recent meta-analysis of 16 intervention studies that found individual treatments to be more effective than family-based treatment for adolescent SUD (effect sizes of 0.75 and 0.46, respectively).[39] Several components of effective individual treatment are described in **Box 3**.

Integration of treatment for co-occurring disorders is an important component of the treatment of SUD. The vast majority (up to 90% in 1 study)[56] of adolescents who receive treatment for substance use have at least 1 co-occurring disorder. Youth who receive treatment at school are even more likely than youth in an outpatient setting to have co-occurring disorders and more likely to have never received mental health treatment.[19–21] The Substance Abuse and Mental Health Services Administration has promoted an integrated treatment strategy in which the treatment of co-occurring disorders includes screening, assessment, treatment planning, service delivery, and continuity of care to address both the substance use and mental health concerns.[56–58]

Recovery High Schools

Some adolescents may continue to struggle to achieve and maintain treatment gains in typical school settings. For these individuals, specialized schools that provide added support for youth in recovery may be appealing. No empirical studies to date

---

Box 3
Components of effective individual treatment

Treatment Component	Description
Motivational enhancement (ME)	This approach aims to reduce ambivalence about engaging in treatment and stopping substance use, and to generate internally motivated change. The clinician uses principles of motivational interviewing to elicit motivational statements from the client and to develop a change plan. After an initial assessment, the clinician provides feedback, generates discussion about substance use, and works to strengthen motivation. Coping skills for risky situations are discussed, cessation strategies are reviewed, and counseling sessions focus on commitment to change or sustained abstinence.
Cognitive–behavioral therapy (CBT)	Cognitive–behavioral approaches aim to replace substance use with other behaviors by identifying antecedents of use (and avoiding those circumstances when possible), and developing coping skills to address problems that lead to increased use. CBT emphasizes changing behavior and thoughts, and teaching and practicing new coping skills. Common skills to consider include: increasing enjoyable activities, resisting peer pressure with assertive communication, and building a recovery support network.
Contingency management (CM)	CM is based on an operant framework, such that substance use is considered operant behavior that is maintained both by the pharmacologic actions of the substance(s) and by social and other nonpharmacologic reinforcement associated with substance use. CM interventions aim to reduce the influence of reinforcement from substance use and its associated features, and to increase the frequency and intensity of reinforcement from healthier alternative activities.

have examined the effect of these programs on adolescent substance use or long-term outcomes. However, a recent qualitative review described 17 recovery high school programs.[59] These programs are small, with an average enrollment of 24 students. Most of the schools had a capacity for more students, but faced challenges with enrollment, including a scarcity of referrals of students, meeting enrollment criteria, and transportation challenges.

SUMMARY

AOD use and SUD are significant public health challenges that affect a great number of youth. Effective strategies have been described that prevent or delay the onset of AOD use at multiple stages of development. Promoting school connectedness, particularly during the middle school years, can be protective in preventing early substance use. In the elementary school years, interventions to improve classroom socialization for youth with aggressive and disruptive behaviors may decrease SUD later in life, although results are modest and may attenuate over time. Some middle school programs that provide education about the potential risks of AOD use, specific refusal skills, and promote self-efficacy, have also proven effective, although the again impact is modest. Early interventions with adolescents who have begun using AOD, but have not developed clinical symptoms, can stall the progression of use and may prevent SUD. In youth who meet criteria for SUD, individual cognitive–behavioral treatment that integrates assessment and treatment of other co-occurring mental health problems is a proven strategy that holds promise for delivery in school settings. The most promising substance abuse treatment intervention for adolescents is MET/CBT, combined with CM/motivational incentives. For youth who continue to struggle to maintain treatment gains, recovery schools may be appealing, but these programs require further investigation to fully understand their impact on long-term outcomes.

REFERENCES

1. Merikangas KR, He J, Burstein M, et al. Service utilization for lifetime mental disorders in U.S. adolescents: results of the National Comorbidity Survey-Adolescent Supplement (NCS-A). J Am Acad Child Adolesc Psychiatry 2011;50(1):32–45.
2. SAMHSA, Substance Abuse and Mental Health Services Administration. Results from the 2013 national survey on drug use and health: summary of national findings. NSDUH Series H-48, HHS Publication No. (SMA) 14–4863. Rockville (MD): U.S. Department of Health and Human Services; 2014.
3. Mills C, Stephan SH, Moore E, et al. The President's new freedom commission: capitalizing on opportunities to advance school-based mental health services. Clin Child Fam Psychol Rev 2006;9(3–4):149–61.
4. Kaplan DW, Calonge BN, Guernsey BP, et al. Managed care and school-based health centers use of health services. Arch Pediatr Adolesc Med 1998;152(1):25–33.
5. Dennis ML. Opportunities for substance abuse prevention and intervention in schools. Presentation at the Joint Meeting on Adolescent Treatment Effectiveness (JMATE). Washington, DC, 2012. Available at: http://www.jmate.org/jmate2012/PastMeetings.aspx.
6. Grant BF, Dawson D. Age of onset of drug use and its association with DSM-IV drug abuse and dependence: results from the National Longitudinal Alcohol Epidemiologic Survey. J Subst Abuse 1998;10(2):163–73.
7. Centers for Disease Control and Prevention. School connectedness: strategies for increasing protective factors among youth. Atlanta (GA): U.S. Department of Health and Human Services; 2009.

8. Durlak JA, Weissberg RP, Dymnicki AB. The impact of enhancing students' social and emotional learning: a meta-analysis of school-based universal interventions. Child Dev 2011;82(1):405–32.
9. Bond L, Butler H, Thomas L, et al. Social and school connectedness in early secondary school as predictors of late teenage substance use, mental health, and academic outcomes. J Adolesc Health 2007;40(4):357.e9–18.
10. Fletcher A, Bonell C, Hargreaves J. School effects on young people's drug use: a systematic review of intervention and observational studies. J Adolesc Health 2008;42(3):209–20.
11. Evans-Whipp T, Beyers JM, Lloyd S, et al. A review of school drug policies and their impact on youth substance use. Health Promot Int 2004;19(2):227–34.
12. Hopfer S, Davis D, Kam JA, et al. A review of elementary school-based substance use prevention programs: identifying program attributes. J Drug Educ 2010;40(1):11–36.
13. Foxcroft DR, Tsertsvadze A. Universal school-based prevention programs for alcohol misuse in young people. Cochrane Database Syst Rev 2011;(5):CD009113.
14. Kellam SG, Wang W, Mackenzie AC, et al. The impact of the good behavior game, a universal classroom-based preventive intervention in first and second grades, on high-risk sexual behaviors and drug abuse and dependence disorders into young adulthood. Prev Sci 2014;15(Suppl 1):S6–18.
15. Kellam S, Brown C, Poduska J, et al. Effects of a universal classroom behavior management program in first and second grades on young adult behavioral, psychiatric, and social outcomes. Drug Alcohol Depend 2008;95(1):S5–28.
16. Faggiano F, Versino E, Zambon A, et al. School-based prevention for illicit drugs use: a systematic review. Prev Med 2008;46(5):385–96.
17. Carney T, Myers BJ, Louw J, et al. Brief school-based interventions and behavioural outcomes for substance-using adolescents. Cochrane Database Syst Rev 2014;(2):CD008969.
18. Carney T, Myers B. Effectiveness of early interventions for substance-using adolescents: findings from a systematic review and meta-analysis. Subst Abuse Treat Prev Policy 2012;7(1):25.
19. Hunter BD, Godley MD, Godley SH. Feasibility of implementing the Adolescent Community Reinforcement Approach in school settings for adolescents with substance use disorders. Advances in School Mental Health Promotion 2014;7(2):105–22. http://dx.doi.org/10.1080/1754730X.201.888224.
20. Hunter SB, Ayer L, Han B, et al. Examining the sustainment of the Adolescent-Community Reinforcement Approach in community addiction treatment settings: protocol for a longitudinal mixed method study. Implementation Science 2014;9(1):104. http://dx.doi.org/10.1186/s13012-014-0104-1.
21. Vincent RM, Belur VK, Ives ML. Feasibility and impact of implementing MET/CBT as a substance use treatment intervention in school-based settings. Presentation at the Joint Meeting on Adolescent Treatment Effectiveness (JMATE). Washington, DC, April 10–12, 2012. Available at: http://www.jmate.org/jmate2012/PastMeetings.aspx.
22. Mitchell SG, Gryczynski J, Gonzales A, et al. Screening, Brief Intervention, and Referral to Treatment (SBIRT) for Substance Use in a School-Based Program: Services and Outcomes. The American Journal on Addictions 2012;21(s1):S5–13.
23. Wilson CR, Sherritt L, Gates E, et al. Are clinical impressions of adolescent substance use accurate? Pediatrics 2004;114(5):e536–40.
24. Winters K, Henly G. Adolescent diagnostic interview (ADI) manual. Los Angeles (CA): Western Psychological Services; 1993.

25. Moberg DP, Hahn L. The adolescent drug involvement scale. Journal of Child and Adolescent Substance Abuse 1991;2(1):75–88.
26. Saunders JB, Aasland OG, Babor TF, et al. Development of the Alcohol Use Disorders Identification Test (AUDIT): WHO collaborative project on early detection of persons with harmful alcohol consumption-II. Addiction 1993;88(6):791–804.
27. Knight JR, Sherritt L, Shrier LA, et al. Validity of the CRAFFT substance abuse screening test among adolescent clinic patients. Arch Pediatr Adolesc Med 2002; 156(6):607–14. Available at: http://www.ncbi.nlm.nih.gov/pubmed/12038895.
28. Tarter R. Evaluation and treatment of adolescent substance abuse: a decision tree method. Am J Drug Alcohol Abuse 1990;16:1–46.
29. Heatherton TF, Kozlowski LT, Frecker RC, et al. The Fagerstrom test for nicotine dependence: a revision of the Fagerstrom tolerance questionnaire. Br J Addict 1991;86:1119–27.
30. Dennis M, Titus J, White M, et al. Global Appraisal of Individual Needs (GAIN): administration guide for the gain and related measures. Bloomington (IL): Chestnut Health Systems; 2002 [Online]. Available at: www.chestnut.org/li/gain/gadm1299.pdf.
31. Vandrey R, Budney AJ, Kamon JL, et al. Cannabis withdrawal in adolescent treatment seekers. Drug Alcohol Depend 2005;78(2):205–10.
32. Winters KC. Development of an adolescent alcohol and other drug abuse screening scale: personal experiences screening questionnaire. Addict Behav 1992;17:479–90.
33. White HR, Labouvie EW. Toward the assessment of adolescent problem drinking. J Stud Alcohol 1989;50:30–7. Available at: http://research.alcoholstudies.rutgers.edu/rapi#sthash.GhBy9PQm.dpuf.
34. White HR, Labouvie EW. Longitudinal trends in problem drinking as measured by the Rutgers alcohol problem index. Alcohol Clin Exp Res 2000;24:76A. Available at: http://research.alcoholstudies.rutgers.edu/rapi#sthash.GhBy9PQm.dpuf.
35. Gossop M, Darke S, Griffiths P, et al. The Severity of Dependence Scale (SDS): psychometric properties of the SDS in English and Australian samples of heroin, cocaine and amphetamine users. Addiction 1995;90(5):607–14.
36. Miller GA. The Substance Abuse Subtle Screening Inventory (SASSI) adolescent manual. Bloomington (IN): The SASSI Institute; 1990.
37. Riggs P. Encompass: an integrated treatment intervention for adolescents with co-occurring psychiatric and substance use disorders. Scientific Proceedings of the American Academy of Child and Adolescent Psychiatry 61st Annual Meeting (AACAP). San Diego, October 23, 2014.
38. Rones M, Hoagwood K. School-based mental health services: a research review. Clin Child Fam Psychol Rev 2000;3(4):223–41.
39. Tripodi SJ, Bender K, Litschge C, et al. Interventions for reducing adolescent alcohol abuse: a meta-analytic review. Arch Pediatr Adolesc Med 2010;164(1): 85–91.
40. U.S. Public Health Service. Report of the surgeon general's conference on children's MH: a national action agenda. Washington, DC: U.S. Department of Health and Human Services; 2000.
41. Waldron H, Turner C. Evidence-based psychosocial treatments for adolescent substance abuse. J Clin Child Adolesc Psychol 2008;37(1):238–61.
42. Walker DD, Stephens R, Roffman R, et al. Randomized controlled trial of motivational enhancement therapy with nontreatment-seeking adolescent cannabis users: a further test of the teen marijuana check-up. Psychol Addict Behav 2011;25(3):474–84.

43. Winters KC, Fahnhorst T, Botzet A, et al. Brief intervention for drug-abusing adolescents in a school setting: outcomes and mediating factors. J Subst Abuse Treat 2012;42(3):279–88.

44. Winters KC, Leitten W. Brief intervention for drug-abusing adolescents in a school setting. Psychol Addict Behav 2007;21(2):249–54.

45. Minozzi S, Amato L, Vecchi S, et al. Psychosocial treatments for drugs and alcohol abusing adolescents (Protocol). Cochrane Database Syst Rev 2011;3: CD00008283.

46. National Institute on Drug Abuse (NIDA). Preventing drug use among children and adolescents: a research guide for parents, educators, and community leaders. 2003. Available at: http://www.drugabuse.gov/sites/default/files/preventingdruguse.pdf. Accessed January 22, 2015.

47. New Freedom Commission on Mental Health. Achieving the promise: transforming mental health care in America, final report (DHHS Pub. No. SMA-03-3832). Rockville (MD): U.S. Department of Health and Human Services; 2003.

48. Budney A, Roffman R, Stephens R, et al. Marijuana dependence and its treatment. Addict Sci Clin Pract 2007;4(1):4–16.

49. Stanger C, Ryan S, Fu H, et al. Parent training plus contingency management for substance abusing families: a Complier Average Causal Effects (CACE) analysis. Drug Alcohol Depend 2011;118(2–3):119–26.

50. Stanger C, Budney A. Contingency management approaches for adolescent substance use disorders. Child Adolesc Psychiatr Clin N Am 2010;19(3):547–62.

51. Dennis M, Godley SH, Diamond G, et al. The Cannabis Youth Treatment (CYT) study: main findings from two randomized trials. J Subst Abuse Treat 2004; 27(3):197–213.

52. Dishion TJ, McCord J, Poulin F. When interventions harm: peer groups and problem behavior. Am Psychol 1999;54(9):755–64.

53. Gifford-Smith M, Dodge KA, Dishion TJ, et al. Peer influence in children and adolescents: crossing the bridge from developmental to intervention science. J Abnorm Child Psychol 2005;33(3):255–65.

54. Kaminer Y. Challenges and opportunities of group therapy for adolescent substance abuse: a critical review. Addict Behav 2005;30(9):1765–74.

55. Brandt NE, Glimpse C, Fette C, et al. Advancing effective family-school-community partnerships. In: Weist MD, Lever NA, Bradshaw CP, et al, editors. Handbook of school mental health. New York: Springer; 2014. p. 209–21.

56. Hawkins EH. A tale of two systems: co-occurring mental health and substance abuse disorders treatment for adolescents. Annu Rev Psychol 2009;60:197–228.

57. Riggs PD. Treating adolescents for substance abuse and comorbid psychiatric disorders. Sci Pract Perspect 2003;2:18–28.

58. Rowe CL, Liddle HA, Greenbaum PE, et al. Impact of psychiatric comorbidity on treatment of adolescent drug abusers. J Subst Abuse Treat 2004;26(2):129–40.

59. Finch AJ, Moberg DP, Krupp AL. Continuing care in high schools: a descriptive study of recovery high school programs. J Child Adolesc Subst Abuse 2014; 23(2):116–29.

Evidence-Based Interventions for Adolescents with Disruptive Behaviors in School-Based Settings

Tarah M. Kuhn, PhD[a],*, Jon S. Ebert, PsyD[a], Kathy A. Gracey, MEd[a],
Gabrielle L. Chapman, PhD[b], Richard A. Epstein, PhD, MPH[a]

KEYWORDS

- Disruptive behavior disorder • School health • Evidence-based practice

KEY POINTS

- Disruptive behaviors in the classroom are a threat to an optimal learning environment. Educators commonly request assistance managing challenging classroom behaviors and these behaviors are a common reason for referral to mental health services.
- Disruptive behavior disorders (DBDs) commonly co-occur with other conditions, thus making defining a course of treatment more challenging. Not all behavior stems from the same emotional/psychosocial source. Interventions need to be individualized and need to consider the underlying and environmental factors contributing to them.
- The primary factor related to effectiveness of interventions for DBDs in adolescents is quality of implementation. Programs with support and established infrastructure, proper training, and ongoing supervision are more effective at reducing disruptive behavior problems.

INTRODUCTION

Approximately 70 million children and adolescents are enrolled in elementary and secondary schools in the United States each year.[1] Elementary and secondary education play a significant role in child and adolescent development. A significant educational task is to create and maintain learning environments that promote optimal learning by providing developmentally appropriate challenges and tasks.[2]

The authors have nothing to disclose.
[a] Department of Psychiatry, Vanderbilt University School of Medicine, 1500 21st Avenue South, Village at Vanderbilt, Suite 2200, Nashville, TN 37211, USA; [b] Peabody Research Institute, Vanderbilt University, 230 Appleton Place, PMB 181, Nashville, TN 37203, USA
* Corresponding author. Department of Psychiatry, Vanderbilt University School of Medicine, 1500 21st Avenue South, Village at Vanderbilt, Suite 2200, Nashville, TN 37211.
E-mail address: tarah.kuhn@vanderbilt.edu

Child Adolesc Psychiatric Clin N Am 24 (2015) 305–317
http://dx.doi.org/10.1016/j.chc.2014.11.005
1056-4993/15/$ – see front matter © 2015 Elsevier Inc. All rights reserved.

childpsych.theclinics.com

Abbreviations	
AACAP	American Academy of Child and Adolescent Psychiatry
ADHD	Attention-deficit/hyperactivity disorder
CD	Conduct disorder
DBD	Disruptive behavior disorder
IED	Intermittent explosive disorder
ODD	Oppositional defiant disorder
PSST	Problem-solving skills training

Disruptive behaviors in the classroom are a common threat to optimal learning environment maintenance and it is not surprising that educators commonly request assistance managing challenging classroom behaviors or that these behaviors are a common reason for referral to mental health services.[3,4] Disruptive behaviors have been shown to impair the school learning environment,[5] take attention away from other students,[6] and increase teacher burnout rates.[7] Teachers who must spend a great deal of time managing challenging classroom behaviors have been shown to have less time for academics and to have students with lower grades and poorer performance on standardized tests.[8]

Disruptive behaviors can include problems, such as defiance, hostility, aggression, and sometimes violence.[9] Although disruptive behavior problems can occur in students of all ages,[10] adolescence is a developmental stage of particular concern because as youths get older, disruptive behavior can become more tied to delinquency, increased risk for substance use, involvement with the juvenile justice system, and other high-risk behaviors. Also, as youths age, disruptive behaviors become more associated with academic underachievement and truancy.[11] Additionally, violence is increasingly prevalent across adolescence,[12] and violence in schools has garnered recent national attention.

There has been an increased recognition by schools of the need to more broadly address students' social and emotional development through the adoption and structuring of social and emotional learning programs that can support the learning of skills needed to be successful.[13] With this recognition has come an increased focus on assisting students in a more formal way with the development of skills, such as regulating affect, staying focused, and navigating social interactions. Schools have adopted varying levels of intervention, including primary, secondary, and tertiary. Primary interventions are focused on prevention that intervenes in behaviors before they become problematic. These are often delivered at a school-wide level. Secondary-level interventions are aimed at addressing problem behaviors before they become severe and are often delivered at a classroom or small group level. Tertiary-level interventions are aimed at youths who have been specifically identified due to problematic behaviors, which are often more intense or frequent and require individualized attention.[14] This clinical review examines existing literature to make recommendations regarding interventions for adolescent disruptive behaviors in school-based settings.

DISRUPTIVE BEHAVIOR PROBLEMS

DBDs are generally defined by a pattern of behaviors that include violation of societal rules and norms that have a negative impact on functioning in the home, community, or school setting.[9] DBDs include oppositional defiant disorder (ODD), conduct disorder (CD), intermittent explosive disorder (IED), and attention-deficit/hyperactivity disorder (ADHD).[9] Criteria for ODD include angry and irritable mood, argumentative and defiant behavior, and vindictiveness. Criteria for CD include aggression and threat of physical harm, deliberate destruction of property, deceitfulness and theft, and serious violation of rules. IED is marked by an inability to control aggressive impulses and includes verbal aggression and physical aggression that is noninjurious or destructive.[9] Although this group of disorders includes ADHD, and some of the behaviors that youths with ODD and CD exhibit may be similar to those of youths with ADHD, these are considered separate diagnoses that can occur independently of one another and have separate treatment pathways.[15,16] This review does not focus on ADHD; rather, it focuses on disruptive behavior problems marked by hostility, defiance, and noncompliance with authority.

DBDs are considered some of the most common psychiatric disorders of adolescence,[16] and the prevalence of disruptive behavior problems more generally is likely higher. The overall prevalence of ODD in children and adolescents is up to 20% and up to 10% for CD.[17] Studies have found that ODD symptoms typically emerge 2 to 3 years earlier in childhood than do CD symptoms, with the average onset for ODD at 6 years compared with 9 years for CD.[18,19] Symptom severity is seen as increasing from ODD to CD, and presentation of these behaviors can be viewed as a developmental progression with increasing age.[20] Approximately one-third of children with ODD subsequently develop CD and, of those who develop CD, approximately 40% later meet criteria for antisocial behavior in adulthood.[21,22]

Epidemiologic research has found significant associations and comorbidity between DBDs and anxiety and depression. Although the ranges of co-occurrence are broad in the literature, 5% to 55% for anxiety and 2% to 50% for depression, this indicates a need for individuals working with youths with disruptive behaviors to consider possible underlying issues.[23] Due to their behaviors, youths with DBDs have difficulty with peer interactions and are also known to struggle with low self-esteem.[24] By preadolescence, ODD has been shown to occur at high rates with major depression.[24] Defining a course of treatment may be more challenging when there are significant comorbidities, because disruptive behaviors are not always intended to purposefully accomplish what the behavior seems to address.[25,26] For example, a youth who is defiant or aggressive in the classroom (eg, displaying disruptive behavior) may have anxiety associated with academic performance or social interactions and the disruptive behaviors may be a means of managing or disguising anxiety. As this example illustrates, it is important to assess co-occurring conditions that may help inform decisions regarding intervention.[26]

Several factors have been shown to increase a young person's risk for disruptive behavior problems.[17,27] Multiple environmental factors, such as parental psychopathology, poverty, problematic family functioning, dysfunctional parent-child interactions, and child abuse, are thought to play a role in the presentation and severity of disruptive behavior problems.[27] In addition to environmental variables, cognitive deficits,[28] social-cognitive information processing,[27] and peer rejection can also be contributing factors.[27] It is important, as with possible comorbidity, to assess for environmental factors contributing to the maintenance of disruptive behaviors. If factors related to parental and family functioning are present, interventions need to be chosen that can address needs on this level. Additionally, assessment of cognitive and social factors that play a role in disruptive factors direct the type and level of intervention that is recommended.

PRACTICE GUIDELINES FOR DISRUPTIVE BEHAVIOR PROBLEMS

General clinical practice guidelines for interventions related to DBDs generally suggest psychosocial interventions, parent training, and pharmacotherapy when needed. This clinical standard is reflected in the American Academy of Child and Adolescent Psychiatry (AACAP) clinical practice guidelines for ODD.[29] The AACAP guidelines include (1) building and maintaining therapeutic alliance with youth and family, (2) cultural awareness and issues, (3) diagnostic interviewing and assessment that include reports from both youth and caregiver, (4) assessment for diagnostic comorbidity of psychiatric disorders, (5) individualized treatment planning, (6) evidence-based parenting interventions, (7) collection of collateral documentation/information, (8) ongoing treatment assessment of treatment dose and intensity, and (9) pharmacotherapy as needed for disruptive behaviors or for comorbid disorders.[29] These guidelines provide a useful framework for outpatient clinical practice but do not provide guidance about a particular psychosocial intervention to use.

INTERVENTIONS FOR ADOLESCENT DISRUPTIVE BEHAVIORS IN SCHOOL SETTINGS

Two recent meta-analyses discussed youth-, program-, and implementation-level characteristics associated with program effectiveness but did not make recommendations about specific, named programs; rather, the recommendations focused on program type.[30,31] Regarding youth-level characteristics, these analyses showed larger effect sizes for youths at high risk for disruptive behavior problems than for youths at low risk and greater reductions in disruptive behaviors for adolescents and young children compared with grade school children.

Specific intervention strategies used to prevent and/or reduce aggressive or disruptive behaviors in the classroom were categorized in the following program types: behavior management, therapy/counseling, cognitive behavior/social competence training, academic services, separate/special school, multimodal programs, and peer mediation. Although behavior management and therapy/counseling programs demonstrated larger effect sizes, the investigators cited similarity in effect size across intervention strategies. One-on-one interventions were only marginally more effective than group interventions, and programs directly targeting aggressive behavior were not significantly more effective than those that were more indirect. Given the similarity of effectiveness across different types of intervention, the primary factor related to effectiveness that these investigators highlight was the quality of the implementation.

Research has shown that the quality of the dissemination and implementation of a program is one of the most significant variables to program effectiveness. In some program implementation initiatives, a well-implemented program of less efficacious research can outperform a more efficacious one that is poorly implemented.[32] The implication is that simply identifying an efficacious approach to disruptive behavior problems is only one part of the process for reducing disruptive behavior problems in school cultures. Attending to the implementation process and following the program model with fidelity over a significant period of time are essential to outcomes. In addition to program model training and fidelity, critical implementation drivers for optimal outcomes include ongoing training and coaching in the program, organizational and infrastructure changes that support the use of the model, and ongoing leadership supports.[33] Therefore, the pairing of an efficacious intervention strategy with quality implementation over time has the best potential to reduce disruptive behavior problems.[34,35]

These meta-analyses suggest a variety of program types effectively reduce adolescent disruptive behavior in classroom settings and that schools should, therefore, focus on choosing programs that they can implement well and support over time. This recommendation is generally consistent with insights from implementation science suggesting that future research focus on service delivery processes and the impact of contextual factors to improve program implementation and sustainability.[33]

SPECIFIC INTERVENTIONS FOR DISRUPTIVE BEHAVIOR PROBLEMS

Although recent reviews find support for various child-, parent-, and family-level interventions, specific guidance about which individual interventions work for which adolescents in specific treatment settings is somewhat lacking.[36,37] When considering the full span of development, there seems to be general support for the utilization of parent training programs as effective for the treatment of disruptive behaviors among young children. In adolescence, the literature recommends youth-focused interventions, a combination of child training and parent training interventions, or multicomponent interventions to treat disruptive behaviors (**Table 1**).[36]

Table 1
Examples of supported evidence-based practice treatment model and description

Treatment Model	Description
Anger control training (Lochman et al,[38] 1999)	Anger control training generally refers to 2 programs, anger coping program and coping power program. Both of these programs are designed for 4th- to 6th-grade youths but can be adapted for older adolescents. Both are cognitive behavior–based programs that conceptualize aggression in youths as linked to increased attribution of hostility in social interactions as well as a heightened attention to hostile cues in the environment. Anger control training interventions use group sessions focused on anger management, perspective taking, social problem solving, emotional awareness, relaxation training, social skills, and goal setting to modify youths' social information processing problems. These interventions are generally done in an 18-session group format but can also be delivered in one-on-one sessions. The coping power program is an extension of the anger coping program, increasing interventions to 34 group sessions and adding a parent group component.
Group assertiveness training (Huey & Rank,[51] 1984)	Group assertiveness training is a manualized group-based intervention that was developed for 8th- and 9th-grade African American boys referred for aggressive behavior. It is based on the verbal response model of assertiveness. Group sessions meet twice weekly and for a total of 8 h. This intervention has been shown effective when delivered by both group and trained peer leaders compared with professional or peer-led discussion group and no treatment controls.
Problem-solving skills training (PSST) (Kazdin,[52] 2003)	PSST is a cognitive behavior intervention that was developed for youths ages 7 to 13 y. PSST is delivered one-on-one with youths over the course of 20–25 sessions. The intervention teaches youths to deal with thoughts and feelings in more constructive ways using modeling, role-playing, token economy, and teaching alternative problem-solving strategies. There are additional extensions of PSST, including PSST plus practice and PSST plus parent management training. PSST plus practice adds a real-life practice component, in which a youth and clinician plan activities aimed at practicing the skills and goals identified in sessions.
Rational emotive mental health program (Block,[53] 1978)	Rational emotive mental health program was implemented with 10th- and 11th-grade students with disruptive behaviors and delivered in a group model. It is based on rational emotive psychotherapy[54] and other work in the area applying rational emotive therapy principles to the education setting.[55] Rational emotive mental health program is based on the principles that thinking evokes emotion, and faulty thinking is linked to negative emotion. The intervention uses lecture, discussion, and repetition to increase positive thought practice with the goal of cognitive restructuring.[56]

(continued on next page)

Table 1 (continued)	
Treatment Model	**Description**
Multisystemic therapy (Henggeler & Lee,[41] 2003)	Multisystemic therapy is a treatment that focuses on reducing antisocial and delinquent behavior in adolescents. Fundamental to the model is a commitment to delivering therapy in the natural or community environment. Cognitive behavior therapy, behavior modification, parent training, family therapy, and medication management are used in the treatment approach.
Multidimensional treatment foster care (Chamberlain & Smith,[57] 2003)	Multidimensional treatment foster care is a community-based, evidenced-based treatment that was originally developed to reduce the effects of severe and chronic delinquent behavior. The model has been used with children and youth ages 3–18 y. Foster families are provided 20 h of preservice psychoeducation in a token reinforcement system and then a child or youth is placed in a home for 6–9 mo with intensive support and in-home therapy services. Concurrently, the biological parents of youths receive intensive parent training in preparation for reunification. Youths participate—at minimum—in weekly individual therapy, consultation once or twice a week with a behavioral support specialist who works with youths and families, and psychiatric consultation. Research reports fewer runaways, decreased arrest rates, decrease in violent activity involvement or incarceration after program completion, and fewer placement failures.
Functional family therapy (Alexander et al, 2000)	Functional family therapy is a treatment that is provided in the home for youths ages 11–18 y to reduce antisocial and delinquent behavior. Treatment focuses on family communication and support and decreasing negativity and dysfunctional patterns of relating. Over approximately 3 mo, the treatment moves through 4 stages—family engagement, building motivation, behavior change, and generalization.
Brief strategic family therapy (Szapocznik et al, 1978)	Brief strategic family therapy treatment is based on 3 basic principles: (1) treatment needs to be a family systems approach, (2) patterns or interactions in the family influence the behavior of each family member, and (3) interventions target the interactional patterns in the family system. Subsequently, youths experience decreases in disruptive behavior and increases in positive family communication and adaptive functioning.

Best Practice Child-Focused Interventions for Disruptive Behavior Problems

Recommended programs working with youths with disruptive behavior problems are generally cognitive behavioral in focus and address social and cognitive deficits contributing to the disruptive behaviors. Some of these programs conceptualize aggression in youths as linked to increased attribution of hostility in social interactions as well as a heightened attention to hostile cues in the environment.[38] The goal of the interventions are to modify youths' social information processing problems, increase skills around assertive versus aggressive communication, and gain better understanding around the relationship between emotions, thinking, and behaviors.[39] Varying best practice interventions delivered at the youth level can take place in the context of a small group and one-on-one. Although many of the youth-focused programs were not designed to be implemented in a school-based setting specifically, the structure of the individual service components (ie, group or individual therapy) makes it possible to consider implementing them in a school-based setting. Child-focused interventions may be more effective for youths whose disruptive behavior is less embedded in environmental factors, such as problematic family functioning (see "Child-Focused Vignette").

CHILD-FOCUSED VIGNETTE

Kyle is a 14-year-old boy who has had a history of defiant behavior in the school setting. He has become increasingly hostile toward teachers during class as evidenced by statements of "don't talk to me" or "I don't have to do what you say" and "leave me alone." When excused from the classroom, Kyle begins to calm down. In addition to his hostility toward authority figures, he has pushed some peers during class transitions. His teachers genuinely want him to be successful but feel confused and puzzled by his threats. His parents are very involved with the school and they make every effort to meet with the teacher and school administration to discuss and problem solve Kyle's noncompliance. Kyle also has 2 older siblings who have navigated junior high school without incident.

Conceptualization

- *Historically, Kyle has been a student who wants to excel but he struggles academically.*
- *Kyle has had difficulty making the transition to high school. The increased pressure to perform academically and to be more self-motivated and sufficient has resulted in an increase of anxiety and low self-esteem. His anxiety has become manifest by increased irritability and hostility.*

Opportunities for intervention

- *Assess, identify, and track difficult situations and/or relationships for the youth to better understand the antecedents to the disruptive behavior (eg, he always becomes hostile in English and history).*
- *Identify thoughts, feelings, and behaviors (cognitive behavioral therapy) associated with these experiences to better understand "hot" cognitions (ie. those thoughts that are driven by strong emotional states) and feelings/behaviors associated with these cognitions (eg, "All these teachers want to do is make me look stupid! So I just leave pissed off").*
- *Support Kyle in the identification of emotional states and teach gradation/intensity of emotion with complementary coping strategies to modulate emotion (eg, feeling thermometer 1–10—deep breathing plan when Kyle feels a "4" frustration with teacher).*
- *With modulation, teach Kyle problem-solving strategies (eg, identification of the problem, potential action steps, potential consequences, selection of healthy action, self-appraisal of problem solving). Build in a structure that provides opportunities to practice in the school and/or home setting.*
- *Identify and provide natural modulation activities (eg, arts, sports, or clubs) to increase prosocial emotion expression and increased sense of competence.*

Multimodal Interventions for Disruptive Behavior Problems

Multicomponent interventions often include a combination of modalities, such as family therapy, parent training, individual therapy, and/or school consultation.[40,41] These programs aim at intervening in environmental risk factors, such as family dysfunction, that have been demonstrated as linked to the development and maintenance of disruptive behavior problems. These interventions take a broader view of the behaviors presented by youths and look at underlying relational dynamics or past familial experiences. The assumption is that by addressing youths within the larger context of family and community system, skills can be developed at the individual, parent, and family levels (see "Multimodal Vignette").

Engaging families and retaining them can be a challenge in the outpatient mental health setting, and these interventions may represent a similar challenge for clinicians operating within the structure of a school-based setting.[42–45] Considering the assumption of multimodal interventions that disruptive behaviors occur in the context of an interpersonal system, such as family, community, and school, it is essential to consider environmental factors in the development and implementation of interventions. When implementing interventions in the school setting, along with attempting to increase family engagement, it is essential to consider the system of the school. School setting and relationships between school staff and youths can serve as a proxy for gains that cannot be made due to lack of access to family in this setting. Given this, it is not sufficient to isolate the focus of treatment planning on youths solely.

When attempting to use the school as a proxy to understand problem behaviors and practice learned skills, it is important to consider other factors in the school setting that can possible influence problematic behaviors. Some examples of ecological factors that can influence disruptive behaviors, both positively and negatively, are teacher characteristics. Characteristics, including but not limited to, self-efficacy, sense of work pressures, sense of autonomy, relationships with parents, discipline problems, and supervisory support, can all have an impact on the teacher/student relationship, thus, an impact on the presentation of disruptive behaviors.[46] Engaging teachers in the contextual and relational components of the disruptive behavior can assist in enhancing the effectiveness of the interventions.

SUMMARY AND PRACTICAL IMPLICATIONS

The nature of disruptive behavior problems intrudes on and prevents youths, and at times peers around them, from focusing on the present educational task or learning. Their behavior disrupts the learning process for the teacher and classroom environment. In an attempt to quickly remediate the disruption, educators deploy behavioral limits (eg, excusing youths from a classroom) to reduce the amount of time taken away from the class focus and distraction created of one student. Although this can be efficient for the greater good of the classroom, the long-term consequence of efficient limits on youths fails to appreciate the underlying reason for the behavior and may be associated with further escalation of behavioral problems.[47] It is essential to consider inclusion of the larger system (ie, classroom and school milieu) in the intervention to facilitate practice, promotion, and transfer of skills outside the structure of the intervention itself.[48] Including factors in consideration of intervention planning, such as the context in which disruptive behavior problems occur in the educational system, is important.

When children or youths enter the ecological system of the school, they bring external systemic stress (internal, family dynamics, socioeconomic, and cultural/religious) that can destabilize the optimal learning environment. It is estimated that one-third of students have psychosocial challenges that have an impact on learning.[49] Youths bring these home environment challenges and ways of interacting into the school setting and act them out in relationship with school personnel in a way that may leave adults confused and with little understanding of the meaning of the behavior. School systems would benefit from routine review and reflective processing of youths' ongoing behavior problems on a team level.

Existing clinical practice guidelines and literature on intervention for adolescent disruptive behaviors suggest that psychosocial interventions can be effective either alone or in combination with pharmacologic interventions in more serious cases.[29,36,37,50] Existing literature on intervention programs for adolescent disruptive behaviors in school-based settings suggests that programs targeting high-risk youths are the most effective at reducing behavioral outcomes. Fidelity to program model and sustainability of program implementation seem even more critical than the type of program modality.

Evidence exists to support child-, parent-, family-, and multimodal psychosocial interventions, although many questions about the comparative effectiveness of these categories of intervention, either alone or in combination with pharmacologic interventions, remain unanswered. Eyberg and colleagues[36] and the Substance Abuse and Mental Health Services Administration[37] review both identify specific evidence-supported programs for adolescents with disruptive behaviors that potentially can be delivered in school-based settings. In general, the literature seems to provide support for multicomponent programs that include parent- or family-level components, but these components present a unique challenge for school-based implementation.[37,50]

Taken together, these two bodies of literature have important practical implications for intervention providers in school-based settings. First, no single model of intervention for adolescents with disruptive behaviors seems unequivocally better than the others.[30,31,36] Second, there is a need to recognize that not all behavior stems from the same emotional or psychosocial source. This means that interventions need to be tailored to individual needs and must also consider the unique constellation of underlying and environmental factors contributing to them. The high prevalence of comorbid internalizing problems reiterates the potential for implementation of evidence-based assessment strategies to aid identification of not only disruptive behaviors but also comorbidities and predisposing factors. Third, all school-based settings planning to implement a program to reduce adolescent disruptive behaviors must give serious consideration to the quality of and support for the implementation and its short-, medium-, and long-term sustainability. Factors, such as infrastructure, administrative and senior leadership support, ongoing training and supervision, and collaboration within the milieu, are essential components to the success of any school-based intervention to reduce disruptive behaviors.

REFERENCES

1. Fast Facts: Back to School Statistics. National Center for Education Statistics. Available at: http://nces.ed.gov/fastfacts/display.asp?id=372. Accessed October 17, 2014.
2. Branford JD, Donovan SM. How students learn: History, mathematics, and science in the classroom. Washington, DC: National Academies Press; 2005.
3. Frick PJ, Lahey BB, Loeber R, et al. Oppositional defiant disorder and conduct disorder: a meta-analytic review of factor analyses and cross-validation in a clinic sample. Clin Psychol Rev 1993;13:319–40.
4. Rose LC, Gallup AM. The 37th annual Phi Delta Kappa/Gallup poll of the public's attitudes toward the public schools. Phi Delta Kappan 2005;87:41–57.
5. Bru D. Academic outcomes in school classes with markedly disruptive pupils. Sch Psych Educ 2009;12:461–79.
6. Finn JD, Pannozzo GM, Voelkl KE. Disruptive and inattentive-withdrawn behavior and achievement among 4th-Graders. Elem Sch J 1995;95:421–34.
7. McCarthy CJ, Lambert RG, O'Donnell M, et al. The relation of elementary teachers' experience, stress, and coping resources to burnout symptoms. Elem Sch J 2009;109:282–300.
8. Shinn MR, Ramsey E, Walker HM, et al. Antisocial behavior in school settings: initial differences in an at-risk and normal population. J Spec Educ 1987;21:69–84.
9. American Psychiatric Association. Diagnostic and Statistical Manual of Mental Disorders. 3rd edition. Washington, DC: American Psychiatric Association; 2013.
10. Keenan K, Wakschlag LS. More than the terrible twos: the nature and severity of behavior problems in clinic-referred preschool children. J Abnorm Child Psychol 2000;28:33–46.
11. Fergusson DM, Horwood LJ. Early disruptive behavior, IQ, and later school achievement and delinquent behavior. J Abnorm Child Psychol 1995;23:183–99.

12. US Centers for Disease Control and Prevention. Injury Prevention and Control: Division of Violence Prevention- Youth Violence. Available at: http://www.cdc.gov/violenceprevention/youthviolence/index.html. Accessed October 17, 2014.

13. Dusenbury L, Zadrazil J, Mart A, et al. State learning standards to advance social and emotional learning. Chicago: CASEL; 2011.

14. Positive Behavior Interventions and Supports. U.S. Department of Education's Office of Special Education Programs (OSEP) Technical Assistance Center. Available at: https://www.pbis.org. Accessed August 01, 2014.

15. Blouin AG, Conners CK, Seidel WT, et al. The independence of hyperactivity from conduct disorder: methodological considerations. Can J Psychiatry 1989;34: 279–82.

16. Abikoff H, Klein RG. Attention-deficit hyperactivity and conduct disorder: comorbidity and implications for treatment. J Consult Clin Psychol 1992;60:881–92.

17. Hinshaw SP, Lee SS. Conduct and oppositional defiant disorders. In: Mash EJ, Barkley RJ, editors. Child psychopathology. 2nd edition. New York: Guilford; 2003. p. 144–98.

18. Loeber R, Farrington DP. Young children who commit crime: epidemiology, developmental origins, risk factors, early interventions, and policy implications. Dev Psychopathol 2000;12:737–62.

19. Lahey BB, Loeber R, Quay HC, et al. Oppositional defiant disorder and conduct disorder. In: Widiger TA, Frances AJ, Pincus HA, et al, editors. DSM-IV Sourcebook, vol. 3. Washington, DC: American Psychiatric Association; 1997. p. 189–209.

20. Loeber R, Keenan K, Lahey BB, et al. Evidence for developmentally based diagnoses of oppositional defiant disorder and conduct disorder. J Abnorm Child Psychol 1993;21:377–410.

21. Loeber R, Green SM, Lahey BB, et al. Findings on disruptive behavior disorders from the first decade of the Developmental Trends Study. Clin Child Fam Psychol Rev 2000;3:37–60.

22. Loeber R, Burke JD, Lahey BB, et al. Oppositional defiant and conduct disorder: a review of the past 10 years, part I. J Am Acad Child Adolesc Psychiatry 2000; 39:1468–84.

23. Maughan B, Rowe R, Messer J, et al. Conduct disorder and oppositional defiant disorder in a national sample: developmental epidemiology. J Child Psychol Psychiatry 2004;45:609–21.

24. Puig-Antich J. Major depression and conduct disorder in prepuberty. J Am Acad Child Adolesc Psychiatry 1982;21:118–28.

25. Hinshaw SP, Greene RW, Doyle AE. Toward a transactional conceptualization of oppositional defiant disorder. Clin Child Fam Psychol Rev 1999;2:129–48.

26. Hinshaw SP. Academic underachievement, attention deficits, and aggression: comorbidity and implications for intervention. J Consult Clin Psychol 1992;60:893.

27. Coie JD, Dodge KA. Aggression and antisocial behavior. In: Damon W, Eisenberg N, editors. Handbook of child psychology, vol. 3. Social, emotional, and personality development. 5th edition. New York: John Wiley & Sons, Inc; 1998. p. 779–862.

28. Moffitt TE, Lynam D. The neuropsychology of conduct disorder and delinquency: Implications for understanding antisocial behavior. In: Fowles DC, Sutker P, Goodman SH, editors. Progress in experimental personality and psychopathology research. New York: Springer; 1994. p. 233–62.

29. Steiner H, Remsing L, Work Group on Quality Issues. Practice parameter for the assessment and treatment of children and adolescents with oppositional defiant disorder. J Am Acad Child Adolesc Psychiatry 2007;46:126–41.

30. Wilson SJ, Lipsey MW, Derzon JH. The effects of school-based intervention programs on aggressive behavior: a meta-analysis. J Consult Clin Psychol 2003;71:136–49.

31. Wilson SJ, Lipsey MW. School-based interventions for aggressive and disruptive behavior: update of a meta-analysis. Am J Prev Med 2007;33:S130–43.

32. Lipsey M. The primary factors that characterize effective interventions with juvenile offenders: a meta-analytic overview. Vict Offender 2006;4:124–47.

33. Fixsen DL, Naoom SF, Blase KA, et al. Implementation research: a synthesis of the literature. Tampa (FL): The National Implementation Research Network; 2005 (FMHI Publication #231).

34. Gottfredson GD, Jones EM, Gore TW. Implementation and evaluation of a cognitive-behavioral intervention to prevent problem behavior in a disorganized school. Prev Sci 2002;3:43–56.

35. Gottfredson GD, Gottfredson DC, Czeh ER, et al. National study of delinquency prevention in schools. Final report for the National Institute of Justice, U. S. Department of Justice, Grant # 96-MN-MV-008. Ellicott City (MD): Gottfredson Associates, Inc; 2000.

36. Eyberg SM, Nelson MM, Boggs SR. Evidence-based psychosocial treatments for children and adolescents with disruptive behavior. J Clin Child Adolesc Psychol 2008;37:215–37.

37. Substance Abuse and Mental Health Services Administration. Interventions for disruptive behavior disorders: characteristics and needs of children with disruptive behavior disorders and thier families. Rockville (MD): Center for Mental Health Services; 2011.

38. Lochman JE, FitzGerald DP, Whidby JM. Anger management with aggressive children. Short-term psychotherapy groups for children. Northvale (NJ): Jason Aronson; 1999. p. 301–49.

39. Digiuseppe R, Kassinove H. Effects of a rational-emotive school mental health program on children's emotional adjustment. J Community Psychol 1976;4(4):382–7.

40. Burns BJ, Schoenwald SK, Burchard JD, et al. Comprehensive community-based interventions for youth with severe emotional disorders: multisystemic therapy and the wraparound process. J Child Fam Stud 2000;9:283–314.

41. Henggeler SW, Lee T. Multisystemic treatment of serious clinical problems. In: Kazdin AE, Weisz JR, editors. Evidence-based psychotherapies for children and adolescents. New York: Guilford; 2003. p. 301–22.

42. Kazdin AE. Dropping out of child psychotherapy: issues for research and implications for practice. Clin Child Psychol Psychiatry 1996;1:133–56.

43. Kazdin AE, Holland L, Crowley M. Family experience of barriers to treatment and premature termination from child therapy. J Consult Clin Psychol 1997;65:453.

44. Yeh M, McCabe K, Hough RL, et al. Racial/ethnic differences in parental endorsement of barriers to mental health services for youth. Ment Health Serv Res 2003;5:65–77.

45. Atkins MS, Frazier SL, Birman D, et al. School-based mental health services for children living in high poverty urban communities. Adm Policy Ment Health 2006;33:146–59.

46. Skaalvik EM, Skaalvik S. Teacher self-efficacy and teacher burnout: a study of relations. Teach Teach Educ 2010;26:1059–69.

47. Garofalo J, Siegel L, Laub J. School-related victimizations among adolescents: an analysis of National Crime Survey (NCS) narratives. Journal of Quantitative Criminology 1987;3(4):321–38.

48. McMahon RJ, Wells KC. Conduct disorders. In: Mash EJ, Barkley RA, editors. Treatment of childhood disorders. New York: Guilford; 1989. p. 73–132.

49. Adelman HS, Taylor L. The School Leader's Guide to Student Learning Supports: New Directions for Addressing Barriers to Learning. Thousand Oaks (CA): Corwin Press; 2006.
50. Brestan EV, Eyberg SM. Effective psychosocial treatments of conduct-disordered children and adolescents: 29 years, 82 studies, and 5,272 kids. J Clin Child Psychol 1998;27:180–9.
51. Huey WC, Rank RC. Effects of counselor and peer-led group assertive training on black-adolescent aggression. J Couns Psychol 1984;31:95–8.
52. Kazdin AE. Problem-solving skills training and parent management training for conduct disorder. In: Kazdin AE, Weisz JR, editors. Evidenced-based psychotherapies for children and adolescents. New York: Guilford; 2003. p. 241–62.
53. Block J. Effects of a rational-emotive mental health program on poorly achieving, disruptive high school students. J Couns Psychol 1978;25:61–5.
54. Ellis A. Reason and emotion in psychotherapy. Oxford, England: Lyle Stuart; 1962. p. 442.
55. Knaus W. Rational emotive education. New York: Albert Ellis Institute; 1974.
56. DiGuiseppe R, Kassinove H. Effects of a rational-emotive school mental health program on children's emotional adjustment. J Couns Psychol 1976;4(4):382–7.
57. Chamberlain P, Smith DK. Antisocial behavior in children and adolescents: The Oregon Multidimensional Treatment Foster Care Model. In: Kazdin AE, Weisz JR, editors. Evidenced-based psychotherapies for children and adolescents. New York: Guilford; 2003. p. 282–300.

Preventing Secondary Traumatic Stress in Educators

Stephen Hydon, MSW[a],*, Marleen Wong, PhD[b],
Audra K. Langley, PhD[c], Bradley D. Stein, MD, PhD[d],
Sheryl H. Kataoka, MD, MSHS[c]

KEYWORDS

- Trauma • Educators • Schools • Secondary traumatic stress • Compassion fatigue
- Posttraumatic stress disorder

KEY POINTS

- A foundational knowledge of secondary traumatic stress (STS), including identification of signs and symptoms and how it affects persons working in schools, is proposed.
- The US Department of Education is conducting training across the country that addresses why STS may be prevalent in the nation's schools.
- Readers are introduced to the evidence-informed intervention, Psychological First Aid: Listen, Protect, Connect, Model, and Teach.

INTRODUCTION

School crisis teams have existed in the United States for more than 3 decades, with school personnel often on the front line in supporting students experiencing a crisis or trauma on campus or in their local community. Although increasing attention has recently been given to the mental health needs of students following traumatic events,[1] there has been a lack of recognition and services for school personnel, such as teachers, administrators, counselors, and others who may hear about a crisis or ongoing traumas of students but do not directly experience such events, despite these

The authors report no disclosures.
This work was supported by Substance Abuse and Mental Health Services Administration Grant SMO61270.
[a] Field Education, University of Southern California School of Social Work, SWC Building, Room 223, Los Angeles, CA 90089, USA; [b] Field Education, University of Southern California School of Social Work, Los Angeles, CA 90089, USA; [c] Department of Psychiatry and Biobehavioral Sciences, UCLA, Westwood Plaza, Los Angeles, CA 90024, USA; [d] RAND Corporation, Pittsburgh, PA, USA
* Corresponding author.
E-mail address: hydon@usc.edu

Child Adolesc Psychiatric Clin N Am 24 (2015) 319–333
http://dx.doi.org/10.1016/j.chc.2014.11.003
1056-4993/15/$ – see front matter © 2015 Elsevier Inc. All rights reserved.

childpsych.theclinics.com

Abbreviations	
PTSD	Posttraumatic stress disorder
STS	Secondary traumatic stress

personnel suffering significant emotional sequelae that ultimately impair functioning. In more recent years, as experts have been called to support school communities after a disaster or major traumatic event, there has been growing recognition of the importance of addressing the stress that teachers and other school staff may experience as a result of their secondary exposure to traumatic events, resulting from their outreach to and care for students.

One example of a school district that was concerned about secondary traumatic stress (STS) of its teachers was in New Orleans. Although there was recognition of the mental health needs of students immediately following this disaster, teachers who supported these students had significant unmet needs. However, when a major oil spill affected whole communities in New Orleans 5 years after Hurricane Katrina, this event compounded the open wounds still healing from the hurricane for both students and teachers. It was this additional traumatic event, which had major economic repercussions to the area, which was the catalyst for district administrators and superintendents from across the greater New Orleans area to address the needs of both students and staff.

Concerned about their staff's well-being, local superintendents reached out to national experts, including Drs Marleen Wong and Robin Gurwitch, to help them better understand the needs of their school communities. During the initial meeting, Dr Wong presented the concept of "compassion fatigue" that Dr Charles Figley had described more than a decade and a half ago that can affect those who are in "helping" professions.[2] There was overwhelming consensus among these superintendents that this conceptual reframing provided an important lens through which they could better understand their teachers' experiences. Subsequent meetings focused on how to support teachers who were experiencing compassion fatigue as a result of exposure to the traumas and stress of their students. Supported by the US Department of Education, Drs Wong and Gurwitch developed a tool kit to support teachers with STS, which led to a series of US Department of Education supported training programs to enhance the response to stressful and traumatic experiences that have occurred in schools and districts throughout the United States.

This article describes what is known about compassion fatigue, otherwise known as STS, and how it may manifest in school personnel. The US Department of Education STS training programs, now considered best practices for supporting educators and other school staff in the prevention, intervention, and postintervention of STS, are then described.

WHAT IS KNOWN ABOUT SECONDARY TRAUMATIC STRESS

STS has been defined as "the natural consequent behaviors and emotions resulting from *knowing* about a traumatizing event experienced by a significant other—the stress resulting from helping or wanting to help a traumatized or suffering person."[3] Charles Figley (1983) initially described the "secondary catastrophic stress reactions" as the empathy that caregivers and family members can experience when a family member experiences a trauma.[3] He notes: "We, too become 'victims' because of our emotional connection with the victimized family member." He later conceptualized compassion fatigue as synonymous with STS, with overlapping symptoms associated with Posttraumatic Stress Disorder, which occurs in various helping professions, including therapists who assist victims of trauma. He comments that "interpersonal networks" such as workgroups can promote recovery within an important organizational system[2] and that these naturally occurring support structures, whether at work or among one's family and friends, are the most common ways by which traumatized persons recover.[4]

The *Diagnostic and Statistical Manual of Mental Disorders* (5th edition) (DSM-5) also recognizes that the stressor leading to symptoms of posttraumatic stress disorder (PTSD) can include stressors beyond direct exposures or witnessing in person life-threatening events to also include secondary exposures such as: "Repeated or extreme indirect exposure to aversive details of the event(s), usually in the course of professional duties (eg, first responders, collecting body parts; professionals repeatedly exposed to details of child abuse). This does not include indirect nonprofessional exposure through electronic media, television, movies, or pictures."[5] Symptom clusters described in STS overlap with those in the criteria for PTSD: intrusive symptoms, avoidance, negative cognitions and mood, and hyperarousal and reactivity.

Although STS and compassion fatigue are often considered synonymous, with similar symptom profiles, 2 additional conditions that are often discussed along with STS are "vicarious trauma" and "burnout." Vicarious trauma has been described as a phenomenon that can occur particularly in psychotherapists who frequently work with trauma survivors. These therapists' cognitive schemas can be permanently disrupted as regards their sense of safety, trust, esteem, intimacy, and control, resulting in a changed view of themselves, others, and the world around them.[6,7] This condition differs from STS in that STS typically describes the emotional and behavioral symptoms that can result from secondary exposure to a victim's trauma. Burnout has been defined as related to the work environment, with chronic occupational stress resulting in diminished job satisfaction. Burnout usually involves general work stress (long hours, high caseloads) and not specifically exposure to direct or secondary trauma, but which nevertheless can result in exhaustion and decreased sense of accomplishment at work.[8]

In addition to "compassion fatigue" that can occur in family members of trauma victims, those in helping professions have also been identified as potentially at increased risk for STS. Much of the STS literature has described the effect of hearing repeated client trauma narratives during the course of providing trauma-focused psychotherapy.[9] In a national survey of trauma therapists, compassion fatigue and burnout were found to be more common in younger and less experienced professionals, and the practice of evidence-based treatments was associated with lower burnout and compassion fatigue, and higher compassion satisfaction (feelings of competence and meaningfulness about trauma-related work).[10] Similarly, child welfare workers who have a high caseload of children with abuse and neglect can be at increased risk for developing STS. Sprang and colleagues[8] found that compared with other behavioral health care providers, social workers had the highest risk for STS and burnout. Disaster mental health workers and first responders, some of whom may have been affected by the disaster themselves, may have brief exposures to trauma victims but still exhibit heightened risk for STS.[11] From a study conducted in New York post-9/11, secure attachment was associated with positive coping and resilience and less compassion fatigue.[12] Professionals potentially at increased risk for STS include those working directly with traumatized individuals and hearing the recounting of traumatic incidents, those who tend to be empathetic, females, those with high caseloads of traumatized clients, and those helping professionals who have unresolved histories of trauma themselves.[13]

Similarly to other helping professions, teachers and school staff can find themselves on the front line responding to a school crisis or community disaster, or more commonly connecting with students who bring to school with them their experiences of trauma and stress. Understanding how STS can manifest in administrators, teachers, and other school personnel, and what can be done to prevent STS, is the subject matter of the remaining part of this article.

TEACHERS AND STUDENT TRAUMA

There are nearly 18,000 local education agencies and almost 100,000 schools in diverse communities across the United States.[14] Schools are a microcosm of society; within its walls vulnerable students spend their days, some of whom have preexisting psychiatric disorders or histories of neglect, in addition to at-risk students living in poverty, with unstable housing situations and extreme economic challenges. When these challenges are compounded with traumatic events, students can experience emotional difficulties and subsequent academic struggles that come to the attention of their teachers.

Unfortunately it is all too common for a student to experience violence. In one nationally representative study of youth aged 10 to17 years, 41% experienced a physical assault in the past year, 14% experienced child maltreatment, and almost one-quarter witnessed violence.[15] According to the US Department of Education, K-12 public schools nationally experienced 1,183,700 violent events on campus, such as fights (with or without a weapon) and threats of physical attacks, at a rate of 25 per 1000 students during the 2009-2010 school year.[16] More violence occurred in middle schools (40 incidents per 1000 students) than in either high schools or elementary schools (21 incidents per 1000 students), with greater numbers of middle schools (39%) reporting daily to weekly incidents of bullying in comparison with other schools (20%).[16]

In addition, whole school communities can be affected by traumatic incidents, such as school shootings, terrorist attacks, natural disasters, or other traumas such as a student suicide. Whether the incident is school-wide or affects particular students, teachers can find themselves in the role of key person in identifying the social-emotional needs of students and recognizing when these traumas affect their ability to learn.

TEACHER STRESS, BURNOUT, AND SECONDARY TRAUMATIC STRESS

For more than 2 decades, researchers have been examining teacher stress and its relationship with job satisfaction, teacher burnout, teaching efficacy, school climate, and student outcomes.[17-19] Although there are many aspects to teacher stress, it has been characterized as resulting from 2 main areas, workload excess and stress related to student behavior and the need for discipline.[18] When stress has resulted from student behavior, studies have shown a reduction in teacher efficacy.[18] Typical teacher education does not often include much mental health education and training, leaving teachers feeling ill-prepared to manage students with psychiatric needs.[20] Ball and Anderson-Butcher[21] found that teachers had less burnout and stress when they had a positive perception about the mental health services available to students. Roeser and Midgley[22] suggested that teachers who feel overwhelmed with students' mental health needs would benefit from skills to help students' access services. Others have found that teacher stress is related to overall school climate.[23]

School staff can be directly and indirectly affected by a school crisis,[24-28] and teachers and school counselors often find themselves in the role of providing social-emotional support for students who have experienced a crisis. However, those same individuals can themselves be at risk for developing compassion fatigue or STS.

Although most STS research to date has been focused on other helping professionals such as social workers and psychologists,[8–11] there has been a growing acknowledgment that teachers, especially those in underresourced communities, are working with traumatized students, and researchers and policy makers have begun to consider the impact of this work on educators' mental health[29] and their relationship with students.[30] **Box 1** defines compassion fatigue, STS, and burnout.

SIGNS OF SECONDARY TRAUMATIC STRESS IN TEACHERS

Margaret is a fourth-grade teacher in a low-income neighborhood. She is a new teacher who has been working at her school for 2 years and genuinely enjoys teaching her students. However, she has begun feeling more and more concerned with the level of violence her students have been talking about that happens in their neighborhood, and she begins feeling unsafe while on campus. She is constantly worrying about her students' safety. One of her students has shared with her that he is haunted by nightmares, and proceeds to describe to her the minute-to-minute details about the shooting that he witnessed on his way home from school 3 days ago, leaving 2 bystanders dead just several blocks away from campus. He writes about it and draws graphic pictures that he shares with her. He is fearful in class, and he has been difficult to keep on task during lessons. Margaret has been working extra hard trying to figure out how to help him, to no avail. After work, Margaret is unable to focus on her personal life and is constantly thinking about the shooting, noticing at times that she is jumpy and having difficulty reading for pleasure. She frequently finds herself getting angry and agitated. One day in her math class, this young boy asks her for help on an equation that she has already explained in class, but he still can't understand how to solve it. Ordinarily Margaret would spend a little extra time with him to explain the difficult concepts. But today is different, today she responds with, "Look, I've already told you how to do it. You're just going to have to figure it out on your own!"

Margaret has begun exhibiting some of the signs of STS, such as increased irritability and intrusive thoughts about her student's trauma narrative. According to the US Department of Education (2012), STS can affect the following bio-psychosocial characteristics: physical, emotional, behavioral, cognitive, interpersonal, spiritual, and professional.[34] As with any characteristic that appears severe, maladaptive, or interferes

---

Box 1
Key definitions

Compassion fatigue: An emotional state with negative psychological and physical consequences that emanate from acute or prolonged caregiving of people stricken by intense trauma, suffering, or misfortune. Compassion fatigue occurs when emotional boundaries become blurred and the caregiver unconsciously absorbs the distress, anxiety, fears, and trauma of the patient (also termed countertransference).[31]

Secondary traumatic stress (STS): The natural consequent behaviors and emotions resulting from knowing about a traumatizing event experienced by a significant other, the stress resulting from helping or wanting to help a traumatized or suffering person.[2]

Burnout: A prolonged response to chronic emotional and interpersonal stressors on the job, defined by the 3 dimensions of exhaustion, cynicism, and inefficacy.[32]

Vicarious trauma: The emotional residue of exposure that counselors have from working with people as they are hearing their trauma stories and become witnesses to the pain, fear, and terror that trauma survivors have endured. A state of tension and preoccupation arising from the stories/trauma experiences described by clients.[33]

with daily functioning and relationships, it is important to seek professional and/or medical guidance. The detailed characteristics of how STS may manifest are as follows.

Physical. Having low energy or feeling fatigued in the classroom; having an upset stomach or nausea; having breathing difficulties; difficulty sleeping because of constant worry about a student.

Emotional. Feeling numb or detached from students; living in denial; feeling anxious; feeling guilty about not doing enough for students or parents; feeling powerless or hopeless that students will succeed; feeling sad or depressed. Perhaps there are feelings of being overwhelmed with grading papers or becoming hypersensitive; feelings of guilt that one is not doing enough to help students succeed; fear and/or anxiety that one may lose one's job.

Behavioral. Changing the routine of things at school and/or at home, such as eating later or not eating at all; becoming withdrawn from other faculty or suffering from sleep disturbances or nightmares about a recent shooting on the school campus. More severe effects can include the use of self-destructive coping mechanisms such as using drugs or alcohol, excessive gambling, or shopping. Some individuals may become accident prone or engage in self-injurious behaviors such as cutting, or become suicidal.

Cognitive. Having diminished concentration affecting the ability to teach for an entire day; difficulty with decision making; decreased self-esteem; self-doubt; blaming others for students not passing exams; becoming hypervigilant or experiencing trauma imagery (ie, seeing events over and over again).

Interpersonal. Becoming physically withdrawn or emotionally unavailable to coworkers or family; decreased interest in intimacy or physical touch; isolation from family, friends, or support systems; becoming impatient or intolerant of students or situations; mistrust or projection of blame onto the school's leadership.

Spiritual. Questioning the meaning of life or losing a sense of purpose in the world; lacking self-satisfaction or becoming angry at a Higher Power; questioning religious or spiritual beliefs.

Professional. Exhibiting poor work effort in classroom instruction; low performance of teaching tasks and responsibilities; low morale at school affecting relationships with other faculty.

The impact of STS on a teacher's personal or professional life can be devastating or debilitating, and acknowledging and recognizing the signs of STS can be one of the first steps in ameliorating its effect.[35]

Similar to other forms of psychological distress, a teacher experiencing STS may recognize symptoms emerging that affect their daily functioning in the classroom or at home. For example, a teacher may have previously experienced a traumatic event, which is triggered by a student's similar traumatic experience,[36] or a teacher may hear about a student's experiences with bullying.[34] Because teachers often reach out to help students and can be at a heightened sense of empathic awareness, they may also be vulnerable to STS. In addition to helping others, they may neglect their own needs and emotions.[34] Each of these scenarios is not uncommon, but could leave a teacher vulnerable to STS. One way to examine this further is to look for signs that STS may be present.

A principal suddenly finds himself responding to a major earthquake that has greatly affected his school community. Although he experiences minor damage to his house from the earthquake, his campus has been badly damaged, and many students are living in emergency shelters. Several teachers tell him about their loss of homes and loved ones, and he hears from students how they felt they would be crushed by falling debris. One student even saw his sister get badly injured from a falling beam. The principal is in crisis mode, trying to resurrect his school single-handedly, with a sense of responsibility that he must fix everything himself. He is not sleeping and worries constantly, feeling a great burden on his shoulders that only he can respond to all the needs of the school. Usually finding comfort in God, the principal has now started questioning his faith and the existence of a God who would allow such tragedy.

Another hallmark of STS in schools can be school personnel pushing themselves too hard to get things done and trying to do it all on their own. Having a close connection to a particular student and fellow educators who had experienced severe trauma, this principal manifested signs of STS, including "intense connections" with those he is trying to help and spiritual doubts. Other STS signs that can manifest in educators include having problems concentrating and focusing even on simple tasks, and experiencing increased physical complaints. It is possible that a person may have a low sense of self-esteem or a feeling of inadequacy; conversely a person may have feelings of grandiosity, overvaluing his or her importance or worth, resulting in a reaction similar to that of the principal in the aforesaid example who felt he had to do everything himself, even though it was impossible. Many of these signs can also be more apparent to others as opposed to the affected individual, especially symptoms such as increased irritability, isolating oneself from others, or becoming easily agitated or annoyed (**Box 2**).

TRAINING THE EDUCATORS

Given the broad spectrum of traumatic events to which students can be exposed and potentially share with their teacher and school staff, in addition to crises that can occur on campus and affect the school staff, the US Department of Education developed a training program for educators, which expands on the STS literature and applies those same concepts to the school environment where teachers can be at risk for developing STS.

Over the past 2 years, the US Department of Education has increasingly recognized the potential for STS in educators across the country, particularly given that schools are frequently experiencing traumatic events or crises such as school shootings or weather catastrophes such as tornados, hurricanes, and mud slides. The purpose of the training is to help school faculty and staff recognize, understand, and orient themselves to the concepts of compassion fatigue, secondary trauma, and resiliency. Trainings are often conducted several months to a year after a major traumatic incident or after a cumulative set of experiences across schools or districts that foster

---

Box 2
Key characteristics of STS

- Previous experience with a traumatic event
- Heightened sense of empathy
- Neglecting one's own needs and emotions
- Pushing oneself too hard to get things done
- Difficulty concentrating
- Low sense of self-esteem
- Feelings of grandiosity

the need to address STS. However, school districts can request these trainings preventively as part of professional development. Each training module bears a stark reminder of the ways in which a traumatic experience can affect educators in profound ways. The following vignette describes one such story described by an attendee at an STS training session.

I am a high school English teacher named Lisa, and while I have only been at my school for a few years, I'd like to think I have been making an impact. I really enjoy teaching and care about all of my students. However, I was especially close to one student named Derek. Derek was a high school sophomore at my school, and he loved to play sports. Basketball, football, you name it; he was one of our school's best. He was also a very popular student, well-liked by me and all of the teachers at our school, and I imagine had more real friends than most Facebook accounts. I knew his family from parent nights, very loving and nurturing, and you could just tell Derek was raised to be respectful and responsible. In a word, he was a superstar, someone we would want all of our children to aspire to be. I recognized Derek's potential and immediately resonated with his enthusiasm to learn and succeed. So when word spread around school one Monday morning that he had taken his own life, I, like the entire school, was shocked. And shock slowly turned into devastation, and it began to trigger some very different emotions. I began to avoid the neighborhood where Derek grew up. I would wake up with nightmares or often get no sleep at all thinking about what had happened, what I could have done to prevent his death. From time to time, I would miss a staff planning meeting or would distance myself from colleagues. I found myself losing focus, daydreaming, or maybe it was something else. One day Joan, a fellow history teacher and good friend, noticed me alone in the break room. I had been unusually quiet and had remained distant from everyone since Derek's suicide. While she did not want to pry, she was concerned about me and so with some hesitancy, she asked if I was doing okay. After some feelings of uneasiness, I finally confided in her that I couldn't shake my sense of loss over Derek's untimely death, that I couldn't stop blaming myself, and that maybe I was in need of some help. Joan validated my feelings and let me know that it was okay to feel this way. That it was understandable and heartbreaking for many of us. She offered to talk with me more and suggested that perhaps I talk with a friend of hers who was a therapist. For Joan, she was reaching out to a colleague. For me, it was a step in the right direction.

This story is one that could happen anywhere. When a major crisis or incident occurs, it can have devastating consequences for many of those affected, including educators. The STS training by the US Department of Education provides education about what STS is, signs and symptoms, how to prevent STS from occurring, and also provides ways that teachers can help other teachers reach out when they recognize that a colleague may be exhibiting signs of STS, as in the example given here. Training for educators can mitigate the effects of trauma.

A MODEL FOR TRAINING ON SECONDARY TRAUMATIC STRESS FROM THE US DEPARTMENT OF EDUCATION
Introduction

The facilitators begin the training with introductions. Although in other trainings this part of the agenda may be formulaic, for this training it can be somewhat cathartic. Attendees are asked not to give specific and graphic details about any traumatic experience, but rather what feelings or experiences they may have had following the event. Many individuals will choose to share their name but also will reflect on why they are in attendance, and describe how they are feeling or what they have been experiencing since the traumatic event. This experience can be a very powerful and emotional one because often it is one of the only times a participant has actually thought about how he or she has been feeling in a safe and comfortable environment.

The facilitators allow the participants space to reflect, and remind them that sharing is optional and, if necessary, individuals have the opportunity to share their experience privately. The overall intent is to help frame the day with the purpose of acknowledging the feelings that they have been keeping to themselves.

Dimensions and Definitions

During this time, facilitators assign conceptual definitions to compassion fatigue, STS, vicarious trauma, and psychological burnout to help diminish any stigma or clarify any ambiguity in terminology. From here, facilitators lead a discussion about how to recognize the signs of STS that a teacher or other school personnel may be experiencing, and the salient conditions that make them vulnerable to such manifestations. In Lisa's case, she began to map her experiences onto all of the symptom clusters described, such as problems focusing on her curriculum and withdrawing from her colleagues.

Impact

During this portion of the day, facilitators describe how STS can affect a teacher in each of the ways described earlier (ie, emotional, behavioral, interpersonal, and so forth). This approach evokes much discussion because people are often experiencing much of the same thoughts and feelings but are afraid to talk about it. For example, male coaches often feel they have to be "strong" and keep up "morale" on the team, but a traumatic incident can take an emotional toll on them as well. It elicits much more human emotions than they feel like they have been allowed to express. This self-disclosure is a process of normalizing and validating that may not have happened otherwise. Lisa began to realize that maybe she was not alone in how she felt. It was helpful for her to understand that what she was experiencing was most likely STS that probably was associated with her reaction to Derek's death.

Self-Care

Self-care refers to "those activities performed with the intention of improving or restoring health and well-being," and must be highly individualized.[37] Facilitators describe self-care as an important step in the healing process. During the training, participants actually engage in a short self-care exercise that can release some of the stored-up tension. Some participants may be reluctant to participate. Participants explore ways to engage in self-care from multiple bio-psychosocial characteristics such as physical, intellectual, environmental, emotional, and even financial self-care (**Fig. 1** details the Self-Care Strategies worksheet); for example, eating lunch off the school campus or taking a walk during a break time. In one such training, several participants considered starting an "exercise-share" whereby anyone interested would meet before school starts and exercise as a group in the gym. During the training, each participant crafts a self-care plan and shares with the rest of the group what they have identified. The facilitators require that each plan be explicit. For example, if a teacher or nurse suggests they will eat healthier meals, the facilitator delves a little deeper. A facilitator might ask, "Which meals? Breakfast, lunch and dinner? And what does "healthier" mean"? This process can be extremely helpful, and allows the group to really become invested in taking care of each other and holding each other accountable for their own self-care.

Psychological First Aid

The second half of the day is an interactive presentation of "Psychological First Aid: Listen, Protect, Connect, Model and Teach."[38] This model is an evidence-informed approach that can be used as a helpful resource for peer-to-peer support among

Social Self-Care. This type of self-care can take on many forms such as belonging to positive social networks; maintain relationships with friends; attending social activities or events. Please list three social self-care activities:

1._____

2._____

3._____

Physical Self-Care. Physical self-care encompasses appropriate exercise; proper eating habits; proper amount of sleep; joining gyms or exercise clubs. Please list three physical self-care activities:

1._____

2._____

3._____

Intellectual Self-Care. Finding opportunities to intellectually stimulate your self can be challenging. Here, this may include reading books; attending work-shops or seminars; learning a new craft or developing a new hobby. Please list three physical self-care activities.

1._____

2._____

3._____

Financial Self-care. Financial self-care is something that takes a disciplined commitment and includes such items as: itemizing bills; monitoring expenses; incorporating expenses for leisure activities; talk with a financial consultant. Please list three financial self-care activities:

1._____

2._____

3._____

Spiritual Self-Care. Often times we resonate with some spiritual being or a Higher Power. Spiritual self-care can be very uplifting and may include taking steps to reconnect with your Higher Power; attending

religious services; participating in study groups; daily reflection on your purpose in life. Please list three spiritual self-care activities:

1._____

2._____

3._____

Environmental Self-Care. This is an opportunity to commit to surrounding yourself with healthy environments such as taking a walk outdoors; creating a specific space in your home that is reserved only for healthy activities or rest; camping or contributing to an environmentally sound cause. Please list three environmental self-care activities:

1._____

2._____

3._____

Fig. 1. Self-care strategies worksheet.

teachers and other school staff on campus in the aftermath of a school crisis, disaster, or other traumatic event. In this model, participants learn simple ways to be a helpful resource to others on their campus when a crisis or traumatic incident occurs. In each step of the model, facilitators describe how participants in their own schools can do the following.

Listen

This section teaches educators how to approach colleagues who may seem upset or withdrawn, and ask them if they would like to share how they are feeling. In Lisa's case, her colleague Joan did not have to be a trained therapist to simply ask, "Lisa, are you doing okay?" Educators during this training are given reassurance and encouragement to find ways to identify when they see changes in their colleagues and how to reach out with support and empathy in a nonjudgmental way. During the training, teachers practice ways of inquiring about one another without feeling uncomfortable or intrusive, and how to practice active listening in a way that validates their colleagues' feelings and avoids trying to "fix" their problems. For each person, the approach and words may be different, so practicing this skill during the training can be an important first step.

Protect

In this phase of the model, participants learn that it is important to help a fellow teacher get back to a regular routine at school. It can help facilitate healing to remove anything in the school environment that may trigger symptoms of STS. It is important that participants understand that any school staff, such as the librarian, custodian, or classroom aide, can be affected by STS from hearing about traumatic events from students.

Connect

The connect phase describes that it can be very powerful for individuals who may be experiencing STS to stay engaged with school colleagues and remain an active member of the school community. All too often, people in despair isolate themselves, and this phase stresses the importance of staying "connected" with those around you. Teachers are reminded that if necessary, they could also encourage their colleague affected by STS to seek professional counseling or guidance. For example, Joan found out how Lisa was doing and then suggested that she find professional help. Involving the affected teacher in group activities at school can also be helpful in ensuring the person stays connected to others.

Model

In this phase, teachers are taught to model calm and optimistic behavior. If appropriate, teachers should help their colleagues look toward the future and reinforce their own resiliency. Facilitating their colleagues in problem-solving ways so that they can cope with day-to-day challenges can help overcome barriers that may seem insurmountable.

Teach

In this last phase of the model, facilitators acknowledge the normalcy of changes that occur in people who have been traumatized, and articulate normal stress symptoms and ways to cope during troubling times.

The trainees participate in a role-play of this model. Role-play gives them an opportunity to experience each stage and affords them a chance to ask about such things as how to frame questions, when to approach a colleague, and with whom this is beneficial.

Recovering From Secondary Traumatic Stress

During the training, teachers learn a strength-based approach that describes how educators can recover from a traumatic incident. Participants are reminded about the following:

- They have the capacity to recover
- They should continue to learn ways to build resilience
- They should take an active role in their own healing and when available, do this with colleagues who may be experiencing similar thoughts, feelings, and emotions

Schools should be a safe place for students and educators, and educators should be equipped with the knowledge that STS is very real and affects the entire school community. In-services, training sessions, workshops, or case presentations focusing on STS should be incorporated into school activities, teacher in-service training, and day-long trainings.

SCHOOL SYSTEM'S ROLE IN SECONDARY TRAUMATIC STRESS PREVENTION

The school environment and availability of resources for the mental health needs of students is critical not only for student learning but also for the well-being and efficacy of teachers.[18] One developing framework for schools is a trauma-informed school systems approach, which promotes social-emotional learning and encourages improving the supports in schools for students who have experienced trauma.[39,40] Cole[40] has outlined specific steps that schools can take in supporting students and teachers regarding trauma, which include:

- School policies to promote a positive and safe school culture
- Staff training about trauma, STS, and how to partner with families and clinicians
- Linkages with mental health professionals who can consult to classrooms and with specific students
- Academic and nonacademic strategies for working with traumatized students[40]

School-wide approaches using Positive Behavior Interventions and Supports, a multi-tiered system of supports to create a positive school environment through proactive strategies, has been associated with improved teacher efficacy and lower teacher burnout.[41,42] Through these types of school system approaches, schools can support teachers in using prevention strategies to minimize stress, burnout, and STS, such as encouraging self-care in groups or individually, and allowing for classroom breaks during the school day if needed. Schools can also encourage activities for staff such as Mindfulness ("paying attention in a particular way; on purpose, in the present moment, and nonjudgmentally"), for which there is preliminary evidence for decreasing stress in teachers, improving attention, and regulating emotion.[43]

SUMMARY

Given the significant toll that STS can take on educators, particularly in schools highly affected by trauma, it is essential that school districts and administrators provide their staff with the tools for preventing STS, such as:

- Normalizing STS and providing a venue for discussion and support
- Organizing professional development sessions at schools to provide important strategies to recognize the signs of STS and proactive ways of mitigating it

- Creating a larger whole-school approach for improving the overall climate of the school
- Providing opportunities for peer support, which can help build collegiality, reduce isolation, and provide important opportunities to vent the difficult feelings often associated with helping others[44]
- Recognizing and understanding the need for self-care

Moreover, schools of education at our colleges and universities nationwide provide the perfect opportunity to offer the necessary skills in STS prevention for our future teachers. Further research is needed to explore the prevalence of STS in educators and other school personnel and its relationship with other types of stress, mental health problems, and teaching efficacy. Examining the effects of a trauma-informed school approach on minimizing the development of STS as well as on student academic outcomes, teacher retention, and job satisfaction, are other key areas for exploration.

ACKNOWLEDGMENTS

The authors would like to thank Arthur Cummins for his ongoing collaboration in this work, and Pamela Vona for her administrative support.

REFERENCES

1. Kataoka S, Langley A, Wong M, et al. Responding to students with PTSD in schools. Child Adolesc Psychiatr Clin N Am 2012;21:119.
2. Figley CR. Compassion fatigue: coping with secondary traumatic stress disorder in those who treat the traumatized. London: Psychology Press; 1995.
3. Figley CR. Catastrophes: an overview of family reactions. In: Figley CR, McCubbin HI, editors. Stress and the family: coping with catastrophe. New York: Brunner/Mazel; 1983.
4. Figley CR. Trauma and its wake: the study and treatment of post-traumatic stress disorder. New York: Brunner/Mazel; 1985.
5. American Psychiatric Association. The diagnostic and statistical manual of mental disorders: DSM 5. Washington, DC: American Psychiatric Publishing; 2013. p. 271.
6. Jenkins SR, Baird S. Secondary traumatic stress and vicarious trauma: a validational study. J Trauma Stress 2002;15:423.
7. McCann IL, Pearlman LA. Vicarious traumatization: a framework for understanding the psychological effects of working with victims. J Trauma Stress 1990;3:131.
8. Sprang G, Craig C, Clark J. Secondary traumatic stress and burnout in child welfare workers: a comparative analysis of occupational distress across professional groups. Child Welfare 2011;90:149.
9. Brady JL, Guy JD, Poelstra PL, et al. Vicarious traumatization, spirituality, and the treatment of sexual abuse survivors: a national survey of women psychotherapists. Prof Psychol Res Pr 1999;30:386.
10. Craig CD, Sprang G. Compassion satisfaction, compassion fatigue, and burnout in a national sample of trauma treatment therapists. Anxiety, Stress & Coping 2010;23:319.
11. Pulido ML. In their words: secondary traumatic stress in social workers responding to the 9/11 terrorist attacks in New York City. Soc Work 2007;52:279.

12. Tosone C, Bettmann JE, Minami T, et al. New York City social workers after 9/11: their attachment, resiliency, and compassion fatigue. Int J Emerg Ment Health 2010;12:103.
13. Baird K, Kracen AC. Vicarious traumatization and secondary traumatic stress: a research synthesis. Couns Psychol Q 2006;19:181.
14. Keaton P. Selected statistics from the common core of data: school year 2011-12. Washington, DC: U.S. Department of Education, National Center for Education Statistics; 2013.
15. Finkelhor D, Turner HA, Shattuck A, et al. Violence, crime, and abuse exposure in a national sample of children and youth: an update. JAMA 2013;167:614.
16. NCES. Indicators of School Crime and Safety. U.S. Department of Education, Institute of Education Sciences, National Center for Education Statistics.
17. Borg MG, Riding RJ, Falzon JM. Stress in teaching: a study of occupational stress and its determinants, job satisfaction and career commitment among primary schoolteachers. Educ Psychol 1991;11:59.
18. Collie RJ, Shapka JD, Perry NE. School climate and social-emotional learning: predicting teacher stress, job satisfaction, and teaching efficacy. J Educ Psychol 2012;104:1189.
19. Friedman-Krauss AH, Raver CC, Morris PA, et al. The role of classroom-level child behavior problems in predicting preschool teacher stress and classroom emotional climate. Early Educ Dev 2014;25:530.
20. Koller JR, Osterlind SJ, Paris K, et al. Differences between novice and expert teachers' undergraduate preparation and ratings of importance in the area of children's mental health. Int J Ment Health Promot 2004;6:40.
21. Ball A, Anderson-Butcher D. Understanding teachers' perceptions of student support systems in relation to teachers' stress. Child Schools 2014. [Epub ahead of print].
22. Roeser RW, Midgley C. Teachers' views of issues involving students' mental health. Elem Sch J 1997;98(2):115.
23. Grayson JL, Alvarez HK. School climate factors relating to teacher burnout: a mediator model. Teach Teach Educ 2008;24:1349.
24. Daniels JA, Bradley MC, Hays M. The impact of school violence on school personnel: implications for psychologists. Prof Psychol Res Pr 2007;38:652.
25. North CS, Nixon SJ, Shariat S, et al. Psychiatric disorders among survivors of the Oklahoma City bombing. JAMA 1999;282:755.
26. North CS, Tivis L, McMillen JC, et al. Psychiatric disorders in rescue workers after the Oklahoma City bombing. Am J Psychiatry 2002;159:857.
27. Schwarz ED, Kowalski JM. Malignant memories: PTSD in children and adults after a school shooting. J Am Acad Child Adolesc Psychiatry 1991;30:936.
28. Sloan IH, Rozensky RH, Kaplan L, et al. A shooting incident in an elementary school: effects of worker stress on public safety, mental health, and medical personnel. J Trauma Stress 1994;7:565.
29. Alisic E. Teachers' perspectives on providing support to children after trauma: a qualitative study. Sch Psychol Q 2012;27:51.
30. Lucas L. The pain of attachment: you have to put a little wedge in there: how vicarious trauma affects child/teacher attachment. Child Educ 2007;84:85.
31. Bush NJ. Compassion fatigue: are you at risk? Oncol Nurs Forum 2009;36:24.
32. Maslach C, Schaufeli WB, Leiter MP. Job burnout. Annu Rev Psychol 2001;52:397.
33. American Psychological Association. Fact Sheet. Available at: http://www.counseling.org/docs/trauma-disaster/fact-sheet-9—vicarious-trauma.pdf?sfvrsn=2. Accessed October 30, 2014.

34. U.S. Department of Education, Office of Safe and Healthy Students and U.S. Department of Health and Human Services. Substance Abuse and Mental Health Services Administration. Resilience strategies for educators: techniques for self-care and peer support. Readiness and Emergency Management for Schools Technical Assistance Center (REMS TA Center) training of trainers. 2012.
35. Bride BE, Walls E. Secondary traumatic stress in substance abuse treatment. J Teach Addict 2006;5:5.
36. Salston M, Figley CR. Secondary traumatic stress effects of working with survivors of criminal victimization. J Trauma Stress 2003;16:167.
37. Stromberg A, Jaarsma T, Riegel B. Self-care: who cares? Eur J Cardiovasc Nurs 2012;11:133.
38. Schreiber M, Gurwitch R, Wong M. Listen, protect, connect—model & teach: psychological first aid (PFA) for students and teachers. Washington, DC: US Department of Homeland Security; 2006.
39. Available at: Traumaawareschools.org. Accessed July 30, 2014.
40. Cole S. Helping traumatized children learn volume 1: a report and policy agenda and helping traumatized children learn volume 2: a guide to creating and advocating trauma-sensitive schools. Boston: Massachusetts Advocates for Children; 2005.
41. Kelm JL, McIntosh K. Effects of school-wide positive behavior support on teacher self-efficacy. Psychol Sch 2012;49:137.
42. Ross SW, Romer N, Horner RH. Teacher well-being and the implementation of schoolwide positive behavior interventions and supports. J Posit Behav Interv 2011. http://dx.doi.org/10.1177/1098300711413820.
43. Gold E, Smith A, Hopper I, et al. Mindfulness-based stress reduction (MBSR) for primary school teachers. J Child Fam Stud 2010;19:184.
44. Hamilton M. Compassion fatigue: what school counselors should know about secondary traumatic stress syndrome. The Alberta Counsellor. Edmonton, Canada: Alberta Teachers Association; 2008,30(1).

School-based Approaches to Reducing the Duration of Untreated Psychosis

Jason Schiffman, PhD[a],*, Sharon Hoover Stephan, PhD[b],
L. Elliot Hong, MD[c], Gloria Reeves, MD[b]

KEYWORDS

- Duration of untreated psychosis • Schools • Psychosis • Early identification
- Early intervention • Stigma

KEY POINTS

- Psychosis is a set of symptoms that includes delusions, hallucinations, disorganized speech, abnormal psychomotor behavior, and negative symptoms.
- Psychosis often first occurs during adolescence, when most youths are in school.
- Shorter time between psychotic illness onset and the receipt of appropriate care is associated with a host of adaptive outcomes.
- Involving schools in efforts to reduce duration of untreated psychosis has the potential to significantly impact the course of illness for affected individuals.
- Through effective screening, psychoeducation campaigns, and a general sensitivity toward the possibility of psychosis in students showing signs, schools and school personnel can be strong contributors to shortened duration of untreated psychosis.

BACKGROUND ON ADOLESCENT PSYCHOSIS

Primary symptoms of psychosis (**Box 1**) include delusions, hallucinations, disorganized speech, abnormal psychomotor behavior, and negative symptoms (eg, avolition,

The authors have no disclosures.
This work was supported in part by funding from the Maryland Department of Health and Mental Hygiene, Mental Hygiene Administration through the Center for Excellence on Early Intervention for Serious Mental Illness (OPASS# 14-13717G/M00B4400241) and the 1915(c) Home and Community-Based Waiver Program Management, Workforce Development and Evaluation (OPASS# 13-10954G/M00B3400369); Baltimore Mental Health Systems; a Research Seed Funding Initiative (RSFI) grant from the University of Maryland, Baltimore County; the Passano Foundation; and the Johns Hopkins Center for Mental Health in Pediatric Primary Care.
[a] Department of Psychology, University of Maryland, 1000 Hilltop Circle, Baltimore County, Baltimore, MD 21250, USA; [b] Division of Child and Adolescent Psychiatry, Department of Psychiatry, University of Maryland School of Medicine, 701 Pratt Street, Baltimore, MD 21201, USA; [c] Department of Psychiatry, Maryland Psychiatric Research Center, University of Maryland School of Medicine, MPRC - Tawes, PO Box 21247, Baltimore, MD 21228, USA
* Corresponding author.
E-mail address: schiffma@umbc.edu

Child Adolesc Psychiatric Clin N Am 24 (2015) 335–351
http://dx.doi.org/10.1016/j.chc.2014.11.004
1056-4993/15/$ – see front matter © 2015 Elsevier Inc. All rights reserved.

Abbreviations

BASC-2	Behavioral Assessment Scale for Children, 2nd edition
DUP	Duration of untreated psychosis
EPIP	Early Psychosis Intervention Program
EPPIC	Early Psychosis Prevention and Intervention Center
KSADS	Kiddie schedule for affective disorders and schizophrenia
TIPS	Treatment and intervention in psychosis

anhedonia, social withdrawal); however, the impact of psychosis goes well beyond psychotic symptoms per se (**Box 2**). People with psychosis are less likely to excel in school, obtain employment, and contribute to the community in ways of their choosing.[1,2] In addition, psychotic illnesses such as schizophrenia are associated with increased mortality because of factors including suicide and elevated prevalence of metabolic and cardiovascular health issues.[3] Thus, psychosis impacts several domains of both health and functioning.

Compared with other mental health conditions (eg, attention deficit hyperactivity disorder, anxiety), psychosis may be perceived by school personnel and parents as an "adult" mental illness.[4] Evidence suggests, however, that psychotic symptoms commonly emerge during adolescence. In a large catchment study, the incidence of the first episode of schizophrenia (the hallmark "psychotic illness") was highest in the 15-year-old to 24-year-old range.[5] Gillberg[6] reported a 0.5% prevalence of first-episode psychosis in 16 to 19 year olds, suggesting that approximately 50% of adults who eventually develop psychosis-related illnesses may experience symptoms by age 19. Although psychosis seen in the schools is relatively uncommon compared with other mental health concerns, school personnel will often have contact with people with psychosis. In one survey of secondary school teachers, approximately one-third of teachers reported having an experience of being concerned about possible psychosis in a student.[7]

Adolescence and early adulthood is a critical time for achieving important milestones, such as completing high school and advancing to college, acquiring life skills (eg, driving), employment, and mastering new social demands (eg, professional and intimate relationships). Progression of psychosis during this time can interfere with these developmental tasks, and young people may be delayed (in some cases, indefinitely) in acquiring important life skills.[8] Furthermore, the impact of psychosis on brain maturation that typically occurs during the teen years seems to have important functional consequences for individuals with early-onset disorders.[9,10]

Box 1
Hallmark psychotic features

- Delusions: beliefs that endure despite conflicting evidence or reason

- Hallucinations: perceptions in the absence of external stimuli

- Disorganized thought/speech: verbal communication that is difficult to follow

- Disorganized or abnormal motor behaviors: unpredictable behavior (eg, childish silliness, agitation, complete lack of motor or verbal activity)

- Negative symptoms: diminished emotional expression, alogia, apathy, anhedonia, avolition

Adapted from American Psychiatric Association. Diagnostic and statistical manual of mental disorders. Fifth edition (DSM-5). Arlington (VA): American Psychiatric Association; 2013.

> **Box 2**
> **Disorders that may present with psychotic features**
>
> - Schizophrenia
> - Schizoaffective disorder
> - Schizophreniform disorder
> - Delusional disorder
> - Mood disorders
> - Substance use
> - Trauma
> - Dementia
> - Certain medical conditions
> - Certain sleep conditions

A range of interventions can help to manage symptoms and promote recovery for people with psychosis[11]; however, there is variability with regard to individual outcomes.[12] Although many prognostic factors are immutable (eg, genetic loading, prenatal complications, gender), one important factor that predicts outcome is the duration of untreated psychosis (DUP).[13] DUP is defined as the duration of time between the onset of psychotic symptoms and the initiation of appropriate treatment and is a potentially modifiable predictor of clinical and functional outcome.[14] As the onset of psychosis most often occurs during adolescence and young adulthood, a time when individuals are likely in high school or college, and DUP is a mutable predictor of course, schools and mental health professionals who work in schools can significantly impact DUP.

DURATION OF UNTREATED PSYCHOSIS
Defining Duration of Untreated Psychosis

Defining the onset of psychotic symptoms as well as the onset of treatment can be an inexact endeavor, as the line between subthreshold and full symptoms is not precise. Most experts think that using standardized rating scales that involve interviewing the client and relevant informants is the best practice. Standardized scales that use a structured or semi-structured interviewing approach can help reduce potential sources of error such as missing milder, but still psychotic-level symptoms; getting misinformation from chart-record reviews; and clarifying discrepancies between reports from students, teachers, and caregivers.[13] On the other end of the DUP timeline, "appropriate treatment" can have various meanings as well. The most common definition of treatment onset is when antipsychotic medications are initiated as part of treatment[15]; however, other definitions of treatment onset include first hospitalization, time until treatment response, and initiation of psychosocial treatments (eg,[16–18]).

The concept of a time-sensitive window for early mental health intervention is a familiar paradigm for schools. For example, there have been strong efforts to optimize early identification of youth with autism and to intervene with behavioral, communication, and academic services (eg,[19]). Schizophrenia, however, is much less common (0.7% of adults have schizophrenia; prevalence of any psychotic disorder estimated at 3%–3.5%[20]) than other mental health conditions often recognized in the schools (eg, autism, depression, substance abuse), so school personnel would be expected to have less experience and knowledge of adolescent psychosis compared with other conditions.[21] School personnel also may have concerns about "mislabeling" an adolescent with psychosis and recommending services prematurely (ie, symptoms may be perceived initially as an "adolescent phase"), and students may experience stigma from school personnel and students alike against psychosis.[22,23]

Impact of Duration of Untreated Psychosis

An influential review of DUP reported that the average DUP was more than 2 years.[24] Relative to those who experience longer DUP, individuals with shorter DUP are likely to have a better response to psychopharmacologic and psychosocial treatments, fewer negative symptoms, higher quality of life, and reduced mortality after illness onset.[13,24–27] Poor social, educational, and occupational functioning, impaired cognitive abilities, and long-term distress are also associated with longer DUP.[24,28–32] Interestingly, although DUP appears linked to poorer responses to treatment at follow-up, it does not appear to be associated with more severe positive symptoms at the time of first treatment. In other words, people who have longer DUP do not typically come into treatment presenting worse off than those with short DUP, and therefore, it is unlikely that longer DUP is a proxy for a more serious and severe illness. Instead, what this research suggests is that it is likely that shortening DUP may be a key component for shaping an individual's long-term trajectory.[24,27]

Factors Contributing to Longer Duration of Untreated Psychosis

Individual factors, such as poor insight, avolition, and poor social integration, have all been noted as contributors to longer DUP.[29] Adolescents may not seek help for psychosis until the symptoms become very impairing and distressing. However, many students in early stages of psychosis seek treatment for a variety of psychosocial difficulties (eg, mood, anxiety, substance use) that are not explicitly tied to psychosis.[33] Ironically, individuals in an early phase of psychosis receiving treatment for other mental health problems can have significantly longer delays in treatment of psychosis than those whose first contact with the mental health system was for psychosis.[33] In these cases, providers may fail to notice emerging psychotic symptoms. Screening and identification of emerging psychosis in schools, therefore, need to strike a balance between engaging youth and families by addressing their chief concerns, but also being mindful of other possible underlying causes such as psychosis if psychosis is suspected.

Contextual factors, such as the availability of mental health services, play an important role in DUP as well. At the system level, better access to mental health assessment and treatment predicts shorter DUP.[34] Teachers, school mental health personnel, and administrators often experience significant logistical challenges in referral for mental health services. Issues such as wait-lists, insurance coverage issues, and caregivers' missed time from work can be significant barriers to mental health referrals. Also, compared with conditions like anxiety and depression, primary care providers may be less willing or capable of providing mental health services for youth with schizophrenia or other psychotic illnesses[4]; therefore, school personnel may have fewer referral options for pharmacologic or psychosocial treatment, an important issue for families who are uncomfortable initiating treatment with a mental health provider.

An advantage schools have as stakeholders in reducing adolescent DUP is that schools can be very effective at outreach to both youth and families. Parent engagement and support are important components of strategies to reduce DUP. Supportive family involvement predicts shorter DUP,[35] and conversely, caregiver strain and fears about stigma have been found to predict longer DUP.[36,37]

Community Outreach

Lack of awareness of signs of illness, concerns about stigma, implications of DUP, and unawareness of and difficulty in accessing specialty treatment facilities may prolong the DUP by delaying recognition of psychosis.[37,38] The need for evidence-based interventions that target mental health stigma in youth and young adults is profound, especially given the negative effects of stigma for people with mental health concerns and the unique effects of stigma on young adults in particular. Stigma for severe mental illness such as psychosis is particularly pronounced and has implications for a host of negative outcomes (eg, treatment delay). In addition, self-stigmatizing attitudes about mental illness and skepticism about treatment effectiveness have been associated with lower help-seeking behavior in transition age youth.[39] Public and self-stigma rates are highest for psychosis relative to other mental health concerns and notably impede critical early intervention and ongoing treatment.[40,41] Increasing public awareness about signs and symptoms of psychosis, and reducing stigma and other barriers to obtaining a clinical evaluation and specialty referral, may in turn reduce DUP.

RESEARCH ON STRATEGIES TO REDUCE DURATION OF UNTREATED PSYCHOSIS THAT INVOLVE SCHOOLS

Although there is a strong theoretic and common-sense rationale to reducing DUP, to date only a handful of controlled trials around the world have reported on DUP reduction, and these suffer from significant methodologic weaknesses.[42] Results from these trials are somewhat mixed, but they offer several implications for school-based interventions for improving identification of students with psychosis and referring these students for treatment.

Norway

The TIPS (Treatment and Intervention in Psychosis) study tested the efficacy of an early detection intervention and found a significant decrease in DUP as well as improved outcomes in long-term follow-up. Publicly funded health care sectors were divided into intervention versus control areas, with a population of 370,000 versus 395,000 each. The intervention consisted of 4 years of early detection initiatives that included intervention teams, public marketing of psychoeducational material, and regular visits to schools to educate students and staff. A total of 874 persons made contact (0.13%); 186 (0.05%) versus 194 (0.07%) cases were qualified for DUP assessment in the intervention versus control arms, or 0.012% [(185 + 194)/ (370,000+395,000)/4 year] annual incidence rate for DUP estimate. The study found a significantly shortened DUP of 5 weeks in the intervention versus 16 weeks in the control sectors, and also better outcomes in 1-year, 2-year, 5-year, and 10-year follow-ups.[43–47] Further supporting its effectiveness, once the campaign discontinued, DUP in the intervention area increased to 15 weeks.[48]

Implications for schools

Outreach and education of students and teachers, not just school mental health personnel, seemed to be a critical ingredient to improving early identification. Universal education also provides the opportunity to reduce stigma and raise awareness in the general population. Similar to antibullying campaigns, universal education about psychosis can also provide guidance to students on appropriate strategies to support affected peers on seeking help.

Australia

This study tested the effect of an awareness and access initiative versus usual care in 2 sectors of Melbourne with a population of 300,000 each and found a similar number of referrals and similar DUP from each group, but the intervention group identified significantly more cases of psychosis with DUP greater than 3 years. In this study, all cases of psychosis were referred to the Early Psychosis Prevention and Intervention Center (EPPIC[49]). The intervention was a 12-month campaign for awareness using promotion of early help-seeking, recognition of psychosis by practitioners and school counselors, easy access to EPPIC, and a mobile early detection team. Forty individuals with early psychosis from the intervention and 58 from the comparison sector were enrolled, yielding 0.02% as the annual incidence rate for DUP estimate. DUP was similar between the 2 sectors. When cases were separated into DUP less than 1 year, 1 to years, and greater than 3 years, 15% of the intervention group had DUP greater than 3 years as compared with 3% in the controls. Long DUP greater than 3 years skewed the comparison, which was possibly due to identification of previously undetected, long DUP cases by the intervention. This finding highlights the complexity of efforts to reduce DUP: it is possible that efforts to decrease DUP may uncover previously undetected and long-standing cases of psychosis.

Implications for schools
Although this project did not demonstrate overall reduction of DUP, one theme from this work is that access to treatment is important to encourage early identification. Because families may be initially uncomfortable seeking services in a mental health setting, the use of co-located school services (eg, school-based mental health specialists, mobile services) may support the initial engagement process.

Canada

The PEPP (Prevention and Early intervention in Psychosis Program) program found that an extensive community awareness campaign did not reduce DUP compared with distribution of information about available services. This study used a 4-year, 2-phase, sequential design trial in a single catchment area of 390,000.[50] The first 2-year phase used distribution of a pamphlet describing the program that included schools, followed by another 2 years of an extensive, blanket community awareness campaign that included regular school visits. After this extensive campaign, 88 and 100 subjects were enrolled in each phase, or 0.027% annual incidence rate. For ages 16 to 30, the rate was 0.05%. The DUP was 21.9 versus 24.3 weeks in phase I versus II. The campaign did not significantly shorten DUP.

Implication for schools
Offering information about available resources and providing specialized clinical personnel who regularly visit schools may be a useful clinical strategy for schools to identify students with untreated psychosis.

Singapore

In the 2-year multifocused EPIP (Early Psychosis Intervention Program) program, mass media, public forums, celebrity endorsements, and hotlines were several of the strategies used to identify people with psychosis and reduced DUP in Singapore, a city with a population of 3.4 million. Regular school meetings, bimonthly newsletters, and workshops were implemented as well. Median DUP in the intervention group was significantly shorter than in the control group, and median DUP was reduced from 12 months to 4 months. There was an increase in both self-referrals and family referrals over the course of the program.[51]

Implications for schools

Public outreach and education campaigns should be structured to be appealing to adolescents. Adolescence is a time when youth generally seek to become independent in their decision-making and become increasingly influenced by input from adults outside the family—public figures, coaches/mentors, and so on. As adolescents have unprecedented access to social media and Internet, there are numerous tools that can be used to disseminate knowledge and engage youth to learn more about this health condition.

Although this literature provides as many questions as answers, at the very least, it appears that the multimodal approaches of certain projects (eg, the TIPS and EPIP programs) seem important for an effective DUP reduction effort. Furthermore, both of these more successful and more rigorously tested interventions involved a school outreach component that might be useful for successful DUP efforts.

POTENTIAL COLLATERAL BENEFITS OF SCHOOL-BASED INTERVENTIONS

Although it is unclear what the essential ingredients for successful reduction of DUP are, it is likely the case that schools can play a useful role. A variety of initiatives within schools may provide potential benefits in terms of creating a more inclusive climate, which may ultimately also reduce DUP.

Reducing Stigma

A major benefit of using schools to promote community-based psychoeducation and outreach about adolescent psychosis is the potential to have a widespread impact on reducing stigma associated with serious mental illness. Brief psychoeducation interventions can be a low-cost, practical, and effective tool to reduce stigma and misconceptions about mental illness. In some cases, a short-term intervention can have sustained impact. For example, a 1-hour classroom workshop for high school students on mental illness stigma resulted in a significant reduction in self-report of stigma (23%) that was sustained 1 month after intervention.[52] In a controlled study of a 2-hour, high school psychoeducation intervention on schizophrenia, students who received the active intervention had significant changes in their beliefs and attitudes that persisted 1 year after intervention.[53] In the "Reaching Out" program, relying heavily on an educational video and including signs and symptoms of schizophrenia, Stuart and colleagues[54] reported that students showed increased knowledge of schizophrenia and reduced desire for social distance.

Education interventions can also be framed as "lesson plans," consistent with existing health education curriculum. In their mental health awareness workshops, Pinfold and colleagues[55] administered a series of lesson plans within schools. Lessons were in some cases cofacilitated by a person with mental health concerns, and the curriculum included a video of a person living with schizophrenia. The authors reported improvements in knowledge and attitudes from pretest to posttest. Watson and colleagues[56] described their evaluation of "The Science of Mental Illness," a 5-lesson lectured-based educational supplement for grades 6 to 8 that emphasizes biological, social, and psychosocial causes of mental health concerns. Results suggested that the curriculum produced improvements in both knowledge and attitudes at posttest.

Despite some promising results within the school mental health awareness literature, significant concerns remain. A recent review by Wei and colleagues[57] was very critical of the scientific rigor used when assessing mental health literacy programs. For instance, the entire field of existing studies, including the studies discussed above,[54–56] were rated "high" for significant risk of bias due to factors such as a lack of randomization, lack of control of possible confounds, lack of validated assessment measures, and a failure to report on attrition, leading some researchers to question the validity and utility of mental health literacy programs. According to Wei and colleagues, most if not all other studies in this area share similar methodologic concerns, leading the authors to conclude that the scientific evidence supporting these types of interventions is not developed enough and that more research is required before actual programs should be implemented. It is clear that the field would benefit from more systematic and rigorous evaluation to provide more confidence in the potential impact of antistigma efforts.

Nonetheless, despite concerns about methodology, based on the studies that show promise as well as knowledge of learning principles, it seems that a combination of structured psychoeducation providing information about signs and treatment, that is youth focused, discussion-oriented, and involves contact with someone with mental health concerns (live or video), while providing tangible resources for specialized referral and meeting regularly over the course of time, may hold promise in reducing stigma, increasing education and awareness, and ultimately facilitating more early help-seeking. Interestingly, an innovative after-school program called "Let's Erase the Stigma" was recently piloted that embraces all these elements through an open-group format and does so outside of school hours.[58] Although the program will require considerably more evaluation, the curriculum seems promising.

ASSESSING PSYCHOSIS IN STUDENTS

Identification of psychotic symptoms in schools is essential toward reducing DUP and requires thorough assessment (**Box 3**). Psychosis can be difficult to diagnose in children and adolescents. Students may be confused about what is happening and have difficulty describing their experiences. In addition, symptoms such as social withdrawal and paranoia can contribute to a reluctance to disclose concerns to parents and clinicians. Furthermore, youth-focused providers may be poorly trained to recognize and treat psychosis, and adult-focused providers may overlook important developmental considerations.[4] Many professionals are unfamiliar with risk symptoms, leading to potentially unreliable or confusing diagnoses during the earlier stages of illness.[59] School personnel, including child psychiatrists and other mental health professionals working in or consulting to schools, can play an important role in identifying signs of psychosis in the service of reducing DUP through their developmental expertise and trusting relationships with students.

Box 3
Potentially important elements of psychoeducation to reduce stigma against psychosis that might lead to reduced duration of untreated psychosis

- Psychoeducation about signs and treatment
- Youth-focused
- Discussion-oriented
- Contact with someone with mental health concerns (live or video)
- Provide tangible resources for specialized referral
- Regular meetings

When considering the possibility of psychosis, the relatively low prevalence of psychotic symptoms among youth highlights the importance of considering more common causes of unusual or disruptive behaviors before considering a psychotic diagnosis (**Box 4**). Consulting with multiple informants (eg, student, teachers, parents) and using multiple methods (eg, standardized questionnaires, observation, interview) can help provide information across different settings and with different people.[60]

When assessing a student with possible psychosis, best practices suggest generating multiple hypotheses regarding the causes of a behavior. Psychosis is only one of many possible explanations for unusual experiences or disorganized behaviors. For instance, as part of adaptive behavior, children often engage in imaginative play, such as talking to imaginary friends or pretending to have superpowers.[61] Other behaviors may resemble psychosis yet be adaptive nonpathological responses to a potentially chaotic life. For example, students who have experienced traumatic events or live in unsafe neighborhoods may show hypervigilance and suspiciousness that if not interpreted in context could be misidentified as psychotic.[62] Cultural considerations should be weighed as well. School personnel may misinterpret certain cultural beliefs and practices (eg, belief in spirits, communication with deceased relatives), making it important to gather information from caregivers regarding alternative explanations for youth behavior.

Another potential cause of diagnostic uncertainty may arise when students are reinforced for reporting psychotic symptoms. If reporting unusual symptoms or engaging in disorganized behaviors secures adult attention and concern, leads to escape of unpleasant tasks, or produces other benefits, students may learn to report symptoms even if they are not experiencing any. A functional assessment to examine antecedents, behaviors, and consequences may help distinguish psychosis from learned behaviors. As diagnoses may change over time for students, periodic re-evaluation of symptoms is often recommended.[60]

Semistructured clinician interviews with both students and their parents can help provide or confirm a diagnosis as well as offer a complete picture of symptoms and functioning. Interviews such as the Kiddie Schedule for Affective Disorders and Schizophrenia (KSADS[63]) have several prompts and useful structures to help guide an informed approach to assessment. The KSADS is free and available on-line at http://www.wpic.pitt.edu/research/AssessmentTools/ChildAdolescent/ksads-pl.pdf.

Specialized assessment tools can help rate the severity of psychotic symptoms in individuals if psychosis is confirmed. The Positive and Negative Syndrome Scale (PANSS[64]) and the Brief Psychiatric Rating Scale (BPRS[65]) include scales for several domains specific to assessment of psychotic symptoms, such as suspiciousness, hallucinations, unusual thought, bizarre behavior, cognitive disorganization, and negative symptoms. It is important to note that these scales require specialized training.

Box 4
Factors (other than psychosis) that may explain unusual experiences or disorganized behaviors

- Adaptive behavior (eg, imaginary friends, pretending to have superpowers)
- Nonpathologic responses to chaotic life (eg, suspiciousness, hypervigilance in response to trauma exposure)
- Cultural beliefs and practices
- Reinforcement for reporting of psychotic symptoms

In addition, behavioral checklists, which in some cases are already administered system-wide in certain school districts (eg, the state of Hawaii), have the potential to help identify students either at risk for or in the early stages of psychosis. These brief questionnaires assess a range of mental health concerns and can be administered quickly to students, caregivers, and teachers. In recent work examining the "atypicality scale" within the Behavioral Assessment Scale for Children, 2nd edition (BASC-2; a commonly administered tool to assess for emotional and behavioral concerns), it was found that both self-report and parent reports of psychosis symptoms were clinically relevant predictors of clinician-determined psychosis/risk among a help-seeking population. The use of tools such as the BASC-2 within schools might be an important step in helping to link students with early psychosis with specialty care.[66–68]

TREATMENT OF STUDENTS WITH PSYCHOSIS

Once psychosis is identified, appropriate treatments must be initiated before DUP can be said to have ended. Treatment of students with psychosis tends to be intensive and involve multiple providers and systems.[69] School personnel may be useful in providing a link between schools, families, and clinical teams. It is important to work early to develop rapport and collaboration with students and families to increase motivation for treatment. Psychopharmacologic treatment is generally the first recommended intervention for psychosis and is widely considered the standard for adequate care from which the end of DUP is pegged. Consultation with a psychiatrist or other specialized prescriber is essential toward creating an appropriate psychopharmacologic plan that is acceptable by prescriber, client, and family. A discussion of side effects and safety issues is also an important part of treatment, and school personnel may be called on to help monitor progress as well as concerns related to medication.[60]

In addition to psychopharmacologic interventions, psychosocial treatment is a part of best practice. Goals for students with psychosis can often focus on educational, social, vocational, and functional well-being in addition to specific symptom management. Given the broad impairment associated with psychosis, treatment of these students is likely to target multiple goals and behaviors.[70]

Treatment goals will also vary depending on illness stage. Among others, McGorry and colleagues[71] have promoted a staging model for intervention based on clinical severity. As illness progresses toward psychosis, attention to clinical symptoms and perhaps response to clinical crises may become pressing. Furthermore, young clients may struggle with feelings of shame or stigma surrounding their experiences and may be at risk of missing milestones or losing friendships as a result of their struggles. Parents, too, may require help processing illness stigma or managing children's anhedonic or oppositional attitudes and behaviors. In this acute phase, crises involving aggressive behavior, suicide attempts, or other behaviors requiring hospitalization may arise. Primary treatment goals for schools might include addressing safety concerns, connecting families with resources, and initiating appropriate medication treatment. Furthermore, across all stages, comorbid conditions can interfere with clinical progress. Having a deep and varied "tool box" of strategies that can be applied across stages and can be individualized to specific clinical needs may be important for effective clinical care. (For a more detailed discussion of treatment of psychosis in students, see[60])

Educational Accommodations

Many students with psychosis will meet eligibility for special education services (Section 504 of the Federal Rehabilitation Act of 1973 or the Emotional Disturbance category of the Individuals with Disabilities Education Improvement Act [2004]).

Thoughtful classroom placement may facilitate the provision of special education services. Individualized decision about appropriate placement is crucial given the variability of symptoms and goals of people with psychosis. It is relevant to note that a study by Frazier and colleagues[72] reported that approximately half of students with schizophrenia are in regular classrooms, with one-third in resource or self-contained classrooms.

Treatment planning may also be informed by psychoeducational testing. Evaluating a student with psychosis may require flexibility in administration, with less note-taking and greater transparency so as not to stoke possible paranoia, more prompts and encouragement for inattention and negative symptoms, and adequate structure for disorganized symptoms. Interpretation of findings can also require substantial judgment as to whether the scores reflect psychiatric illness or the student's ability level.[60]

Role of School Professionals

This review suggests that the development of specialized programs in schools holds promise for positive outcomes such as increasing early identification; however, existing school-based mental health providers are already positioned to have an important impact on DUP. Educators, administrators, and mental health professionals in schools can work from a prevention framework with access to all students, not just those with known emotional or behavioral concerns. Equipped with the right knowledge of signs, school personnel can monitor or intervene with students showing distress or deterioration, such as changes in academic and social functioning, rather than waiting until problems become more impairing and acute. Furthermore, school personnel can actively work to reduce stigma associated with mental health treatment by normalizing care and encouraging families and teachers to engage with mental health services. School personnel can also impact issues associated with access to or knowledge about care, by providing interventions within the school setting or serving as a knowledgeable referral source for families who might benefit from receiving mental health care in a more traditional clinical setting. Despite this potential, some research suggests that the comfort level and knowledge related to psychosis among individuals trained to work with youth are significantly less than that of professionals trained to work with adults.[4] Child psychiatrists and other specialty mental health professionals can assist schools in these supporting roles by providing education about signs and monitoring, offering training in screening and stigma reduction, facilitating community referrals, and consulting about specific students that may be exhibiting signs of psychosis.

CLINICAL VIGNETTE

Carlos is a 17-year-old Hispanic adolescent, currently attending his junior year of high school. His English teacher referred him to the school counselor after noticing "odd" behavior that caused her concern. His teacher said she would have referred him sooner, but previously he had refused, saying he did not want to talk to anyone. Carlos's mother was eager to get help as well, but did not know where to turn. She initially thought that Carlos was just going through a typical adolescent "phase," but thought that before she knew it, he was in a place well outside typical development. Carlos was referred to a school psychologist for a thorough evaluation. On inquiry, Carlos's mother reported that his father has resided in a psychiatric hospital in Mexico for years for "strange" behavior, including hearing voices. She said that recently, Carlos has not spoken much to anyone. She reported that approximately a year ago, he started being particularly picky about his food, and more recently, he blamed the neighbor of trying to poison him to take him "out of the picture." His mother reported that there was no evidence for this and that the neighbor was a close family friend, but that Carlos has become very angry in the past when she has attempted to challenge his beliefs. Related, several of Carlos's teachers reported that he is frequently agitated at school because he feels other teenagers are plotting against him. They report that although there is not likely a plot to cause Carlos serious harm, he is sometimes bullied for unusual behaviors, such as talking to himself and for having bad hygiene. Carlos initially refused to talk, but later opened up, saying in a slow, flat voice that he felt depressed, that the world was "so cruel," and that he would "probably die soon" from other people's actions. However, he could not provide specific details on why he thought this. He said that he found it very difficult to do anything and to express himself. He has been in all special education classes for several years, and his mother was considering withdrawing him from classes because he was not progressing in his work and he was reporting such distress at school. Carlos reported that he very occasionally has 1 or 2 beers and has used marijuana, but denies other substances. Medical tests did not produce any significant findings. Despite a variety of challenges, Carlos also had several notable strengths including having several friends who still cared about him despite the recent changes in his behavior. He also had an interest in drawing and reported that he enjoys art as a way to express himself.

The school had no programs in place for the identification of psychotic symptoms in students. Carlos's situation, however, sensitized them to the potential benefits of efforts that could help Carlos as well as other students with similar challenges. The first implemented change was to encourage all students who went to the counselors or other mental health professionals for services to fill out a self-report checklist that provided information on a broad swath of mental health concerns (BASC-2). Counselors were encouraged to pay attention to the "atypicality" scale as a possible indication of psychotic symptoms. During a school-wide professional development, a speaker came to discuss early signs of psychosis and to address misconceptions of the illness. The training was attended by the entire staff (teachers, counselors, maintenance, administration) and included helpful local specialized referral information for the school. In addition, one of the counselors started a mental health awareness and antistigma afterschool club. Carlos's friends were specifically invited to join. The meetings focused in part on helping students identify warning signs about mental health concerns and encouraging them to see the counselors if they wanted to talk about anyone or themselves. The club also provided a place where students could share concerns, learn about others, and just generally know that it is OK to talk about issues related to mental health. The efforts helped to reduce stigma and misconceptions faced by Carlos and also created a school climate more apt to identify students in the future who might have psychotic symptoms.

FUTURE DIRECTIONS

With a limited number of studies and a variety of methodologic flaws, the effectiveness of current efforts to reduce DUP can be considered provisional at best.[42] Even fewer studies have addressed efforts that focus on or involve school-based efforts toward reducing DUP. Future research is needed to support schools in optimizing early identification and treatment of adolescent psychosis in students.

A variety of clinical research priorities await future efforts to uncover effective ways to maximize school resources to reduce DUP. Additional research could be applied to improving psychoeducational approaches to reducing DUP. Although short-term education seems to have positive effects on factors such as reducing stigma among students, longer curriculums that involve education (including both factual and experiential information) and contact with people with mental health concerns may unlock promising avenues for DUP reduction. Lloyd-Evans and colleagues[42] emphasize the need for youth-focused approaches that are developmentally sensitive. Involving youth in the creation of programs that aim to reduce DUP in schools seems like an obvious strategy to help make efforts more youth-oriented and informed. In addition, standardization of DUP definition is important to compare outcomes across intervention models. Measurement tools that are sensitive to subthreshold symptoms and applicable to school settings might help facilitate more valid and reliable DUP

> **Box 5**
> **Ways to help reduce duration of untreated psychosis in schools**
>
> - Offer stigma reduction programs
> - Provide psychoeducation to teachers and school personnel
> - Conduct community outreach and education
> - Involve families in early treatment
> - Offer sensitive, thorough, and valid mental health assessments
> - Increase awareness of "at-risk" symptoms to identify individuals before psychosis develops
> - Reduce barriers to specialized care

recognition. Greater attention to screening efforts seem like a viable approach to reducing DUP in the schools as well. Screeners have been shown to be effective in a variety of settings, and tools that are already commonly used in schools that include psychosis items might be one means for relatively easy integration of screening in some schools.[60,66,68,73,74]

In addition to research, there are many clinical needs that remain inadequately addressed. Improving access to a well-trained mental health providers can reduce DUP,[75] but finding quality specialized care is often a challenge. Although attention to these issues continues to grow, the need for more providers who are well versed in early identification and evidence-based care for people in their earliest phases of psychosis remains a mental health care system priority. Ultimately, if identification efforts are successful, pathways to appropriate specialized care will be required to appropriately match those with psychosis to the right care.[76]

SUMMARY

Students with psychosis often experience delays in diagnosis and treatment, leading to longer-than-necessary DUP. Given the variety of negative consequences of DUP, there is an imperative to reduce DUP to the smallest possible window. School settings have tremendous potential to contribute to this effort. Through education, screening, assessment, treatment, and in some cases, referrals, schools can play powerful roles in reducing DUP. Although a great deal of research remains, school personnel, including child psychiatrists and other specialty mental health providers working with schools, are already poised to reduce DUP and can make an important difference for students with emerging psychosis (**Box 5**).

REFERENCES

1. Cohen A, Patel V, Thara R, et al. Questioning an axiom: better prognosis for schizophrenia in the developing world? Schizophr Bull 2008;34(2):229–44.
2. Harris MG, Henry LP, Harrigan SM, et al. The relationship between duration of untreated psychosis and outcome: an eight-year prospective study. Schizophr Res 2005;79(1):85–93.
3. Saha S, Chant D, McGrath J. A systematic review of mortality in schizophrenia: is the differential mortality gap worsening over time? Arch Gen Psychiatry 2007; 64(10):1123–31.
4. Kline E, Davis B, Schiffman J. Who should treat youth with emerging psychosis? Schizophr Res 2014;157:301–11.

5. Amminger GP, Leicester S, Yung AR, et al. Early-onset of symptoms predicts conversion to non-affective psychosis in ultra-high risk individuals. Schizophr Res 2006;84(1):67–76.

6. Gillberg C. Teenage psychoses: epidemiology, classification and reduced optimality in the pre-, peri- and neonatal periods. J Child Psychol Psychiatry 1986; 27(1):87–98.

7. Collins A, Holmshaw J. Early detection: a survey of secondary school teachers' knowledge about psychosis. Early Interv Psychiatry 2008;2(2):90–7.

8. Röpcke B, Eggers C. Early-onset schizophrenia: a 15-year follow-up. Eur Child Adolesc Psychiatry 2005;14(6):341–50.

9. Paus T, Keshavan M, Giedd JN. Why do many psychiatric disorders emerge during adolescence? Nat Rev Neurosci 2008;9(12):947–57.

10. Vidal CN, Rapoport JL, Hayashi KM, et al. Dynamically spreading frontal and cingulate deficits mapped in adolescents with schizophrenia. Arch Gen Psychiatry 2006;63(1):25–34.

11. Dixon LB, Dickerson F, Bellack AS, et al. The 2009 schizophrenia PORT psychosocial treatment recommendations and summary statements. Schizophr Bull 2010;36(1):48–70.

12. Perkins D, Lieberman J, Gu H, et al. Predictors of antipsychotic treatment response in patients with first-episode schizophrenia, schizoaffective and schizophreniform disorders. Br J Psychiatry 2004;185(1):18–24.

13. Marshall M, Harrigan S, Lewis S. Duration of untreated psychosis: definition, measurement and association with outcome. The recognition and management of early psychosis: a preventive approach. 2nd edition. Cambridge (United Kingdom): Cambridge University; 2009. p. 125–45.

14. Compton MT, Carter T, Bergner E, et al. Defining, operationalizing and measuring the duration of untreated psychosis: advances, limitations and future directions. Early Interv Psychiatry 2007;1(3):236–50.

15. Norman RM, Malla AK. Duration of untreated psychosis: a critical examination of the concept and its importance. Psychol Med 2001;31(3):381–400.

16. Bottlender R, Sato T, Jäger M, et al. The impact of the duration of untreated psychosis prior to first psychiatric admission on the 15-year outcome in schizophrenia. Schizophr Res 2003;62(1):37–44.

17. de Haan L, Linszen DH, Lenior ME, et al. Duration of untreated psychosis and outcome of schizophrenia: delay in intensive psychosocial treatment versus delay in treatment with antipsychotic medication. Schizophr Bull 2003;29(2): 341–8.

18. Malla AK, Norman RM, Manchanda R, et al. One year outcome in first episode psychosis: influence of DUP and other predictors. Schizophr Res 2002;54(3): 231–42.

19. Ehlers S, Gillberg C, Wing L. A screening questionnaire for Asperger syndrome and other high-functioning autism spectrum disorders in school age children. J Autism Dev Disord 1999;29(2):129–41.

20. American Psychiatric Association. DSM 5. Arlington, VA: American Psychiatric Association; 2013.

21. Whitley J, Smith JD, Vaillancourt T. Promoting mental health literacy among educators: critical in school-based prevention and intervention. Can J Sch Psychol 2013.

22. Liu CC, Chang LR, Tseng HH, et al. Differential propensity in recognition of prepsychotic phenomena among psychiatrists, clinical psychologists and school counsellors. Early Interv Psychiatry 2010;4(4):275–82.

23. Boydell KM, Volpe T, Gladstone BM, et al. Youth at ultra high risk for psychosis: using the Revised Network Episode Model to examine pathways to mental health care. Early Interv Psychiatry 2013;7(2):170–86.
24. Marshall M, Lewis S, Lockwood A, et al. Association between duration of untreated psychosis and outcome in cohorts of first-episode patients. Arch Gen Psychiatry 2005;62(9):975–83.
25. Barrett EA, Sundet K, Faerden A, et al. Suicidality before and in the early phases of first episode psychosis. Schizophr Res 2010;119(1–3):11–7.
26. Farooq S, Large M, Nielssen O, et al. The relationship between the duration of untreated psychosis and outcome in low-and-middle income countries: a systematic review and meta analysis. Schizophr Res 2009;109(1–3):15–23.
27. Granö N, Lindsberg J, Karjalainen M, et al. Duration of untreated psychosis is associated with more negative schizophrenia symptoms after acute treatment for first-episode psychosis. Clin Psychol 2010;14(1):10–3.
28. Black K, Peters L, Rui Q, et al. Duration of untreated psychosis predicts treatment outcome in an early psychosis program. Schizophr Res 2001;47(2–3):215–22.
29. Drake RJ, Haley CJ, Akhtar S, et al. Causes and consequences of duration of untreated psychosis in schizophrenia. Br J Psychiatry 2000;177:511–5.
30. Harrigan SM, McGorry PD, Krstev H. Does treatment delay in first-episode psychosis really matter? Psychol Med 2003;33(1):97–110.
31. Larsen TK, Melle I, Auestad B, et al. Substance abuse in first-episode non-affective psychosis. Schizophr Res 2006;88(1–3):55–62.
32. Lester H, Birchwood M, Freemantle N, et al. Redirect: cluster randomised controlled trial of GP training in first-episode psychosis. Br J Gen Pract 2009; 59(563):e183–90.
33. Rietdijk J, Hogerzeil SJ, van Hemert AM, et al. Pathways to psychosis: help-seeking behavior in the prodromal phase. Schizophr Res 2011;132(2–3):213–9.
34. Large M, Farooq S, Nielssen O, et al. Relationship between gross domestic product and duration of untreated psychosis in low-and middle-income countries. Br J Psychiatry 2008;193(4):272–8.
35. Morgan C, Abdul-Al R, Lappin JM, et al. Clinical and social determinants of duration of untreated psychosis in the AESOP first-episode psychosis study. Br J Psychiatry 2006;189:446–52.
36. Compton MT. Barriers to initial outpatient treatment engagement following first hospitalization for a first episode of nonaffective psychosis: a descriptive case series. J Psychiatr Pract 2005;11(1):62–9.
37. Franz L, Carter T, Leiner AS, et al. Stigma and treatment delay in first-episode psychosis: a grounded theory study. Early Interv Psychiatry 2010;4(1):47–56.
38. Merritt-Davis OB, Keshavan MS. Pathways to care for African Americans with early psychosis. Psychiatr Serv 2006;57(7):1043–4.
39. Eisenberg D, Golberstein E, Gollust SE. Help-seeking and access to mental health care in a university student population. Med Care 2007;45(7):594–601.
40. Couture S, Penn D. Interpersonal contact and the stigma of mental illness: a review of the literature. J Ment Health 2003;12(3):291–305.
41. Schiffman J, Dixon L. Treatment issues and challenges facing young adults with chronic mental illness. The Maryland Psychologist 2011;56:19–21.
42. Lloyd-Evans B, Crosby M, Stockton S, et al. Initiatives to shorten duration of untreated psychosis: systematic review. Br J Psychiatry 2011;198(4):256–63.
43. Hegelstad WT, Larsen TK, Auestad B, et al. Long-term follow-up of the TIPS early detection in psychosis study: effects on 10-year outcome. Am J Psychiatry 2012; 169(4):374–80.

44. Larsen TK, Melle I, Auestad B, et al. Early detection of first-episode psychosis: the effect on 1-year outcome. Schizophr Bull 2006;32(4):758–64.
45. Larsen TK, Melle I, Auestad B, et al. Early detection of psychosis: positive effects on 5-year outcome. Psychol Med 2011;41(7):1461–9.
46. Melle I, Larsen TK, Haahr U, et al. Prevention of negative symptom psychopathologies in first-episode schizophrenia: two-year effects of reducing the duration of untreated psychosis. Arch Gen Psychiatry 2008;65(6):634–40.
47. Melle I, Larsen TK, Haahr U, et al. Reducing the duration of untreated first-episode psychosis: effects on clinical presentation. Arch Gen Psychiatry 2004; 61(2):143–50.
48. Joa I, Johannessen JO, Auestad B, et al. The key to reducing duration of untreated first psychosis: information campaigns. Schizophr Bull 2008;34(3):466–72.
49. Krstev H, Carbone S, Harrigan SM, et al. Early intervention in first-episode psychosis–the impact of a community development campaign. Soc Psychiatry Psychiatr Epidemiol 2004;39(9):711–9.
50. Malla A, Norman R, Scholten D, et al. A community intervention for early identification of first episode psychosis: impact on duration of untreated psychosis (DUP) and patient characteristics. Soc Psychiatry Psychiatr Epidemiol 2005;40(5):337–44.
51. Chong SA, Mythily S, Verma S. Reducing the duration of untreated psychosis and changing help-seeking behaviour in Singapore. Soc Psychiatry Psychiatr Epidemiol 2005;40(8):619–21.
52. Ke S, Lai J, Sun T, et al. Healthy Young Minds: The Effects of a 1-hour Classroom Workshop on Mental Illness Stigma in High School Students. Community Ment Health J 2014. [Epub ahead of print].
53. Economou M, Peppou LE, Geroulanou K, et al. The influence of an anti-stigma intervention on adolescents' attitudes to schizophrenia: a mixed methodology approach. J Child Adolesc Ment Health 2014;19(1):16–23.
54. Stuart H. Reaching out to high school youth: the effectiveness of a video-based antistigma program. Can J Psychiatry 2006;51(10):647–53.
55. Pinfold V, Toulmin H, Thornicroft G, et al. Reducing psychiatric stigma and discrimination: evaluation of educational interventions in UK secondary schools. Br J Psychiatry 2003;182(4):342–6.
56. Watson AC, Otey E, Westbrook AL, et al. Changing middle schoolers' attitudes about mental illness through education. Schizophr Bull 2004;30(3):563–72.
57. Wei Y, Hayden JA, Kutcher S, et al. The effectiveness of school mental health literacy programs to address knowledge, attitudes and help seeking among youth. Early Interv Psychiatry 2013;7(2):109–21.
58. Murman NM, Buckingham KC, Fontilea P, et al. Let's erase the stigma (LETS): a quasi-experimental evaluation of adolescent-led school groups intended to reduce mental illness stigma. In: Murman NM, Buckingham KC, Fontilea P, et al, editors. Child & youth care forum. New York: Springer; 2014. p. 1–17.
59. Jacobs E, Kline E, Schiffman J. Practitioner perceptions of attenuated psychosis syndrome. Schizophr Res 2011;131(1):24–30.
60. Kline E, Denenny D, Reeves G, et al. Early identification of psychosis in schools. In: Weist M, Lever N, editors. Handbook of school mental health: research, training, practice, and policy. New York: Springer; 2014. p. 323–38.
61. Taylor M, Cartwright BS, Carlson SM. A developmental investigation of children's imaginary companions. Dev Psychol 1993;29:276–85.
62. Whaley AL. Cultural mistrust: an important psychological construct for diagnosis and treatment of African Americans. Prof Psychol Res Pract 2001; 32(6):555.

63. Kaufman J, Birmaher B, Brent D, et al. Schedule for affective disorders and schizophrenia for school-age children - present and lifetime version (KSADS-PL): initial reliability and validity data. J Am Acad Child Adolesc Psychiatry 1997;36:980–8.

64. Kay SR, Fiszbein A, Opfer LA. The positive and negative syndrome scale (PANSS) for schizophrenia. Schizophr Bull 1987;13(2):261–76.

65. Overall JE, Gorham DR. The brief psychiatric rating scale. Psychol Rep 1962;10: 799–812.

66. Thompson E, Kline E, Reeves G, et al. Using parent and youth reports from the behavior assessment system for children, to identify individuals at clinical high-risk for psychosis. Schizophr Res 2014;154(1):107–12.

67. Thompson E, Kline E, Reeves G, et al. Identifying youth at risk for psychosis using the behavior assessment system for children. Schizophr Res 2013;151(1): 238–44.

68. Tsuji T, Kline E, Sorensen HJ, et al. Premorbid teacher-rated social functioning predicts adult schizophrenia-spectrum disorder: a high-risk prospective investigation. Schizophr Res 2013;151(1):270–3.

69. Schiffman J, Daleiden EL. Population and service characteristics of youth with schizophrenia-spectrum diagnoses in the Hawaii system of care. J Child Psychol Psychiatry 2006;47(1):58–62.

70. Schiffman J, Chorpita BF, Daleiden EL, et al. Service profile of youths with schizophrenia–spectrum diagnoses. Child Youth Serv Rev 2008;30(4):427–36.

71. McGorry PD, Hickie IB, Yung AR, et al. Clinical staging of psychiatric disorders: a heuristic framework for choosing earlier, safer and more effective interventions. Aust N Z J Psychiatry 2006;40(8):616–22.

72. Frazier FA, McClellan J, Findling RL, et al. Treatment of early-onset schizophrenia spectrum disorders (TEOSS): demographic and clinical characteristics. J Am Acad Child Adolesc Psychiatry 2007;46:979–88.

73. Nugent KL, Kline E, Thompson E, et al. Assessing psychotic-like symptoms using the BASC-2: adolescent, parent and teacher agreement. Early Interv Psychiatry 2013;7(4):431–6.

74. Kline E, Schiffman J. Psychosis risk screening: a systematic review. Schizophrenia Research 2014;158(1):11–8.

75. Friis S, Vaglum P, Haahr U, et al. Effect of an early detection programme on duration of untreated psychosis: part of the Scandinavian TIPS study. Br J Psychiatry 2005;187(Suppl 48):s29–32.

76. Birchwood M, Singh SP. Mental health services for young people: matching the service to the need. Br J Psychiatry 2013;202(s54):s1–2.

School-Based Suicide Prevention

Content, Process, and the Role of Trusted Adults and Peers

Shashank V. Joshi, MD[a,*], Samantha N. Hartley, BA[b],
Moira Kessler, MD[a], Maura Barstead, BA[a]

KEYWORDS

- Suicide prevention • School mental health • School-based suicide prevention
- Supporting alliance • Child/adolescent • Suicide/self-harm • High-risk behaviors

KEY POINTS

- Suicide accounts for more deaths among youth and young adults in the United States than do all natural causes combined.
- Most deaths by suicide occur in people who have had mental health conditions, such as depression or severe anxiety, for at least a year.
- Prevention efforts must focus on school-based mental health education and promotion.
- Currently available programs focus on varying areas, including (1) Awareness/Education Curricula; (2) Screening; (3) Gatekeeper Training; (4) Skills Training; and (5) Peer Leadership.
- *Behavior change* for either self or a friend with regard to help-seeking for suicidal behaviors is an important focus for research.
- Process considerations are paramount and guide the nurturing of relationships and the building (and maintenance) of trust with school staff and administrators in enacting school-based strategies that highlight not only suicide prevention, but also health/wellness promotion and structural changes where indicated.

BACKGROUND

Suicide accounts for more deaths among 10 to 24 year olds in the United States than do all natural causes combined.[1] At the time of this publication in the United States, 5% to 8% of all adolescents attempt suicide annually, and up to one-third of these

The authors have no conflicts of interest to disclose.
[a] Lucile Packard Children's Hospital at Stanford University, Palo Alto, CA, USA; [b] School Mental Health Team, Lucile Packard Children's Hospital at Stanford University, 401 Quarry Road, Stanford, CA 94305, USA
* Corresponding author. Division of Child & Adolescent Psychiatry, 401 Quarry Road, Stanford, CA 94305.
E-mail address: svjoshi@stanford.edu

Abbreviations	
AFSP	American Foundation for Suicide Prevention
BFFD	Break Free from Depression
BPR	Best Practice Registry
CAP	Child and Adolescent Psychiatry
CARE	Care, Assess, Respond, Empower
CAST	Coping and Support Training
FAQs	Frequently asked questions
GBG	Good Behavior Game
LEADS	Linking Education and Awareness of Depression and Suicide
MTS	More than Sad
QPR	Question, Persuade, Refer
SOS	Signs of Suicide
SPRC	Suicide Prevention Resource Center

attempts result in an injury requiring medical intervention.[2] Suicidal youths may be more attracted to death and less able to generate alternatives to suicide when faced with severe stress, feeling that suicide is their only option, also leaving communities at a loss.[3,4] The risk of suicide contagion, a phenomenon defined by the Centers for Disease Control and Prevention as a process by which exposure to the suicide or suicidal behavior by one or more people influences others to commit or attempt suicide, is especially high in adolescents. Estimates are that more than 100 to 200 teens die in suicide clusters each year, accounting for about 1% to 5% of all teen suicides annually.[5,6]

To address this public health problem, school-based suicide prevention and education programs have become more common as an efficient and cost-effective way to reach adolescents in the context of their daily lives, given that most youth spend most of their waking hours in school.[7] Other investigators have conducted a detailed and thoughtful review of established prevention and education programs.[8] In this paper, the authors focus on new and emerging school-based programs, with a focus on classroom curricula and peer leader programs. The authors also describe important steps to create buy-in from administrative personnel and build trust with school staff.

CONTENT: EDUCATIONAL CURRICULA AND PROGRAMS THAT AIM TO PREVENT COMPLETED SUICIDES

Prevention efforts must take into account the important link between suicide and mental health conditions, such as mood disorders and substance abuse, as 75% to 90% of deaths by suicide occur in people who have had such disorders for at least a year.[9] Numerous depression education curricula and school-based suicide prevention programs have been developed over the past 10 years, and Katz and colleagues[8] recently reviewed 16 of the most commonly used. Most of these programs focus on increasing students' and school staffs' knowledge about, and attitudes toward, depression and suicide. The investigators found that few of these programs were rigorously evaluated for their effectiveness in actually reducing suicide attempts. However, most were able to show a reduction in suicidal ideation overall, improve general life skills, and change gatekeeper behaviors. Any comprehensive suicide prevention plan should include the 4 components of health promotion, prevention/education, intervention, and postvention.[10-12] Several useful tool kits are readily available to address these components.[11-14] The report by Katz and colleagues[8] comprehensively reviews the research and supporting evidence of many suicide prevention programs in current use and gives recommendations regarding the most thoroughly evaluated and best-practice programs. The broad categories include (1) awareness/education curricula, (2) screening, (3) gatekeeper training, (4) skills training, and (5) peer leadership. All 16 programs reviewed are included in **Table 1**. Note that these were graded by the investigators using the Oxford Center for Evidence-based Medicine Criteria (2009) and are more of an evaluation of the research thus far on particular programs rather than an evaluation of the programs themselves. As noted in **Table 1**, a grade of D does not necessarily indicate an ineffective program but rather a lack of conclusive evidence or a poorly designed study.

Programs with the most rigorous evaluations are summarized in the following section.

Awareness/Education Curricula

The goal of these programs is to help students become more knowledgeable of the signs and symptoms of suicide so they can recognize these in themselves and in others.[8] These programs are designed to facilitate self-disclosure, especially to other peers.[15] Suicide awareness and (often) depression education can be incorporated into the regular school curriculum, within the forum of a life skills, science, physical education, or health education course. Although programs of this nature have demonstrated some improvements overall, the results are mixed in terms of changing attitudes, knowledge, and behavior. Currently, the design of these typically resembles a hybrid model that includes both screening and gatekeeper components, increasing the likelihood of identifying at-risk students. Limitations continue, however. For example, though designed to deglorify suicide and destigmatize the use of mental health services, knowledge and attitude changes are not necessarily correlated with changes in behavior, which can be difficult to measure.[8] Also, students who are at highest risk for suicide often lack a broad peer network, limiting the scope of these programs.[16]

An example of an awareness campaign (that also includes a screening component), is Signs of Suicide (SOS). SOS is a universal (school-wide) program that promotes the idea of suicide being directly related to mental illness rather than a normal reaction to stress or emotional distress. The program includes suicide awareness, mental health education, and a self-screening component. Through video and guided classroom discussions, students learn to acknowledge the signs of suicide displayed by others and to take them seriously, to let their peers know that they care, and to tell an adult. Secondary to the awareness education is the screening component of the program, which uses the Brief Screen for Adolescent Depression. Students identified as at risk are encouraged to seek further help.[17] In the evaluation by Katz and colleagues,[8] because of the high quality of the conducted trials on suicide attempt outcomes, SOS received a favorable designation. However, it has yet to show statistically significant results for decreasing suicidal ideation. Other challenges include the need for active consent, which may discourage at-need youths from participating, and the word suicide in the title of the program can sometimes dissuade administrators from embracing the screening portion of the program.

Emerging Curricula

Previous investigators[18–20] have proposed an adapted framework for how a teen may pass through a series of filters before accessing care for mental health concerns. The first filter involves symptom recognition. In this framework, adolescents will not seek treatment if they do not first recognize that they are suffering from symptoms worthy of professional attention or if they think that adults from whom they seek assistance will be able to help them.[21,22] Therefore, the educational objectives of any depression curriculum must addresses this first filter, not only for the affected teen but also for their

Table 1
School-based suicide prevention programs

Program	Attitude/ Knowledge	General Skills Training (Decreased Risk/Increased Protective Factors)	Gatekeeper Behavior	Help-Seeking Behavior	Suicide Behavior Ideation	Suicide Behavior Attempts
ASAP	C	C	D	—	—	—
CAST/CARE	B	B	—	—	D	D
CD-ROM (team up to save lives)	D	—	—	—	—	—
Psychoeducational program	C–	—	—	—	—	—
QPR	B	—	D	—	—	—
RAPP	C	—	—	—	—	—
Reconnecting youth	B	B	—	—	—	—
SEHS	C	—	—	—	—	—
SOAR	C	—	C	—	D	—
SOS	B	—	—	D	D	B
Sources of Strength	B	—	B	—	—	—
TeenScreen (Columbia Suicide Screen)	B	—	—	—	—	—
The Good Behavior Game	—	—	—	—	B	B
Yellow Ribbon Suicide Prevention Program	—	—	—	D	—	—
YSPP	C	—	—	—	—	—
Zuni/American Indian Life Skills Development	—	C	—	—	C	—

The authors note that, for example, a grade of D does not necessarily indicate an ineffective program but rather a lack of conclusive evidence or a poorly designed study evaluating the program.

Abbreviations: ASAP, Adolescent Suicide Awareness Program; CAST/CARE, Coping and Support Training/Care Assess Respond Empower; QPR, Question, Persuade, Refer; RAPP, Raising Awareness of Personal Power; SEHS, South Elgin High School Suicide Prevention Program; SOAR, Suicide, Options, Awareness, and Relief; SOS, Signs of Suicide; YSPP, Youth Suicide Prevention Program.

From Katz C, Bolton S, Katz LY, et al, the Swampy Cree Suicide Prevention Team. A systematic review of school-based suicide prevention programs. Depress Anxiety 2013;30:1032; with permission.

community of friends to whom they might turn for guidance in whether or not to seek care.[19]

The following section provides information on 3 emerging school-based depression/suicide prevention awareness and educational curricula: *More than Sad: Teen Depression*; *More Than Sad: Preventing Teen Suicide* (American Foundation for Suicide Prevention), *Break Free from Depression* (BFFD) (Boston Children's Hospital Neighborhood Partnerships), and *Linking Education and Awareness of Depression and Suicide* (LEADS) (Suicide Awareness Voices of Education). These programs have all been listed in the Best Practice Registry (BPR) compiled and maintained by the American Foundation for Suicide Prevention (AFSP) and the Suicide Prevention Resource Center (SPRC). The purpose of the BPR is to identify, review, and disseminate information about best practices that address specific objectives of the National Strategy for Suicide Prevention.[23]

Best practice registry structure
The BPR is organized into 3 sections:

- *Section I: Evidence-based programs* include interventions that have undergone formal evaluation and demonstrated statistically significant positive outcomes.
- *Section II: Expert and consensus statements* summarize the current state of knowledge in the suicide prevention field and provides best practice recommendations to guide program and policy development.
- *Section III: Adherence to standards* lists suicide prevention programs that have been reviewed for the factual accuracy of their content, likelihood of meeting suicide prevention objectives, and adherence to program design standards but that have not undergone the process of formal evaluation required for Section I inclusion.

The AFSP/SPRC BPR includes only those materials and programs that have been submitted and reviewed according to the designated criteria described earlier and, therefore, does not represent a comprehensive inventory of all suicide prevention initiatives. The creation of the BPR was guided by the belief that suicide prevention efforts can be improved by incorporating new knowledge as the field advances and that, although programs should undergo rigorous process and outcome evaluation whenever possible (Section I designation), the field can benefit from the dissemination of programs and practices whose content has been reviewed by content experts for accuracy, safety, and program design standards (Section III inclusion). The hope is that future research may focus on the evaluation of emerging curricula to ensure that suicide prevention efforts in schools may continue to be evidence based.

More than Sad: Teen Depression and More than Sad: Preventing Teen Suicide
More than Sad (MTS) is an approximately 75-minute program developed by the AFSP for high school students (*More than Sad: Teen Depression*) and for their teachers (*More Than Sad: Preventing Teen Suicide*). It was approved for Section III BPR inclusion in January 2010.

The MTS program consists of a 26-minute video followed by a group discussion, delivered in either a single 75-minute period or over the course of two 40-minute classes. The program's materials include the student video DVD, a second film for parents/school staff that provides an overview of common adolescent mental health concerns, and a brief facilitator's guide (including a suggested lesson plan, potential discussion questions, responses to questions frequently asked by students, and informational handouts).

The student film features vignettes of 4 fictional teens experiencing symptoms of depression or anxiety, interspersed with narration summarizing common symptoms, the brain-based/medical nature of depression, and various pathways by which a depressed teen may enter treatment (eg, concerned friends/parents, school counselor, physician, mental health hotlines). Particular emphasis is given to the treatable nature of depression and the importance of seeking help when teens notice symptoms of depression in either themselves or their friends, but the film does not include an in-depth discussion of the nature of various treatment options.

The nature of the postvideo group discussion section is largely determined by the instructor, who may use the questions given as suggested examples in the facilitator's guide or questions/reflections submitted by students to either reemphasize core themes from the film or to touch on related topics not covered in the film (eg, how to approach a friend who may be depressed, school- and community-based resources, mental health treatment options, stigma, perceived barriers to help-seeking, nonsuicidal self-injury, the distinction between what is normal vs clinically relevant, suicide and its link to depression, and so forth). A productive, informative discussion relies on the instructor's ability to accurately provide explanations to student questions. Unless the classroom teacher delivering the curriculum is confident in his/her knowledge-base concerning adolescent mental health, a counselor or outside mental health professional may need to assist in order to fill the information gaps not covered by the program's frequently asked questions (FAQs) guide. The authors have found this to be a wonderful opportunity for child and adolescent psychiatry (CAP) residents to team up with CAP faculty to provide a much-needed community service as well as a scholarly focused activity regarding depression education, suicide prevention, and community engagement.

Among teachers and school administrators, MTS is an appealing curriculum option because of its relatively minimal demands on classroom time, potential for customized discussion, and general coverage of depressive symptoms (minimizing any risk of triggering students who have personal experience with depression). For these reasons, the authors think that MTS could be considered not only for high schools but also as an introduction to mental health education for younger, middle school audiences. Older students may value less scripted, more detailed discussion of teen depression and suicide prevention that would make this curriculum best paired with a mental health expert or school nurse who is versed in the topical areas of depression, anxiety, substance use, and suicide prevention.

More information about *More than Sad: Teen Depression*, and *More Than Sad: Preventing Teen Suicide* can be accessed at: http://www.morethansad.org/. A revised and more detailed version of the latter is scheduled for release in 2014.

Break Free From Depression

BFFD is a 4-session (approximately 4 hours) curriculum developed by Boston Children's Hospital for delivery in a high school setting; it has been classified under Section III of the BPR, as of September 2012.

The goal of BFFD is to increase student awareness and knowledge of adolescent depression and suicide risk factors and to promote the acceptability of help-seeking behaviors for themselves and others. The curriculum is delivered in a variety of formats, including PowerPoint (Microsoft Corporation, Redmond, WA)-assisted lectures, interactive student activities, a documentary film, and guided small-group discussions. Included in the BFFD curriculum is a detailed facilitator's guide with step-by-step instructions for each of the 4 sessions, the documentary DVD, and a second disc containing all of the handouts, forms, surveys, and PowerPoint presentations discussed in the facilitator's guide. In addition to thorough lesson plans, the facilitator's guide includes a discussion of the rationale for creating the curriculum and the need for adolescent suicide education and prevention efforts in schools, logistical considerations for program implementation, suggestions for engaging parents, a related school staff training, supplementary activities for students centered on building/practicing healthy stress-management and coping techniques, and suggested discussion points for FAQs from students, staff, and parents. The facilitator's guide is comprehensive and easy to follow and allows for a wide range of instructor skill sets and experience in delivering the curricular material as long as the instructor undergoes the proper training to best deliver the program with fidelity.

The 4 modules of BFFD consist of (1) a lecture providing an overview of key topics in adolescent depression/suicide (eg, causes and symptoms of depression, statistics, common misconceptions and sources of stigma, warning signs of depression and suicide in teens); (2) a 35-minute documentary featuring the unscripted stories of actual teens who have struggled with depression (It includes a discussion of their personal experience with depression, anxiety, self-harm, suicide, and treatment, and what has helped them to cope.); (3) a small-group discussion about the film; and (4) a final section that offers students strategies and options for seeking help for themselves and others, including a discussion about the influence of stigma, barriers to help-seeking and how to overcome them, treatment options, and ways to access help. Throughout the program, students are provided the opportunity to discretely request an appointment with a counselor or to request immediate individual assistance. Therefore, although only one instructor is required to deliver the curriculum, school counselors or a partnered community mental health resource should be aware of the schedule on which BFFD is being taught and available for students who choose to self-refer.

BFFD provides an engaging, comprehensive depression/suicide prevention-focused educational curriculum for high school students. The variety of content-delivery modalities, lecture, discussion, film, interactive activities, helps maintain student interest and focus in spite of the program's length. The documentary's use of an economically and racially diverse group of adolescents comfortable with candidly speaking on their own experiences delivers a compelling message to students that depression is a serious condition that can affect anyone, which, in the authors' experience delivering this program, deeply resonates with students, teachers, and parents alike. Although it is not uncommon for the film's realness to be emotionally evocative for students, the program protects against fears that it may be triggering for or put struggling students at additional risk by building in frequent opportunities for students to request assistance from a counselor or mental health professional, without drawing undue attention to themselves in class. More information on BFFD can be found at http://www.childrenshospital.org/breakfree.

Linking Education and Awareness of Depression and Suicide (LEADS) for youth
The LEADS program is a 3-day (approximately 1 hour per day) classroom curriculum developed for high school students. It was approved for Section III BPR inclusion in February 2008 and qualified for a Section I listing in January 2012.

The goal of the LEADS program is to improve knowledge of depression and suicidal behavior, increase awareness of suicide prevention resources, decrease the stigma of mental health problems, and promote help-seeking behaviors among adolescents. The curriculum is available on a CD-ROM containing a detailed facilitator's guide that covers step-by-step lesson plans, presentation materials and PowerPoint slides, and handouts for each activity and assignment; an extended teacher's guide; an overview of the evaluations the program has undergone to earn its Section I BPR listing; and recommendations for school-based crisis management. Although ideally

Table 2
Summary of 3 emerging curricula in suicide prevention

	Time Required[a,b]	Target Audience	Main Staff Required	Additional Staff	Materials Included	Teaching Tools	Examples
MTS[24]	75 min	8th–12th Grade (staff development version also included and may be used as part of parent education)	2–3 Informed discussion leaders	Not required	Suggested lesson, FAQ	Docudrama film, discussion	Simulated
BFFD[25]	4 h	9th–12th Grade	1 Instructor (nonrestrictive)	On-call counselor or mental health professional	Facilitators guide (detailed)	Documentary film, PPT presentation, activities, discussions	Nonscripted, actual teen stories
LEADS[26]	3 h	9th–12th Grade	1 Instructor (nonrestrictive)	Not required	Facilitator guide (detailed)	PowerPoint presentation, activities, discussions, homework	Simulated

a Previous research[19,27] has led to recommendations against 1-and-done presentations, as they may not be effective in changing behavior. Moreover, students (and school staff or parents) ought to have opportunities for questions, reflection, and follow-up; all 3 of these curricula should be delivered over multiple sessions.

b This table is not meant to represent a comprehensive list of newer curricula that have yet to undergo Oxford Criteria Evaluation. For example, the Adolescent Depression Awareness Program[19] is another such program that has shown positive outcomes.

Table 3 Program content coverage			
	MTS	**BFFD**	**LEADS**
Symptoms	2	3	3
Causes of depression	2	2	2
Nonsuicidal self-injury	0	3	0
Suicide	1*,3*	3	3
Treatment	2	2	2
Existing stigma	1-2	3	3
Common misconceptions	1-2	3	3
Destigmatizing efforts	1-2	3	3
Getting help	2	2	3

Scoring guide: 0, briefly mentioned/not covered; 1, minimal explanation/coverage; 2, good explanation/coverage; 3, excellent explanation/coverage; 1*- MTS, Teen Depression; 3*-MTS, Preventing Teen Suicide.

delivered by an instructor who is knowledgeable about mental health issues in teens, the thorough nature of the LEADS facilitator's guide makes it appropriate for less experienced instructors with an interest in the topic.

LEADS lessons cover key aspects of adolescent depression and suicide, including the nature of depression as a medical illness caused by a chemical imbalance in the brain; how clinical depression differs from having the blues or feeling sad; symptoms and treatment options for depression; stigma surrounding suicide and mental illness; risk factors, protective factors, and warning signs of suicide; barriers to getting help; how teens can get help for a friend; and examples of school, community, and national mental health resources. The homework assignment on day 2 asks students to apply what they have learned about identifying symptoms/risk factors and talking to friends about getting help through the use of realistic online communications.

Lessons are delivered using a combination of PowerPoint presentations, class discussion, small group activities, and homework assignments. In the absence of a film component, LEADS relies on classroom discussions to maintain student focus and engagement during the PowerPoint-based lessons; therefore, it would be an especially good match for an actively participatory class or a teacher skilled at facilitating classroom discussions. More information on LEADS for youth can be found at: https://www.save.org/leads (**Tables 2** and **3**).

SCREENING

Screening is a specific technique in suicide prevention designed to detect high-risk individuals. The method typically involves online or paper/pencil questionnaires for mental health symptoms, either for all students or for at-risk students only, noting those at increased risk and recommending further treatment. The availability of referral sites or clinicians before screening occurs is an important factor that needs addressing, in addition to any potential shortage of clinicians with expertise in treating suicidal youths or those in crisis.[8] Screening tools typically assess for risk factors, such as depression, drug and alcohol abuse, and past suicidal behavior, with the goal of identifying at-risk students who may otherwise go unidentified or undertreated. Until 2012, TeenScreen was the primary screening program in the United States and was used in both outpatient and school-based settings.

Although not in current use, a brief overview is presented next, as the program is undergoing an administrative revision as of the time of this publication.

TeenScreen

The TeenScreen tool was a universal self-report tool that assessed risk factors for suicide. The tool had evolved for use in schools, primary care, and other settings.[8,28–30] Although some of the forms of this screening tool are broader, TeenScreen is focused on school-based screening. A nonrandomized cohort study was conducted, demonstrating its validity and reliability in identifying at-risk students. All students who had obtained parental consent were given this screening tool plus the Beck Depression Inventory. Students who endorsed key risk factors were interviewed further. The tool has shown a sensitivity of 75% to 100% in student populations.[28,31] However, the benefit of the tool was time dependent; this method could potentially fail to identify students who were not actively at risk. Its success depended on subsequent referral.[8] Challenges to using this type of intervention include the need for active parental consent, and this can dissuade those at highest risk from assenting (or their parents from consenting) to be screened. This challenge has been observed in communities that have experienced a suicide cluster, where there may be the misguided perception that merely asking these questions may plant the ideas of suicide and self-harm into vulnerable youth.[32]

GATEKEEPER TRAINING

Gatekeeper training takes those considered to be natural helpers (both adults and/or youths) and aims to impart knowledge and teach skills to recognize signs and symptoms of suicide.[8] The principle is that suicidal youths, in general, may be underidentified and training school staff to recognize warning signs can enhance identification.[16] In addition, adults are trained on how to respond effectively. The ultimate success of this type of program also depends on the local availability of clinical expertise and subsequent service use of those identified at risk.[8] Question, Persuade, Refer (QPR) is one of the main gatekeeper programs used in schools at the time of this writing.

Question, Persuade, Refer

The QPR gatekeeper program may be conducted in communities or in schools. The school-based version trains students and school staff to recognize suicide risk factors in peers or students, respectively. It can be delivered in-person or online. The in-person version allows for role-play activities among participants and can help to desensitize students regarding the language of suicide prevention and intervention.[12] The program is based on 4 steps: (1) training and education to recognize suicide warning signs, (2) training all school staff in QPR, (3) training school counselors to properly assess at-risk students, and (4) organizing access to professional assessment and treatment.[33,34] The expected outcomes of this program include increasing school personnel awareness of suicide and their abilities to not only intervene by recognizing the warning signs, but also by responding appropriately.[8]

In a randomized controlled trial of 249 school staff, QPR demonstrated a benefit with regard to suicide knowledge, skills, and attitudes.[35,36] School staff participated in one of 2 contrasting gatekeeper-training models. Positive effects were shown on general knowledge, perceived preparedness, self-evaluated knowledge, and efficacy outcomes, including increased self-reported knowledge about suicide, appraisals of efficacy, and access to services. Although gatekeepers demonstrated improvements in knowing how to identify those at risk, only the gatekeepers who typically approached students to seek help felt comfortable doing so.[8] Notably, this program did not show an effect on subsequent mental health service use, a crucial component of any gatekeeper program. In a second study, Tompkins and colleagues[37] compared the effectiveness of training 78 school staff in QPR with a 24-person control group. In that study, QPR resulted in increased knowledge about suicide, and desirable changes in attitudes were also seen. Because of the high-quality randomized controlled trial (RCT), QPR was given a favorable grade for the knowledge and attitudes outcome in the review by Katz and colleagues.[8] The program has also been adapted to train youths as training initiatives that focuses solely on adults can result in a lack of help-seeking from teens to adults.[35]

On (adult) gatekeeper behavioral outcomes, such as asking students about suicide, increased number of referrals, and better connections with students, the study found no positive effects. Furthermore, a large evaluation in Georgia found no behavior change among youths in a large community where most of the adults were trained (and teens were not trained).[35] In several communities in Northern California, the authors of this paper have combined the practice of training adults on campus with training youths in QPR as well, using a modified version that is more applicable to youths.[12] This system has yet to be formally evaluated but has resulted in a much higher number of youths being referred to trusted adults by youths themselves. This combined approach also uses BPR-listed curricula, such as BFFD or MTS, and uses what Katz and colleagues[8] hypothesized "that one program may not be sufficient on its own to cover the breadth of suicide prevention required in schools, and that a combination of programs may be most effective."[8(p1037)]

Skills Training

The skills-training approach aims to increase protective factors by using a risk-reduction strategy for suicide prevention. These programs teach general life skills, such as coping, problem solving, decision making, and enhancing cognitive skills. Although the programs do not focus on suicide directly, they do target risk factors and aim to give youth important skills in order to prevent the development of suicidal behavior.[8]

Examples of promising programs in this arena include the American Indian Life Skills Development, which can be adapted to other cultural groups as well; The Care, Assess, Respond, Empower/Coping and Support Training Program; the Reconnecting Youth Program; and the Good Behavior Game (GBG).[17,38–40] The GBG, in particular, is robust as a primary prevention approach and has been found to substantially reduce later high-risk behaviors in teens, including suicide attempts. The GBG is a universal program for early elementary school students and is a classroom-based, teamwork, and behavior management approach to help children develop intrinsic self-regulation by rewarding teams that meet the behavior standards set by a teacher. The goal of the program is to create a positive classroom environment where students support one another and can learn in an environment without aggression or disruptive behavior. Students are grouped into teams with equal distribution of those with disruptive and aggressive behavior histories. The teacher posts the rules of the game regarding student behavior, and all teams who accumulate 4 or fewer infractions of acceptable student behavior are rewarded.[8,41]

When the GBG was implemented in first- or second-grade urban classrooms, a well-designed RCT found that there were reduced suicidal ideation and attempts (by 50%) and also a substantial reduction in substance use and antisocial and risky behaviors 15 years later in the same cohort.[41] This finding demonstrates the potential suicide prevention impact from promoting and teaching self-regulatory processes through early and intentional universal interventions.[8,41]

Peer Leadership Training

These programs seek to understand the role of peers and peer leader influences in schools. They are considered to be school-wide health promotion programs (as well as suicide prevention programs) that provide training for student peer leaders. *Sources of Strength* is the newest and best studied of these and focuses on training a diverse group of *both* peer leaders and adult advisors.[42] These students then conduct focused peer-to-peer prevention and messaging activities on campus, designed to build social and ecological protective influences across the full student population.[1,43] In an 18-school RCT, Wyman and colleagues[1] demonstrated that the training of peer leaders with the *Sources of Strength* program led to changes in norms across the full population of high school students after 4 months of school-wide messaging. Youth opinion leaders from diverse social cliques, including at-risk adolescents, were trained to change the norms and behaviors of their peers by conducting well-defined social messaging activities with close adult guidance. Peer leaders were nominated by administration and faculty, and the training consisted of 4 hours of interactive training for peer leaders and adult advisors. There was a focus on 8 protective 'sources of strength' and skills for increasing those resources for themselves and other students.[42] The 2 social norms most strongly enhanced through the intervention were (1) students' perceptions that adults in their school can provide help to suicidal students and (2) the acceptability of seeking help from adults. The largest, most positive increases in perceptions of adult help for suicidal youths occurred among students with a history of suicidal ideation. In the larger high schools studied, *Sources of Strength* training also increased peer leaders' referrals of friends to adults because of concerns about suicide. By training a diverse group of peer leaders within each school, the program was able to provide well-adapted students with opportunities to influence at-risk students, thereby reducing possible iatrogenic effects that may occur by grouping at-risk adolescents.[44] The investigators proposed that because adolescents are far more likely to be aware of suicidal behavior in their friends than adults are,[45] then increasing students' partnering with adults to help suicidal peers may be a key process for reducing adolescent suicidal behavior.[1] They also highlight that the protective factors pertaining to help seeking, connectedness with adults, and school engagement cannot only lower the risk for suicidal behavior[35,46,47] but are also associated with a reduced risk for school dropout,[48,49] depression, and substance use problems.[50–52] The overlap of suicide prevention objectives with other school-based educational and health promotion goals, such as keeping students enrolled in school and increased academic achievement, can increase the attractiveness and feasibility of disseminating this peer leader intervention.[1]

FROM IMPROVED PERCEPTIONS OF ADULT HELP TO BEHAVIOR CHANGE IN SEEKING HELP

What is currently unclear in the literature is whether school-based programs lead to *behavior change* for either self or a friend with regard to help seeking for mental health problems. Cigularov and colleagues[21] and Aseltine and DeMartino[53] suggested that appropriate help-seeking skills be taught as a major goal in any school-based or community-based suicide prevention education program. Previous investigators[54] have proposed that "help-seeking itself can be a self-threatening experience associated with feelings of inadequacy, inferiority, incompetence, embarrassment and dependency, as well as fears of being stigmatized, especially for problems that are central to one's esteem and self-concept."[54]

Other studies have examined adolescent barriers to seeking help specifically for suicidal behavior[55–58] and in school-based settings.[21] Research thus far indicates that adolescents might be more willing to *refer others for help* than to seek *help for themselves* for both severe and minor problems because the former is a less threatening experience. Cigularov and colleagues[21] showed that the most prominent barriers for seeking help for self were the inability to discuss problems with adults, self-overconfidence (feeling that they could handle crises on their own), fear of hospitalization, and lack of closeness to school adults. The most prominent barriers for troubled friends were friendship (loyalty) concerns, unavailability of adults at school, fear of friend's hospitalization, and underestimating friend's problems.

From a developmental theory perspective, the stakes associated with help seeking may be especially high to adolescents because they tend to be cognizant and sensitive to being perceived negatively by others.[21,59] These psychological costs may then become barriers to seeking help that limit adolescents' intent or willingness to seek help for mental health problems, including depression or suicidal thinking in either oneself or peers.[21,58,60–63]

Thus, it would be difficult to achieve the goals of a suicide prevention program unless critical barriers that impede effective responses to depressive symptoms or suicidal behaviors are recognized and reduced. It reinforces the need for examining the barriers to help seeking that may be perceived by adolescents. Several types of barriers have emerged from the adolescent help-seeking literature. These types include (1) concerns about confidentiality and privacy; (2) stigma about mental health conditions and feelings of embarrassment, shame, low self-confidence, and helplessness; (3) negative perceptions of adult helpers as being judgmental, unavailable, inaccessible, unhelpful and not caring, listening, understanding, or deserving trust; (4) problem avoidance and denial; (5) fears of hospitalization, forced treatment, and negative consequences; (6) self-reliance for problem solving; (7) negative previous experiences with help seeking; (8) influence from significant others (peers, family members, teachers); and (9) practical constraints (affordability, location of services, transportation, time conflict with other activities).[21]

For adolescents in particular, the stigma associated with receiving treatment of mental health conditions often poses a significant obstacle to seeking care,[64,65] particularly in the school setting.[66] In general, we know little about youths' subjective experiences with stigma as mental health consumers[67] and even less about the factors that relate to greater risk for self-stigmatization among youths. This stigma is very relevant to suicide prevention work, as stigma has the potential of being especially detrimental to youths who are navigating important developmental terrain, including the consolidation of identity, which motivates youths to fit in socially and maximize independence or autonomy.[68–70] Future research in this area must produce recommendations that will add to a growing evidence base that highlights the crucial roles that adolescent peers (with adult mentoring) can play in improving knowledge, changing attitudes, decreasing stigma, and enhancing the coping of teens with depression or other conditions that can increase the risk of suicidal behaviors.

PROCESS CONSIDERATIONS

Before introducing a suicide prevention program or curriculum, mental health providers would be wise to be mindful of seminal work in this area, which offers guidance on nurturing working relationships and building (and maintaining) trust with school staff and administrators,[71–74] especially in the face of such tragic events as a suicide of someone in the school community. Bostic and Rauch's 3R's of school consultation model[71] include the *relationships* that need to be cultivated and fostered, the *recognition* of human motivation during an important or sensitive time, and the *responses* to challenges. For a school mental health consultant, each face-time contact with administration is an opportunity to improve the school system and its response to those in greatest need and also to strengthen the system as a whole. First, the consultant strengthens the *relationships* of professionals allied around students, parents, and the greater school community, building bridges among them. This partnership among parents, staff, and therapists for school mental health has been termed the *supporting alliance in school mental health* and has been described previously.[75] Second, the school consultant can foster *recognition* of human motivation and the resistance that may impede healthy changes in the case of suicide prevention. Guiding principles include determining the wishes and motives of the student, parent, teacher, and administrator and dismantling resistance to change. The reluctance to embark on universal suicide prevention strategies often stems from a place of fear (eg, that such programs may plant the idea of suicide not only in vulnerable youth but also in those who had not considered suicide previously). Third, the school consultant can help the staff create *responses* to challenges. Guiding principles include providing staff new skills to reach and teach distressed students and finding common goals to unite students in the school, to reach parents in the community, and to determine the developmental steps toward shared goals.[71] Finally, the school consultant can leverage the trust they have built with school administration and school district leadership to advocate for school climate and other structural changes that have an emerging research base in support of youth mental health. These changes include later school start times to improve total sleep[76]; detailed self-study into the sources of major and daily stressful life events for youths,[77] such as severe academic stress in communities where youths may see themselves as being evaluated solely in terms of their academic performance and the pressure to excel is an important measure of their success in school[78,79]; and the adoption of formal suicide prevention policies with administrative regulations by local school boards.[12] The aforementioned empowering principles allow therapeutic skills used in individual and family therapies to provide strategies that can assist education professionals, students, and the larger school community simultaneously.

SUMMARY

In summary, there are several emerging programs and approaches that can be used to implement suicide prevention in schools. In this paper, the authors try to highlight not only the content of such programs but also the process of school stakeholder buy-in. Several studies have highlighted that peers, teachers, and other school staff are actively interested in understanding suicide risk factors, learning how to implement practical tools for responding to students in need, developing classroom management strategies for those in crisis, and disseminating strategies to connect with students in need and refer them to resources. Several emerging curricula and interventions were reviewed, with a highlight on the AFSP/SPRC's BPR curricular programs and peer-leader training with guidance by trusted adults, as promising strategies for primary prevention. Programs such as the GBG in elementary schools and *Sources of Strength* in secondary schools can be used as school-wide positive behavior and suicide prevention programs and may also have important downstream prevention benefits in reducing adolescent risk-taking behaviors more broadly.

REFERENCES

1. Wyman PA, Brown CH, LoMurray M, et al. An outcome evaluation of the Sources of Strength suicide prevention program delivered by adolescent peer leaders in high schools. Am J Public Health 2010;100(9):1653.

2. Centers for Disease Control. Youth risk behavior surveillance, United States 2013. MMWR Surveill Summ 2014;63(4):1–168. Available at: http://www.cdc.gov/mmwr/pdf/ss/ss6304.pdf. Accessed September 1, 2014.
3. Brent DA. Preventing youth suicide: time to ask how. J Am Acad Child Adolesc Psychiatry 2011;50(8):738–40.
4. Orbach I, Rosenheim E, Hary E. Some aspects of cognitive functioning in suicidal children. J Am Acad Child Adolesc Psychiatry 1987;26:181–5.
5. Gould MS, Wallenstein S, Kleinman MH, et al. Suicide clusters: an examination of age-specific effects. Am J Public Health 1990;80(2):211–2.
6. Hacker K, Collins J, Gross-Young L, et al. Coping with Youth Suicide and Overdose: One Community's Efforts to Investigate, Intervene, and Prevent Suicide Contagion. Crisis 2008;29(2):86–95.
7. Miller DN, Eckert TL, Mazza JJ. Suicide prevention programs in the schools: a review and public health perspective. Sch Psychol Rev 2009;38(2):168–88.
8. Katz C, Bolton S, Katz LY, et al, the Swampy Cree Suicide Prevention Team. A systematic review of school-based suicide prevention programs. Depress Anxiety 2013;30:1030–45.
9. Bertolote JM, Fleischmann A. Suicide and psychiatric diagnosis: a worldwide perspective. World Psychiatry 2002;1(3):181–5.
10. Gould M, Velting D, Kleinman M, et al. Teenagers' attitudes about coping strategies and help-seeking behavior for suicidality. J Am Acad Child Adolesc Psychiatry 2004;43(9):1124–33.
11. AFSP/SPRC American Foundation For Suicide Prevention and the Suicide Prevention Resource Center. After a suicide: a toolkit for schools. 2011. Available at: http://www.sprc.org/sites/sprc.org/files/library/AfteraSuicideToolkitforSchools.pdf. Accessed August14, 2014.
12. Joshi SV, Hartley SN, Lenoir L, et al. A comprehensive suicide prevention toolkit. Palo Alto (CA): PAUSD Press; 2013. p. 166. Available at: http://pausd.org/parents/services/health/downloads/ComprehensiveSuicidePreventionToolkitforSchools.pdf. Accessed September 1, 2014.
13. Allison PD. Missing data: quantitative applications in the social sciences. Br J Math Stat Psychol 2002;55:193–6.
14. Kerr MM, Brent DA, McKain B, et al. Postvention standards manual: a guide for a school's response in the aftermath of sudden death. 4th edition. Pittsburgh, PA: University of Pittsburgh Medical Center, Western Psychiatric Institute and Clinic, Services for Teens at Risk (STAR-Center); 2011. Available at: http://www.sprc.org/library_resources/items/postvention-standards-manual-guide-schools-response-aftermath-sudden-death. Accessed September 1, 2014.
15. Kalafat J, Elias M. An evaluation of a school-based suicide awareness intervention. Suicide Life Threat Behav 1994;24(3):224–33.
16. Gould MS, Greenberg T, Velting DM, et al. Youth suicide risk and preventive interventions: a review of the past 10 years. J Am Acad Child Adolesc Psychiatry 2003;42(4):386–405.
17. SAMHSA. NREPP: SAMHSA's national registry of evidence- based programs and practices. 2011. Available at: http://www.nrepp.samhsa.gov. Accessed September 1, 2014.
18. Goldberg D, Huxley P. Mental illness in the community: the pathway to psychiatric care. New York: Tavistock; 1980.
19. Swartz KL, Kastelic EA, Hess SG, et al. The effectiveness of a school-based adolescent depression education program. Health Educ Behav 2010;37(1):11–22.

20. Zwaanswijk M, Verhaak PF, Bensing JM, et al. Help seeking for emotional and behavioural problems in children and adolescents: a review of recent literature. Eur Child Adolesc Psychiatry 2003;12(4):153–61.

21. Cigularov K, Chen PY, Thurber BW, et al. What prevents adolescents from seeking help after a suicide education program? Suicide Life Threat Behav 2008;38(1):74–86.

22. Cialdini RB, Reno RR, Kallgren CA. A focus theory of normative conduct: recycling the concept of norms to reduce littering in public places. J Pers Soc Psychol 1990;58(6):1015–26.

23. U.S. Surgeon General's Office. National strategy for suicide prevention: goals and objectives for action. 2012. Available at: http://www.surgeongeneral.gov/library/reports/national-strategy-suicide-prevention/overview.pdf. Accessed September 1, 2014.

24. American Foundation For Suicide Prevention and Suicide Awareness Voices of Education. More than Sad: teen depression, More than Sad: preventing teen suicide. New York: American Foundation For Suicide Prevention; 2009.

25. Cambridge Neighborhood Partnerships and Children's Hospital Boston. 2011

26. Suicide Awareness Voices of Education. Linking education and awareness of depression and suicide: for youth. Bloomington (MN): Suicide Awareness Voices of Education; 2008.

27. Centers for Disease Control and Prevention. Characteristics of an Effective Health Education Curriculum. Available at: www.cdc.gov/healthyyouth/SHER/characteristics/index.htm. Accessed February 18, 2015.

28. Shaffer D, Scott M, Wilcox H, et al. The Columbia Suicide Screen: validity and reliability of a screen for youth suicide and depression. J Am Acad Child Adolesc Psychiatry 2004;43(1):71–9.

29. Singer JD, Willett JB. Applied longitudinal data analysis: modeling change and event occurrence. Oxford University Press; 2003.

30. SPRC/AFSP Suicide Prevention Resource Center/American Foundation for Suicide Prevention. Best practice registry for suicide prevention. 2008. Available at: http://www.sprc.org/bpr. Accessed September 1, 2014.

31. Scott MA, Wilcox HC, Schonfeld IS, et al. School-based screening to identify at-risk students not already known to school professionals: the Columbia Suicide Screen. Am J Public Health 2009;99(2):334–9.

32. Gould MS, Marrocco FA, Kleinman M, et al. Evaluating iatrogenic risk of youth suicide screening programs: a randomized con- trolled trial. JAMA 2005;293(13):1635–43.

33. QPR for schools. Spokane, WA: QPR Institute; 2011.

34. Raudenbush SW, Bryk AS. Hierarchical linear models: applications and data analysis methods, vol. 1. Sage Publications, Inc; 2002.

35. Wyman P, Hendricks Brown C, Inman J, et al. Randomized trial of a gatekeeper program for suicide prevention: 1-year impact on secondary school staff. J Consult Clin Psychol 2008;76(1):104–15.

36. Wyman PA, Gaudieri PA, Schmeelk-Cone K, et al. Emotional triggers and psychopathology associated with suicidal ideation in urban children with elevated aggressive-disruptive behavior. J Abnorm Child Psychol 2009;37(7):917–28.

37. Tompkins TL, Witt J, Abraibesh N. Does a gatekeeper suicide prevention program work in a school setting? Evaluating training outcome and moderators of effectiveness. Suicide Life Threat Behav 2009;39(6):671–81.

38. Hooven C, Herting JR, Snedker KA. Long-term outcomes for the promoting CARE suicide prevention program. Am J Health Behav 2010;34(6):721–36.

39. LaFromboise T, Howard-Pitney B. The Zuni life skills development curriculum: description and evaluation of a suicide prevention program. J Couns Psychol 1995;42(4):479–86.

40. Lapinski MK, Rimal RN. An explication of social norms. Commun Theory 2005; 15(2):127–47.
41. Wilcox HC, Kellam SG, Brown CH, et al. The impact of two universal randomized first- and second-grade classroom interventions on young adult suicide ideation and attempts. Drug Alcohol Depend 2008;95(Suppl 1):S60–73.
42. LoMurray M. Sources of strength facilitators guide: suicide prevention peer gatekeeper training. Bismarck (ND): The North Dakota Suicide Prevention Project; 2005. Available at: http://www.sourcesofstrength.org. Accessed September 01, 2014.
43. Wyman PA. Developmental approach to prevent adolescent suicides: research pathways to effective upstream preventive interventions. Am J Prev Med 2014; 47(3S2):S251–6.
44. Dishion TJ, McCord J, Poulin F. When interventions harm: peer groups and problem behavior. Am Psychol 1999;54(9):755–64.
45. Gould MS, Klomek AB, Batejan K. The role of schools, colleges and universities in suicide prevention. In: Wasserman DW, editor. Oxford textbook of suicidology and suicide prevention: a global perspective. 1st edition. New York: Oxford University Press; 2009. p. 551–60.
46. Borowsky IW, Ireland M, Resnick MD. Adolescent suicide attempts: risks and protectors. Pediatrics 2001;107(3):485–93.
47. McKeown RE, Garrison CZ, Cuffe SP, et al. Incidence and predictors of suicidal behaviors in a longitudinal sample of young adolescents. J Am Acad Child Adolesc Psychiatry 1998;37(6):612–9.
48. DuBois DL, Silverthorn N. Natural mentoring relationships and adolescent health: evidence from a national study. Am J Public Health 2005;95(3):518–24.
49. DuBois DL, Silverthorn N. Characteristics of natural mentoring relationships and adolescent adjustment: evidence from a national study. J Prim Prev 2005;26(2):69–92.
50. Resnick MD, Bearman PS, Blum RW, et al. Protecting adolescents from harm. Findings from the national longitudinal study on adolescent health. JAMA 1997; 278(10):823–32.
51. Resnick MD, Harris LJ, Blum RW. The impact of caring and connectedness on adolescent health and well-being. J Paediatr Child Health 1993;29(Suppl 1):S3–9.
52. Rhodes JE, Contreras JM, Mangelsdorf SC. Natural mentor relationships among Latina adolescent mothers: psychological adjustment, moderating processes, and the role of early parental acceptance. Am J Community Psychol 1994;22(2):211–27.
53. Aseltine RH Jr, DeMartino R. An outcome evaluation of the SOS suicide prevention program. Am J Public Health 2004;94(3):446.
54. Nadler A. Esteem, relationships and achievement explanations of help seeking behavior. In: Karabenick SA, editor. Strategic help seeking: Implications for learning and teaching. Mahwah, NJ: Erlbaum; 1998. p. 61–96.
55. Goffman E. Stigma: notes on the management of spoiled identity. Touchstone; 1963.
56. Nadler A. Help-seeking behavior as a coping resource. Learned resourcefulness: on coping skills, self control, and adaptive behavior. New York: Springer; 1990. p. 127–62.
57. Wahl OF. Mental health consumers' experience of stigma. Schizophr Bull 1999; 25(3):467.
58. Geis BD, Edlavitch S. Adolescent barriers to seeking help for suicide: a cognitive-behavioral science of prevention? Poster presented at the National Conference of the American Association of Suicidology. Broomfield (CO), April 2005.
59. Bell JH, Bromnick RD. The social reality of the imaginary audience: a grounded theory approach. Adolescence 2003;38:205–20.
60. Helms JL. Barriers to help seeking among 12th graders. J Educ Psychol Consult 2003;14(1):27–40.

61. Kuhl J, Jarkon-Horlick L, Morrissey RF. Measuring barriers to help-seeking behavior in adolescents. J Youth Adolesc 1997;26(6):637–50.

62. Lindsey CR, Kalafat J. Adolescents' views of preferred helper characteristics and barriers to seeking help from school-based adults. J Educ Psychol Consult 1998; 9(3):171–93.

63. Wilson CJ, Deane FP. Adolescent opinions about reducing help-seeking barriers and increasing appropriate help engagement. J Educ Psychol Consult 2001; 12(4):345–64.

64. Austin JK, MacLeod J, Dunn DW, et al. Measuring stigma in children with epilepsy and their parents: instrument development and testing. Epilepsy Behav 2004;5(4):472–82.

65. Corrigan PW, Lurie BD, Goldman HH, et al. How adolescents perceive the stigma of mental illness and alcohol abuse. Psychiatr Serv 2005;56(5):544–50.

66. Wang-Kraus SD, Loftus PD, Chu IM, et al. Acculturative Family Distancing (AFD) in secondary school students: an examination of family cohesion, ruminations, and help-seeking behaviors in relation to high distress. Presented at the Amer Acad of Child & Adol Psychiatry, Ann Meeting. San Diego, 2014.

67. Hinshaw SP. The stigmatization of mental illness in children and parents: developmental issues, family concerns, and research needs. J Child Psychol Psychiatry 2005;46(7):714–34.

68. Leavey JA. Youth experiences of living with mental health problems: emergence, loss, adaptation and recovery (ELAR). Can J Commun Ment Health 2005;24(2):109–26.

69. Moses T. Being treated differently: stigma experiences with family, peers, and school staff among adolescents with mental health disorders. Soc Sci Med 2010;70(7):985–93.

70. Wisdom JP, Clarke GN, Green CA. What teens want: barriers to seeking care for depression. Adm Policy Ment Health 2006;33(2):133–45.

71. Bostic JQ, Rauch PK. The 3 R's of school consultation. J Am Acad Child Adolesc Psychiatry 1999;38(3):339–41.

72. Waxman RP, Weist MD, Benson DM. Toward collaboration in the growing education-mental health interface. Clin Psychol Rev 1999;19(2):239–53.

73. Weist MD, Lowie JA, Flaherty LT, et al. Collaboration among the education, mental health, and public health systems to promote youth mental health. Psychiatr Serv 2001;52(10):1348–51.

74. Nadeem E, Kataoka S, Chang VY, et al. The Role of Teachers in School-Based Suicide Prevention: A Qualitative Study of School Staff Perspectives. School Mental Health 2011;3:209–21.

75. Feinstein NF, Fielding K, Udvari-Solner A, et al. The supporting alliance in child and adolescent treatment: enhancing collaboration between therapists, parents and teachers. Am J Psychother 2009;63(4):319–44.

76. American Academy of Pediatrics (Adolescent Sleep Working Group, Committee on Adolescence, and Council on School Health). School start times for adolescents. Pediatrics 2014;134:642–9.

77. Wagner BM, Cole RE, Schwartzman P. Psychosocial correlates of suicide attempts among junior and senior high school youth. Suicide Life Threat Behav 1995;25(3):358–72.

78. Ang RP, Huan VS. Relationship between academic stress and suicidal ideation: testing for depression as a mediator using multiple regression. Child Psychiatry Hum Dev 2006;37:133–43.

79. Anthony RW, DeMaso DR, Dennery S, et al. Break free from depression curriculum. Boston: Cambridge Neighborhood Partnerships; 2012.

Supporting the Transition from Inpatient Hospitalization to School

Catharine L. Weiss, PhD*, Angela M. Blizzard, BA,
Courtney Vaughan, LCSW-C, Tierra Sydnor-Diggs, LCSW,
Sarah Edwards, DO, Sharon Hoover Stephan, PhD

KEYWORDS

- Psychiatric hospitalization • Schools • Families • Youth
- Cross-system collaboration

KEY POINTS

- Transitioning out of an inpatient psychiatric stay presents a variety of challenges for youth and their families.
- Limited family support and lack of coordination with school personnel may increase risk for hospital readmission.
- Families commonly express a need for increased information and support during transition from inpatient psychiatric care to school.
- The School Transition Program developed at University of Maryland provides support and care coordination through Family Connectors, School Transition Specialists, and mobilizing resources within the school.
- Having a transition specialist or advocate who can attend school meetings with families and collaborate on individualized plans may promote cross-system communication and improve outcomes.

SUPPORTING THE TRANSITION FROM INPATIENT HOSPITALIZATION TO SCHOOL

Inpatient psychiatric hospitalization is the most restrictive intervention available for youth with emotional and behavioral challenges and targets youth with the most severe psychiatric difficulties.[1,2] These hospitalizations are costly to the mental health

Funding Source: 1915c Demonstration Waiver (Grant Number: 13-10954G/M00B3400369): Community Alternatives to Psychiatric and Residential Treatment Facilities Demonstration Waiver Program Management, Workforce Development and Program Evaluation.
Conflict of Interest: The authors have no conflicts of interest to report.
Division of Child and Adolescent Psychiatry, University of Maryland School of Medicine, 701 West Pratt Street, Baltimore, MD 21201, USA
* Corresponding author. University of Maryland School of Medicine, 701 West Pratt Street, 4th floor, Baltimore, MD 21201.
E-mail address: cweiss@psych.umaryland.edu

Child Adolesc Psychiatric Clin N Am 24 (2015) 371–383
http://dx.doi.org/10.1016/j.chc.2014.11.009
1056-4993/15/$ – see front matter © 2015 Elsevier Inc. All rights reserved.

childpsych.theclinics.com

Abbreviations	
C & R	Connect And Reflect
FC	Family Connector
IEP	Individualized Education Program
SC	School Connector
STP	School Transition Program
STS	School Transition Specialist

system, with annual costs estimated at $3.9 billion.[3] In addition to financial costs to the system and individual families, hospitalizations result in increased stress for youth and families.[4] With readmission rates ranging from 30% to 50%, youth are also at risk of cycling through multiple hospitalizations in a short period of time.[5,6] The emotional consequences to children and families and the financial costs incurred by frequent readmissions have led hospitals to place an increased focus on better supporting families during transition from inpatient care, and on reducing readmissions.[7]

Limited family support and lack of coordinated care may heighten the risk for readmission to inpatient psychiatric care.[8] Specifically, high caregiver burden and low levels of parent involvement in treatment are associated with a greater risk for readmission.[5,9,10] However, few studies have examined caregivers' perceptions of their child's hospitalization or their needs after the hospitalization. Caregivers report mixed feelings related to their child's hospitalization, expressing a desire for their children to improve, but also expressing concerns related to stigma.[11] A study examining the needs of caregivers during their child's hospitalization found that many caregivers felt supported by hospital staff during the stay, but desired more support related to behavior management strategies and information about their child's needs.[12]

Although prior research has examined the transition from hospital to school after a physical illness,[13–15] there has been far less empirical examination of the transition from inpatient psychiatric hospitalization to school. This is concerning, given that youth and families face various academic and emotional challenges when returning to school after inpatient psychiatric care. A number of common fears are reported by youth during this transition. Hospital therapists reported the fears youth experienced most frequently after discharge were related to peer relationships (88%), followed by personal coping skills, academic performance, and relationships with school personnel (range, 67%–61%).[16] The most frequently reported difficulty was anxiety (67%) followed by disruptive behavior (49%).[16] Academic challenges experienced upon return to school may reduce academic self-efficacy without proper school supports and intervention.[17]

Clinical providers also report that many hospitalized youth have difficulties transitioning back to an outpatient setting. Inpatient settings can feel safe for children, both physically, with a secure unit and highly structured routines, and emotionally, with respite from family/social stressors impacting their psychiatric functioning (eg, a time away from bullying, parent–child conflict). At discharge, many youth worry about the stigma of mental illness; they worry about family and friends being judgmental and may also wrestle with their own internal stigma with feelings of guilt, shame, and embarrassment. Families frequently struggle during this transition period with worries about relapse, guilt and fear that their actions caused their child's illness, and worries about keeping their children safe. Without acknowledging and addressing these important concerns, youth are at heightened risk for relapse and rehospitalization. Families may require support to learn different ways of managing challenging behaviors as well as approaches and skills to increase the kinds of behavior that will allow children to be successful in their home and school setting. However, fueled by the quick pace of crisis stabilization, discharge planning often does not address these factors and consists only of scheduling outpatient appointments or recommending outpatient providers. Youth and families are then left to navigate this transition alone and are at risk for not connecting with aftercare mental health services.

Few programs exist with the goal of helping youth and families transition to the school and community after an absence for an emotional or behavioral crisis. The majority of existing programs target youth exiting residential treatment. Of 6 programs identified in the literature, only 1 focused on the transition from acute inpatient care back to school.[18] This pioneering program aimed to Improve the transition from inpatient care back to the community through the creation of an individualized, family-focused crisis and transition plan. Findings demonstrated high levels of family satisfaction, decreased lengths of inpatient stay, and decreased readmissions to inpatient units. Given that acute inpatient stays tend to be significantly shorter than residential stays, and consequently there is less time for stabilization and planning, there should be an increased focus on implementing similar programs and strategies to help youth and families during this transition. Moreover, increased focus should be paid to how to augment cross-system collaboration to include schools. Most recently, Savina and colleagues[19] provided an ecological overview of the transition from intensive psychiatric care to school. Based on a review of the existing literature, they recommended implementing a school reintegration plan for youth returning to the school after a psychiatric hospitalization. They also advocate for additional research examining best practices for engaging hospital-based staff and families in the reintegration process.

THE SCHOOL TRANSITION PROGRAM

In 2012, with funding support from the State behavioral health authority, a team from the University of Maryland developed *The School Transition Program* (STP), an intervention designed to provide support to children and their families for 3 months after an inpatient psychiatric stay and to promote communication across school, home and hospital. Based on the Double ABCX Model,[20] the intervention aims to increase youth and caregiver empowerment, support, and access to resources during the transition, and ultimately to decrease unnecessary readmission to inpatient psychiatric care. Program components were developed to match the needs and context of this group (**Table 1**), and were informed by qualitative interviews with families as their children were discharged from inpatient psychiatric care.

Family Needs During Transition from Inpatient Psychiatric Care to School

To inform the ongoing development of the STP, our team conducted brief qualitative interviews with caregivers of children exiting inpatient care about their needs at home and school, as well as why they were interested in participating in the STP (Blizzard A, BA, Weiss C, PhD, Wideman R, BA, personal communication, 2015). At home, caregivers identified wanting to increase parenting knowledge, improve the caregiver–child relationship, increase emotional support for themselves, and gain access to additional child and family services. Not knowing the next steps to take to help their children or to secure aftercare services was noted as causing distress (eg, "I am trying to figure out the best path for me and my child. I don't know all the options I have and

Table 1 School Transition Program (STP) needs and components	
Family Need	**STP Component**
Cross-system communication and care coordination	Consultation with hospital and school staff Participation in school meetings
School-based resources and interventions	Transition support plan
Guidance on common after transition concerns	Family education Peer-to-peer support
Engagement in school and aftercare services	Development of communication and advocacy skills and problem-solving barriers Connection to community resources
Emotional support for caregiver	Peer-to-peer support
School connectedness and support	Brief daily check-ins with student and daily feedback to family on coping

I'm feeling lost, so I'm seeking all the help I can get"). Some youth were not connected to mental health services after discharge and some caregivers voiced wanting a change in or expansion of services. For some, it was difficult to get appointments with outpatient providers, including psychiatrists, because of their insurance and/or their child's symptom severity limited who would accept them. Caregivers often expressed current difficulty handling their children's behavior and wanting help with improving their family environment and their children's condition by learning better management strategies and establishing household rules. They often perceived that what they were lacking in resources and parenting skills may be contributing to their child's difficulties, but did not know how to address this on their own. Caregivers expressed concern regarding how their children's continued mental health difficulties had stressed the caregiver–child relationship, and they desired increased emotional support.

School challenges were most often the reason caregivers cited for enrolling in the program ("He has missed so much school time and needs help with working with the school and I heard that STP will work hand in hand with school, which is what I need"). Identified concerns fell into 4 areas at school: their child's social–emotional functioning, learning, access to increased school services, and advocacy. The return to school after hospitalization was generally described as a stressful event. Caregivers voiced a need for support to face the challenges that arose from the disruption of hospitalization and their child's ongoing difficulties (eg, "I don't think [my son] is ready to go back to regular school directly after an inpatient admission. He still has issues he needs to work on and we need a good transition or we will go back to square one"). The hospitalization was often viewed as a reason that the school needed to change their child's placement or offer more services. Many caregivers expressed concerns about the school environment related to their children being teased or bullied at school and desired a stronger school response. A portion of caregivers described that their children did not want to return to school or had significant anxiety about returning, because of concerns about how to explain their hospitalization and the stigma attached to mental illness. Caregivers also noted concerns about how their children would catch up with missed work and how the absences would affect their grades, and this was intensified if their children had preexisting learning problems. They reported feeling that school policies about making up academic work were unclear.

In addition, caregivers conveyed a need for assistance in advocating for themselves and their children in the school setting (eg, "help guide us through the process of returning to school, instead of throwing him back into school"). Some described the frustration that they have had in trying to communicate with the school and getting answers to their questions and concerns. Through their efforts alone, many caregivers felt they were not experiencing change, not being heard, and that the school did not share the same goals for their children. As a result, they desired that someone external to the school help them to navigate school procedures by attending reentry meetings with them.

School Transition Program Components

Families participating in the STP are assigned to a Transition Team, consisting of a Family Connector (FC) and School Transition Specialist (STS). The FCs implement an adapted version of the evidence-based Parent Connectors program,[21] and are legacy family members of a child with emotional or behavioral difficulties. FCs have experience navigating the mental health and education systems and have been trained to provide peer-to-peer support. The FC provides the child's caregiver with emotional and informational support through structured, weekly phone calls that can last up to 1 hour. They share their personal stories with caregivers as appropriate, work to help build caregivers' communication and advocacy skills, and encourage caregivers to become actively engaged in their child's school and mental health services.

The STS are social workers with extensive experience working with youth and families in school and community settings. The STS work with the family and school staff to create transitions plans for the school and home that address child and family strengths and needs, and then to monitor implementation of this plan during the 3-month program. Their role is distinct from a therapist or counselor, because they do not provide therapy to the family, but rather, they help to map out specific goals and corresponding strategies to support the transition. Core program components implemented by the STS include collaborating on the development of transition plans, providing psychoeducation to families, and connecting families to mental health and community resources. STS meet monthly with families, participate in at least 2 school meetings, and call periodically to facilitate engagement with mental health services and progress on the home and school transition plans.

TRANSITION PLANS

STS meet with caregivers upon program enrollment to discuss the youth's return to school and home. They review the hospital discharge plan, the youth's mental health history, and assess engagement in and barriers to mental health services. They discuss the caregiver's relationship with the school and their perceptions of the appropriateness of current school services for their child. A transition plan for the home is created that outlines the caregiver's goals, family and youth strengths and resources, and a crisis plan. Based on these discussions, families are also recommended community resources. Either before a child returns to school or as soon as possible afterward, STS work with families to schedule reentry meetings at the school. STS attend meetings with families and school staff to develop a transition plan. The youth's existing services and supports in addition to any hospital discharge recommendations are reviewed. The school's crisis protocol is discussed and adapted, if appropriate, for the particular student. An individualized transition form is completed that includes discussion of the youth's strengths, needs, and desired goals in emotional/behavioral, social, and academic functioning (**Table 2**).

Table 2
Information to be included in school transition plan

Relevant background information	
Current medications and medical history	
Family values and beliefs that may inform the plan	
Contact information for all providers (primary care and mental health)	
Domains of school functioning	**Areas to address within each domain**
Academic	Student's current functioning
Social skills	Student's strengths and needs
Behavioral/emotional	Goals for student
	Action plan
	School and family role in action items

PSYCHOEDUCATION AND RESOURCES

Caregiver education modules were developed by the STP team to address common transition and reentry issues reported by youth and families in the areas of mental health, education, and self-care. At meetings with caregivers, topics are presented to them as a menu of options that are matched to caregiver interest and needs. Some examples of these topics are how to address homework/workload concerns, communication with school staff, peer questions about hospitalization, and coping and relaxation strategies for caregivers.

The team has also developed psychoeducation content and other tools for school staff. Experience implementing the program emphasized the importance of educating school staff about hospitalization and alternatives to hospitalization that are available. Some school staff felt that if the youth's problems had not been resolved that they should be returned to the hospital quickly. Also, our team felt there was a need to increase school awareness about a family's experience of psychiatric hospitalization and return to school. Specifically, STS devoted time with school personnel to discussing possible experiences of families during this transition, including feeling significant stress, having questions and concerns about school issues, and possibly having difficulty connecting to mental health services. Student-specific psychoeducation is also presented at the reentry meetings or at subsequent meetings with key staff, such as the classroom teacher. Some examples of psychoeducation that have been provided include modules on specific diagnoses and symptoms, such as psychosis and Autism Spectrum Disorder, and appropriate classroom interventions. Schools are now provided with information sheets that describe what to expect after a hospitalization, area resources that may be alternatives to hospitalization, and typical family concerns and needs (see **Table 2**). Recommended guidelines for how to the content and process of reentry meetings are now regularly provided to school staff (**Table 3**).

Another component introduced during transition meetings is the Connect and Reflect program (C & R). The C & R program was developed based on the concept of the Check & Connect program, a more intensive intervention that involves an adult consistently "checking in" with a student during the school day to promote increased school connectedness and academic outcomes.[22] The goal of C & R is to increase connectedness with a supportive adult ("School Connector" [SC]) at the school and to monitor the youth's mood and coping by conducting brief, daily check-ins at specified times during the school day (typically 2–3 scheduled). It also aims to increase student responsibility, feeling identification, utilization of coping skills, and

Table 3
Common family questions for school staff after hospitalization

Question	School Strategies
What can the school do to help make sure my child is safe and supported?	Create or adapt school crisis plan Identify "student connector" in school to encourage and check in with child Identify "safe space" for student (eg, specific area in classroom, resource room)
How will my child make up missed work and will she/he be penalized for their absence?	Provide family with district/school policies Outline steps for missed learning and work
Who can I contact if I have questions or concerns about my child's progress after returning to school?	Identify one point person at school Set up schedule for regular feedback
What plan will be put in place to address my child's academic and behavioral/emotional needs?	Collaborate with relevant school staff to create a transition place that addresses child's strengths and needs
How will my child discuss his/her absence with peers and school staff?	Make plan with family that addresses youth and family concerns and values

problem-solving skills. A school staff member (eg, teacher, student support staff, administrator) is identified as the SC, taught how to implement the program, and encouraged to use it if deemed appropriate for the youth.

During each C & R check-in, the assigned SC encourages the student to identify how they are feeling and to reflect on why they are feeling that particular way. The SC will then assist the student on coming up with a strategy or plan to cope while in school. SCs are provided with feelings faces and a toolbox sheet to which students can refer for options of possible coping strategies. Each contact is logged on a form, with a duplicate sent home daily to increase home/school communication. Caregivers reported that the C & R process helped to reduce their worries about stepping down their youth from the structure and supervision of the inpatient setting. The C & R logs provided a reassuring, daily report of their child's progress and emotional functioning and a contact at school who knew their child well and with whom they could consult.

To illustrate the strategies used by the STSs and FCs, 2 families who participated in and completed the program will be presented. Pseudonyms have been used and identifying details have been altered to protect the privacy of these families.

VIGNETTE #1

Background

Jordan was a 12-year-old Caucasian boy who had 1 inpatient hospitalization before participating in the STP. Jordan was diagnosed with mood disorder, not otherwise specified, attention deficit/hyperactivity disorder, and reactive attachment disorder. Jordan was born in Bulgaria and was adopted by his parents when he was a toddler. After prompting from his therapist and psychiatrist, Jordan's parents agreed to admission to a child inpatient unit because of escalating verbal and physical aggression at home. Jordan had thrown objects, broken furniture, eloped from the home, locked his mother in the basement, and physically and verbally assaulted his parents.

Jordan attended a neighborhood public school and had an Individualized Education Program (IEP) for a learning disorder in math. His mother believed that Jordan also had delays in reading comprehension, but stated she had not felt comfortable in the past to speak up about this concern at school meetings. Jordan had started refusing to go to school over the last few months and was only attending sporadically. He was becoming very aggressive each morning with his parents. Although a Pupil Personnel Worker was involved from the school district to address his attendance problems, his mother reported that this had not helped and that the school staff was not aware of his school refusal and aggressive behavior, and that there were no behavior problems perceived by school. Jordan had been seeing a psychiatrist for medication management for 2 years. He had also participated in individual and family therapy twice per week at his home for the previous year.

During the first meeting with the family, the STS worked with Jordan's mother to determine their family's needs at home and school and strategies that could be implemented to help address these needs.

Caregiver Needs

- Education on effective ways to encourage Jordan to attend school and complete his homework.
- Enrollment in new health insurance owing to the husband's recent unemployment and loss of benefits. How will the change in insurance affect his ability to see his established mental health providers?
- Education/training on establishing rules, rituals, structure, and a behavior system within the home and managing oppositional and aggressive behaviors. How can she set limits effectively at home without increasing his aggression?
- Emotional support for the parents and access to support groups.
- Increased knowledge about school resources and communication with staff. Should she discuss concerns that she has about Jordan's educational needs and advocate for supportive accommodations?

Child Needs

- Determination of what contributes to his school avoidance and what factors may promote attendance. Is he feeling disconnected from school staff?
- Significant worry about school performance and how will he explain absences to classmates. How will he complete the school work he missed from his hospital stay and the days he refused to attend? What will people say when he comes back?
- Additional testing for reading, writing, and comprehension to determine need for interventions.
- Assistance with class assignments as needed.
- More opportunities for success at home and school, and to be rewarded when demonstrating desired behaviors.

School Needs

- Increased communication between the family and school staff. Jordan's mom had never met with the team or discussed his mental health history.
- Information about Jordan's mental health diagnosis and its impact on school performance and attendance.
- Assessment of Jordan's academic skills and adjustment of workload expectations to address missed time.

Strategies Implemented by the School Transition Program

- Facilitated meeting with hospital clinical staff (including the social worker, psychiatrist, and nursing staff), who provided pertinent discharge information to relay to school staff for continuity of care.

- Coordinated transition meeting at school with his teachers, administrator, and support staff. His mother discussed for the first time her son's mental health difficulties and her concerns about his learning.

- Classroom teacher began using C & R as part of the daily school routine. Jordan enjoyed the positive attention from his teacher, and mother appreciated receiving daily feedback regarding Jordan's emotional status and coping skills utilization.

- Developed with school staff a school crisis plan to be used as needed, especially during Jordan's arrival to school.

- Collaborated on a transition plan that addressed attendance and a plan for missed work and learning.

- Spoke with mom about how she wanted Jordan to discuss his absence with peers and made a script that she role played with him and communicated this to school staff.

- Aided in process of applying for medical assistance so that Jordan could continue to participate in therapy and obtain his prescribed psychiatric medication.

- Developed a crisis plan for the home, especially when Jordan becomes violent. Identified examples of situations when the police should be called and/or Jordan should be taken to the hospital.

- Provided mother with information about the county 24-hour "Warm Line" to obtain info about mental health services.

- Provided mother with information about local psychiatric rehabilitation program services to review with Jordan's therapist for a referral. Jordan was able to get connected before discharge from STP.

- Psychoeducation to address household routines and ways to implement incentives for compliant behaviors. Connected mom with support groups for adoptive caregivers and a mental health advocacy group.

VIGNETTE #2

Background

Brian was a 10-year-old African-American boy who had participated in mental health services (therapy and medication) since age 5 and had 4 psychiatric hospitalizations in his lifetime. School staff initiated a hospitalization after he was verbally and physically aggressive with a teacher and administrator, and ran through the halls slamming doors. He was diagnosed with attention deficit/hyperactivity disorder, oppositional defiant disorder, and mood disorder, not otherwise specified. According to his mother, Brian always had difficulty sitting still and paying attention and became irritated easily. She stated that as he gets older, especially within the past 1 to 2 years, his mood had worsened; he had become increasingly aggressive toward his parents and sibling, and displayed volatile and destructive behavior both at home and at school.

Brian always did well academically and was in all advanced classes at his public middle school. He received a 504 plan at the beginning of the school year to address attention deficit/hyper-activity disorder symptoms; however, his mother was concerned that that her son needed more intensive services at school, and appropriate accommodations to address frequent anger outbursts in the classroom, elopement, and aggression. School staff contacted his mother most days about Brian's behaviors, asking her to come to the school and take him home, which led to her missing a significant amount of time from work. She voiced that she felt helpless and did *not know what to do for her son, and felt frustrated with school staff that they expected her to leave work frequently and remove her son from the school.*

During the family meeting, the STS worked with Brian's mother to determine their needs and what strategies could be used to address these needs at school and home.

Caregiver Needs

- *Increased support from others owing to concerns about feeling isolated and judged because of her son's behaviors.*
- *Advocacy for her son at school and figuring out what services are available and are most appropriate for Brian.*
- *Information about Special Education Laws, specifically the difference between a 504 Plan and an IEP. What services does her son qualify for? What are the steps to take to initiate these processes?*
- *Assistance in explaining to school staff and administration her son's mental health diagnosis. What does the diagnosis mean and how does it affect his behavior and interactions with others?*
- *Help in figuring out what role she should play when her son's behavior is problematic at school. Can staff encourage mother to take her son home?*
- *More balanced feedback and support from her son's school; a desire to hear from school staff when her son does something positive as opposed to receiving only negative feedback.*

Child Needs

- *Identification of school staff member to talk to or somewhere to go during the school day when he becomes frustrated or upset to process his feelings and calm down.*
- *Consistency with all staff members regarding how they respond to him as his behaviors escalate.*
- *Help with certain schoolwork, particularly math, because he was falling behind and becoming frustrated.*
- *More positive interactions with peers and school staff and administrators.*
- *Support in using coping skills to better manage difficult feelings.*

School Needs

- *Improved understanding of Brian's mental health diagnoses and how it affects his behavior.*
- *Identification of how best to address this student's needs both behaviorally and academically—what level of services does he need for him to succeed academically and what can the school do to promote emotional stability?*
- *Identification of the factors that contribute to his problem behavior.*
- *Development of a specific crisis plan to use with Brian when he does not respond to the school's universal interventions.*

Strategies Implemented by STP

- *Conducted family session focused on education around special education: what services are available, family rights, what mother can expect at school team meetings.*
- *Assisted mother in composing letter to the team at Brian's school requesting an initial meeting and for Brian to be assessed by the team to determine eligibility for an IEP.*
- *Connected mother with a caregiver support group in her area where she and her husband could meet with other adults to discuss caring for a child with emotional and behavioral needs.*
- *Initiated a discussion between Brian's outpatient therapist and key school staff members on Brian's mental health diagnoses and specific strategies and interventions that have been successful with Brian.*

- Translated hospital discharge recommendations from the child and adolescent psychiatrist at the hospital to the school staff working with Brian.
- Consulted with the staff at the inpatient unit to modify their "Daily Success Sheet" that was used effectively with Brian while he was admitted, to apply to his current school. Specifically, wanted to use the same language, certain interventions, and incentives so that there was consistency and easier for him to follow.
- Consulted with Brian, mother, outpatient therapist, psychiatrist, and school staff to create a crisis plan specific to Brian's needs. Copies were made and handed out to all of his teachers.
- Identified SC who implemented C & R on daily basis. Brian developed a positive relationship with the SC (one of school's support staff) who conducted the check-ins. Previously, he had only spoken to school staff on nonacademic issues when he was having an issue, or had gotten into trouble.
- Performed classroom observation, identified factors that contributed to problem behaviors, and provided consultation to school staff.
- Facilitated process to determine eligibility through IEP, which was completed in less than 2 months.
- Weekly individual and group counseling sessions were included when developing Brian's IEP to address his emotional and behavioral needs.
- IEP team moved Brian to a math class that better addressed his academic needs.
- School staff verbalized having a better understanding of Brian's mental health disorders, and were able to implement appropriate strategies outlined in Brian's IEP and crisis plan. Mother received fewer calls regarding Brian's negative behaviors and more positive feedback from school staff.

Box 1
Strategies for Helping Families after Psychiatric Hospitalization

- Acknowledge family's experience with mental health challenges and concerns about transition.
- Identify one point of contact for family (eg, school administrator, social worker).
- Obtain hospital records, medical history, and discharge plans.
- Schedule a school team meeting with parent (and youth, if appropriate) before reentry.
- Create a transition plan (see **Table 2**).
- Set up brief daily check-ins with student.
- Provide feedback to family about positive behavior.
- Create or adapt a crisis plan specific to the youth's needs.
- Incorporate the youth and family's strengths into the plan.
- Encourage staff participation in professional development related to mental health.
- Consider alternatives to rehospitalization if symptoms persist or worsen.

Box 1 provides a helpful list of strategies that can be implemented for aiding families following psychiatric hospitalization.

SUMMARY

This article outlines the challenges faced by youth and their families transitioning back to school and community after an inpatient psychiatric stay. It describes development of the STP, an intervention designed specifically to help support youth, families, and school staff and to promote cross-system communication and collaboration. Findings from the first year of implementation indicate that caregivers experience diminished caregiver strain and increased empowerment (compared with baseline scores) and a very high level of satisfaction with the program. Related to an increasing interest in population health initiatives and these positive outcomes, one of the hospitals involved in the pilot year added the program as a clinical service offered to families exiting treatment.

Because inpatient stays are very short and focus primarily on stabilization, upon discharge youth are at risk of entering a "revolving door" of hospitalizations. Findings from the literature and the challenges voiced by families highlight the need for targeted interventions that may not be typically offered by school and mental health providers. Promising interventions for this population include increasing emotional support and psychoeducation to caregivers, identifying family and youth unmet needs and matching resources, and providing a transition specialist who can attend school meetings with families, make an individualized plan, and help to bridge communication across systems.

REFERENCES

1. Stroul BA, Friedman RM. A system of care for severely emotionally disturbed children & youth. Washington, DC: Georgetown University Child Development Center; 1986.
2. Romansky JB, Lyons JS, Lehner RK, et al. Factors related to psychiatric hospital readmission among children and adolescents in state custody. Psychiatr Serv 2003;54(3):356–62.
3. Ringel JS, Sturm R. National estimates of mental health utilization and expenditures for children in 1998. J Behav Health Serv Res 2001;28(3):319–33.
4. Causey DL, McKay M, Rosenthal C, et al. Assessment of hospital-related stress in children and adolescents admitted to a psychiatric inpatient unit. J Child Adolesc Psychiatr Nurs 1998;11(4):135–45.
5. Blader JC. Symptom, family, and service predictors of children's psychiatric rehospitalization within one year of discharge. J Am Acad Child Adolesc Psychiatry 2004;43(4):440–51.
6. Fontanella CA. The influence of clinical, treatment, and healthcare system characteristics on psychiatric readmission of adolescents. Am J Orthop 2008;78(2):187–98.
7. Kocher RP, Adashi EY. Hospital readmissions and the affordable care act: paying for coordinated quality care. JAMA 2011;306(16):1794–5.
8. Parmelee DX, Cohen R, Nemil BM, et al. Children and adolescents discharged from public psychiatric hospital: evaluation of outcome in a continuum of care. J Child Fam Stud 1995;4(1):43–55.
9. Blader JC. Which family factors predict children's externalizing behaviors following discharge from psychiatric inpatient treatment? J Child Psychol Psychiatry 2006;47(11):1133–42.

10. Brinkmeyer MY, Eyberg SM, Nguyen ML, et al. Family engagement, consumer satisfaction and treatment outcome in the new era of child and adolescent inpatient psychiatric care. Clin Child Psychol Psychiatry 2004;9(4):553–66.
11. Scharer K, Jones DS. Child psychiatric hospitalization: the last resort. Issues Ment Health Nurs 2004;25(1):79–101.
12. Puotiniemi TA, Kyngäs HA, Nikkonen MJ. The resources of parents with a child in psychiatric inpatient care. J Psychiatr Ment Health Nurs 2002;9(1):15–22.
13. Deidrick KK, Farmer JE. School reentry following traumatic brain injury. Prev Sch Fail 2005;49(4):23–33.
14. Kaffenberger CJ. School reentry for students with a chronic illness: a role for professional school counselors. Sch Couns 2006;9(3):223–30.
15. Shaw SR, McCabe PC. Hospital-to-school transition for children with chronic illness: meeting the new challenges of an evolving health care system. Psychol Sch 2008;45(1):74–87.
16. Simon JB, Savina EA. Facilitating hospital to school transitions: practices of hospital-based therapists. Resid Treat Child Youth 2007;22(4):49–66.
17. Clemens EV, Welfare LE, Williams AM. Tough transitions: mental health care professionals' perception of the psychiatric hospital to school transition. Resid Treat Child Youth 2010;27(4):243–63.
18. Drell M. Innovations: child & adolescent psychiatry: sweet are the uses of adversity: a transition program for children discharged from an inpatient unit. Psychiatr Serv 2006;57(1):31–3.
19. Savina E, Simon J, Lester M. School reintegration following psychiatric hospitalization: an ecological perspective. Child Youth Care Forum 2014;43:1–18.
20. Hill R. Generic features of families under stress. Soc Casework 1958;49:139–50.
21. Kutash K, Duchnowski AJ, Green AL, et al. Effectiveness of the parent connectors program: results from a randomized controlled trial. School Ment Health 2013; 5(4):192–208.
22. Christenson SL, Stout K, Pohl A. Check & connect: a comprehensive student engagement intervention. Minneapolis (MN): University of Minnesota; 2012.

Engaging Youth and Families in School Mental Health Services

Kimberly D. Becker, PhD[a],*, Sara L. Buckingham, MA[b],
Nicole Evangelista Brandt, PhD[c]

KEYWORDS

- Engagement • Barriers • School mental health • Families • Youth

KEY POINTS

- Engaging youth and families in children's mental health treatment is challenging.
- School mental health services increase access to care for youth; however, there are unique barriers to engaging families in treatment.
- Strategies to effectively engage families have been identified based on a review of the extant literature and findings from focus groups with consumers.
- Providers can thoughtfully decide which engagement strategies will address their clients' barriers.

Estimates suggest that 20% to 40% of youth have a psychiatric disorder[1] and may be in need of mental health services. Yet, national survey data show that as many as 75% of youth in need of mental health services do not enroll in treatment.[2,3] Schools are the primary entry point for children and adolescents who receive mental health services,[4] and more youths receive mental health services in schools than in any other setting.[5] Across school and specialty mental health settings, treatment engagement remains low relative to the needs of youth. Of those few children and adolescents who enroll in services, approximately 55% do not attend the first session,[6,7] and 50% to 70% terminate treatment prematurely.[8,9]

Funding Source: 1915c Demonstration Waiver: Community Alternatives to Psychiatric and Residential Treatment Facilities Demonstration Waiver Program Management, Workforce Development and Program Evaluation.
Conflict of Interest: The authors have no conflicts of interest to report.
[a] Division of Child and Adolescent Psychiatry, University of Maryland School of Medicine, 737 West Lombard Street, Room 424, Baltimore, MD 21201, USA; [b] Human Services Psychology Program, University of Maryland, Baltimore County, 1000 Hilltop Circle, Math/Psych Room 312, Baltimore, MD 21250, USA; [c] Department of Psychology, Columbus State Community College, 550 East Spring Street, Room 335B, Columbus, OH 43215, USA
* Corresponding author.
E-mail address: kbecker@psych.umaryland.edu

Child Adolesc Psychiatric Clin N Am 24 (2015) 385–398
http://dx.doi.org/10.1016/j.chc.2014.11.002
1056-4993/15/$ – see front matter © 2015 Elsevier Inc. All rights reserved.

childpsych.theclinics.com

Abbreviations	
BSPS-DV	Barriers to Service Participation Scale for Caregivers and Children Who Experience Domestic Violence
BTPS	Barriers to Treatment Participation Scale
SMH	School mental health

Many factors influence youth and family engagement in mental health services.[10–13] One of the most obvious factors is the availability and accessibility of services. The delivery of mental health services in schools has the potential to fundamentally enhance treatment engagement by increasing access to care for youth in need.[14–16] Such accessibility allows for children's mental health problems to be identified early by school personnel (ie, problems often manifest as poor academic or behavioral performance in the classroom), who can provide more efficient referrals for school mental health (SMH) treatment. Mandatory school attendance and the naturalistic setting of SMH services may mitigate both practical (eg, transportation issues, scheduling conflicts) and psychological (eg, stigma) barriers.[17–20] Further, youth who receive SMH treatment learn skills that may be better generalized, because the skills are taught in a natural, social setting.[21]

Although there are certainly advantages to SMH services related to better access to care and follow through with referrals, there are unique barriers to engagement.[6,22] Enrollment in SMH services requires identification of youth who could benefit from mental health services, and many teachers report a lack of training and experience in this area.[23] Adolescents in particular have many issues that may prevent them from seeking care, such as perceiving that they should handle mental health problems on their own, failing to recognize that their mental health problems require treatment, not believing that mental health services would be useful, and paying greater attention to peers' views and worrying about stigma, privacy, and confidentiality.[22,24] Although housing mental health services in schools increases accessibility for youth, it can hinder families from engaging in treatment. For example, the timing of the services often coincides with caregivers' work schedules.[25] In addition, caregivers vary in the extent to which they are involved with or connected to their children's schools; thus, SMH may not be desirable for all caregivers.[26,27] Hence, SMH services cannot fully mitigate all barriers to treatment engagement. It therefore falls within the role of the mental health provider to use additional strategies to manage the many obstacles that youth and families continue to face. In our own work as scientist-practitioners, we have taken a 2-pronged approach to identifying strategies to enhance treatment engagement by (1) reviewing the empirical literature (ie, Refs.[28,29]) and (2) querying consumers of mental health services (ie, Brandt NE, Buckingham SL, Becker KD, et al. Youth and family perspectives about children's mental health services: barriers to and facilitators of engagement, manuscript in preparation).

There is a burgeoning literature that can guide providers on how to reduce barriers and enhance treatment engagement. Over the past decade, multiple investigators (eg, Refs.[30–34]) have published qualitative reviews of engagement intervention studies, presenting strategies for better engaging families in services. Another approach to reviewing the literature involved a quantitative review of 40 randomized controlled trials testing engagement interventions in child and adolescent mental health services using a distillation method[35] to identify practices commonly used in effective engagement interventions (eg, appointment reminders, reinforcement, motivational enhancement). Lindsey and colleagues[28] concluded that the practices most frequently used in effective engagement interventions include assessment, accessibility promotion, psychoeducation about services, homework assignment, and assessing barriers to treatment.

Expanding on this work, Becker and colleagues[29] examined whether practices varied according to the engagement outcome of interest in the study: attendance, cognitive preparation (eg, understanding of and expectations for treatment, motivation for change), and adherence (eg, session participation, out-of-session practice, contact with referrals; **Fig. 1** shows engagement practices mapped onto the outcomes). Results showed that certain practices, such as accessibility promotion, assessment, and psychoeducation about services, were frequently used across multiple outcomes.[29] In contrast, assessment of barriers to treatment was frequently used in interventions successful at increasing attendance. Homework assignment was common in interventions targeting adherence, whereas modeling and instilling hope were used in interventions targeting cognitive preparation. This comprehensive literature review suggests that certain engagement practices were more frequent than others and that their use varied according to the engagement outcome of interest. Armed with this knowledge, providers can make decisions to use more strategies that work to strategically enhance cognitive and behavioral domains of treatment engagement that are tailored for each client.

To explore the validity of these engagement practices, our team conducted focus groups to examine youth's and families' experiences with children's mental health

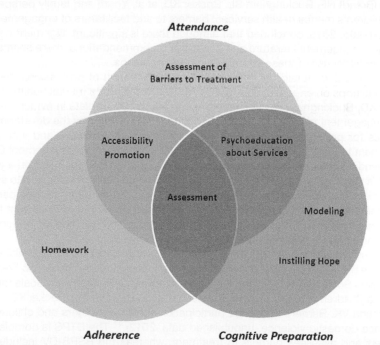

Attendance

Assessment of
Barriers to Treatment

Accessibility
Promotion

Psychoeducation
about Services

Assessment

Modeling

Homework

Instilling Hope

Adherence   *Cognitive Preparation*

Fig. 1. Engagement practices by engagement outcome. A literature review[29] identified adherence (*lower left*), attendance (*top*), and cognitive preparation (*lower right*) as 3 frequent engagement outcomes measured in children's mental health services research. Some engagement practices (eg, assessment of barriers to treatment) situated within 1 circle in the figure were uniquely associated with a particular engagement outcome (eg, attendance). In contrast, other practices (eg, psychoeducation about services) situated within overlapping circles in the figure were associated with multiple engagement outcomes (eg, attendance, cognitive preparation).

treatment, and perspectives on providers' engagement techniques (Brandt NE, Buckingham SL, Becker KD, et al. Youth and family perspectives about children's mental health services: barriers to and facilitators of engagement, manuscript in preparation). During 4 focus groups, consumers of children's mental health services (ie, youth and young adults [$n = 11$]; caregivers [$n = 20$]) described their involvement in treatment, challenges to their participation in treatment, and strategies that providers had used or could use to engage them in services. Participants reported many attitudinal and practical barriers to treatment engagement (eg, poor relationship with provider, perceptions that therapy was unfocused, location). They noted several strategies that providers had used to address these barriers and improve engagement. Although these strategies frequently coincided with the literature (**Table 1**), participants recommended additional engagement strategies. For example, they recommended that providers connect and empathize with their clients, strive to truly understand their clients, and build a relationship with their clients to encourage the families to have a strong voice and choice in treatment (ie, rapport building, cultural acknowledgment, compassion, empowerment, and youth-directed and family-directed services). Focus group participants also suggested that providers use a collaborative approach to goal setting, coordinate with other service providers to achieve treatment goals, continually assess progress toward treatment goals, and provide consumers with clear expectations for treatment (ie, goal setting, progress monitoring, service coordination, managing expectations). Brandt and colleagues (Brandt NE, Buckingham SL, Becker KD, et al. Youth and family perspectives about children's mental health services: barriers to and facilitators of engagement, unpublished data, 2015) concluded that although there is significant alignment between the extant engagement literature and consumer recommendations, there seems to be a gap in provider use of these strategies in clinical settings.

This empirical work laid the groundwork for the creation of professional development workshops on engaging youths and families in children's mental health services (Becker KD, Buckingham SL, Brandt NE, et al. Training therapists in evidence-based family engagement practices, unpublished data, 2015), as well as the development of resources for providers seeking to assess treatment engagement and incorporate engagement techniques into their clinical practice. The Strategic Engagement Checklist (Appendix 1) guides providers through a series of questions to reflect on a youth's or family's treatment engagement. Indicators of low engagement are linked to specific engagement practices that a provider could implement to address that particular engagement issue. This checklist can be used at the beginning of treatment to promote engagement or throughout the course of treatment to monitor engagement and manage new issues that arise.

Questionnaires are available in the literature to assist providers with determining what barriers are likely to impede treatment engagement, including the Barriers to Treatment Participation Scale (BTPS)[36–40] and the Barriers to Service Participation Scale for Caregivers and Children Who Experience Domestic Violence (BSPS-DV) (Becker KD, Mueller CW, Kanuha VK. Barriers to service participation scale for mothers and children who experience domestic violence, unpublished data, 2012).[41] The BTPS is completed by caregivers and assesses barriers to treatment, whereas the BSPS-DV includes both caregiver and youth versions, consisting of items measuring barriers to and facilitators of treatment engagement. With knowledge of the barriers facing youth and their families in treatment, a provider can use the Strategic Engagement Checklist (Appendix 1) to further consider what engagement strategy might be used to address one of several common barriers. The 4 case vignettes that follow show the integration of these resources and the application of engagement practices within the context of SMH services. At the end of each case vignette is a corresponding checklist of engagement strategies.

Table 1 Engagement strategies		
Commonly Suggested By	**Strategy**	**Definition**
Literature review	Homework assignment	Therapeutic tasks given to youth/families to complete outside sessions to reinforce/facilitate knowledge and skills
	Modeling	Demonstration of a desired behavior to promote imitation and performance of that behavior by client
	Motivational enhancement	Exercises designed to increase readiness to participate in additional therapeutic activity or programs
Focus groups	Compassion	Expression of empathy for the youth/family and their situation
	Cultural acknowledgment	Asking questions designed to explore the client's culture; adapting therapeutic practices to incorporate youth/family's culture (eg, race/ethnicity, age, sexual orientation, religion)
	Empowerment and youth-directed/family-directed services	Validation of youth/family experiences, roles, and perspectives; supporting self-efficacy by providing opportunities for choice and involvement in decisions; collaboration with the family
	Goal setting	Selection of a therapeutic goal for the purpose of working toward achieving that goal
	Managing expectations	Discussion or provision of corrective information to help the family have realistic expectations for treatment (pace, duration, improvement progress)
	Progress monitoring	Repeated review of a target process or behavior throughout treatment to regularly assess progress, homework completion, satisfaction with services, or youth/family's perception of therapeutic relationship, with the goal of eliciting feedback or information so that the provider can address potential problems
	Rapport building	Enhancement of the quality of the relationship between the youth/family and the provider
	Service coordination	Coordination and oversight of formal supports; communication with the youth/family's other providers
Literature review and focus groups	Accessibility promotion	Any strategy used to make services convenient and accessible (eg, offering evening hours, transportation, coming to the house, child care, reduced fees); providing around-the-clock access to services
	Assessment	Information gathering about the youth's strengths and needs through the use of a variety of methods (including interviews, questionnaires, observations) at the beginning of treatment
	Assessment of barriers to treatment	Open discussion about barriers to participation in treatment (eg, practical issues, previous experiences, stigma)
	Instilling hope	Facilitation of positive expectations for change
	Psychoeducation of services	Review of information about services or the service delivery system (eg, session frequency/content, roles of provider and youth/families)

VIGNETTE 1: PROMOTING ENGAGEMENT FOR ALL YOUTHS AND FAMILIES
Case Background

Mr Hart was the first SMH provider at his school, and found that most students and families did not understand his role as an SMH provider and the services that he could provide. In addition, his impression was that the families and surrounding community were distrustful of mental health providers. Several teachers had approached Mr Hart and informed him that several students were showing severe disruptive behaviors; the teachers wanted him to help immediately. Although Mr Hart knew that many students could benefit from mental health services right away, he had been unsuccessful reaching caregivers to schedule an intake and enroll them in services. To identify the most appropriate engagement strategies, Mr Hart used the Strategic Engagement Checklist (see Appendix 1) and determined that he would use school-wide engagement strategies to increase the visibility of his services in the school and to build rapport with school staff, students, and families.

Rapport Building and Psychoeducation About Services

Mr Hart capitalized on opportunities to make connections and build rapport with all youths, families, and school staff during school-wide events. To develop these relationships, he attended school-sponsored family events, such as back to school night or a science fair, and participated in parent-teacher organization meetings. During these events, he had an informational table on hot topics that concerned caregivers, were not stigmatizing, and were culturally appropriate (eg, stress management for parents, tips for Internet safety and children, how to manage homework time). Mr Hart also attempted to reduce mental health treatment stigma by showcasing and providing information about SMH services during these school-wide events and alongside other school programs (eg, band, chess, athletic teams). These outreach efforts allowed him to build relationships with all families (regardless of their need for SMH services), reduce stigma about mental health, connect with families who may be interested in SMH services, and provide education about SMH services. By showing that he was committed to the students and families at the school, Mr Hart forged strong relationships with other school staff. When Mr Hart was unable to reach a caregiver whose child could benefit from SMH services, he reached out to his colleagues on the school staff to help facilitate communication with the family. In these ways, Mr Hart earned a reputation among the school staff and community members that he was kind, sincere, and trustworthy, which helped caregivers to feel comfortable enrolling their child for SMH services.

*In addition to connecting with caregivers, Mr Hart also conducted classroom-wide prevention activities to reach many students in the school. The prevention activities introduced the students to Mr Hart, reduced the stigma of mental health, and provided an entry into future services. In these ways, Mr Hart proactively built rapport and engaged youths and families before connecting with them about SMH services (**Box 1**).*

Box 1
Tips for promoting engagement for all youths and families

- Attend school-sponsored family events
- Organize an informational table showing parenting topics or strategies
- Provide information about SMH services in a nonstigmatizing manner
- Participate in school-wide events with youth
- Conduct classroom-wide prevention activities
- Collaborate with school staff to facilitate communication with families

VIGNETTE 2: FOSTERING ENGAGEMENT WHILE CONDUCTING BUSINESS
Case Background

Maria, a 13-year-old Latina student nearing the end of eighth grade, was referred by the art teacher for depressed mood and decreased performance. Ms Boyd, the SMH provider, scheduled an intake with Maria and her mother.

Empowerment

Ms Boyd knew that it was easy to fall into using an expert approach and not be collaborative with families. This approach might negatively affect the family's engagement in treatment. Expert and noncollaborative approaches often lead families to feel misunderstood, devalued, and unimportant. Instead, Ms Boyd used a collaborative approach during the intake and worked carefully to let the family take the lead and tell their story. Ms Boyd briefly discussed her experience in working with youth to improve emotional and behavioral functioning; yet, she emphasized that Maria and her mother were experts on their family (as opposed to Ms Boyd being the expert). She explained that they would work as a team to help improve Maria's mood and academic performance. This approach empowered the family by encouraging their voice to be heard and allowing them to guide treatment from the beginning.

Assessment

As requested by Ms Boyd, Maria and her mother completed questionnaires to assess Maria's mood and related concerns. Although Ms Boyd did not have time to score all of the questionnaires, she provided initial feedback and discussed how some of the family's responses might suggest depression and anxiety that would benefit from treatment. She informed the family that comprehensive feedback about the assessment would be presented at the next meeting.

Psychoeducation About Services

At a meeting after the assessment, Ms Boyd provided comprehensive psychoeducation about the services, including information about the nature of services (eg, theoretic approach, availability of psychiatry services), treatment demands (eg, frequency, cost, activities), and the responsibilities of the provider, Maria, and her mother. Ms Boyd educated the family about issues particularly relevant to the school setting. For example, she discussed confidentiality issues, highlighting the fact that the family could complete a release of information form that allowed school staff and Ms Boyd to exchange information. She also reassured them that therapy sessions would be short (ie, 30 minutes) and missed instruction time in classroom would be minimized. She discussed scheduling and availability of services during the summer. Ms Boyd comprehensively described her role, Maria's role, and her mother's role in treatment, emphasizing the importance of Maria's mother's engagement. During this conversation, Ms Boyd solicited their feedback regarding their role in treatment, helped to establish reasonable expectations, and provided flexible options for the mother's participation and engagement. For example, she offered flexible scheduling, home visits, and telephone sessions. Toward the end of the session, she elicited the family's understanding of treatment, corrected any misperceptions, and provided ample time for their questions to be answered.

Assessing Barriers to Treatment, Instilling Hope, and Coordination

While providing psychoeducation about services, Ms Boyd elicited the family's perspective about treatment and their previous experiences with SMH services. She learned that Maria received SMH services in elementary school, but the family discontinued services. Ms Boyd probed about why they terminated services and learned that it was because of high provider turnover (ie, 3 providers in 2 academic years). Ms Boyd responded by providing empathy and communicating her genuine interest in helping Maria and her family. She proactively discussed Maria's transition to high school, the services available there, and how she could coordinate services with a new provider. Ms Boyd then explained that she had successfully helped youth with similar problems and conveyed her belief that Maria would also improve. By eliciting the family's perspective about treatment, providing ideas about coordinating future care, and being hopeful, Ms Boyd improved the family's attitude about treatment.

Using several engagement strategies, Ms Boyd created a safe and empowering environment for Maria and her mother to share their perspectives, yet she also accomplished the business aspects of conducting an intake. Through dialogue, Ms Boyd helped the family gain hope and clarity about SMH services (Box 2).

Box 2
Tips for fostering engagement while conducting business

- Use a collaborative approach
- Use active listening skills
- Allow youths and families to guide treatment
- Collect data to inform treatment and provide feedback to families
- Instill hope, provide empathy, and show genuine interest
- Coordinate care after school transitions or transfers
- Provide psychoeducation about services, particularly focusing on issues unique to mental health services provided in school
- Provide flexible scheduling, such as evening hours
- Offer home visits and telephone sessions

VIGNETTE 3: CONNECTING AND MOTIVATING TO PROMOTE BEHAVIOR CHANGE
Case Background

Jim, a 15-year-old Native American student in ninth grade, was referred by the principal for suspected marijuana use. Jim and his grandfather (his legal guardian) attended an intake with Mr Tom and were beginning treatment. Mr Tom sensed that the family had several barriers to engagement, which they were uncomfortable sharing.

Assessing Barriers to Treatment

Mr Tom normalized barriers, noting that all families have things that get in their way of participating in treatment from time to time. Although Jim and his grandfather initially denied any obstacles, Mr Tom encouraged them to complete the BTPS to explore possible barriers.[38] Jim and his grandfather endorsed items related to the relevance of treatment, suggesting that they perceived that treatment might not be necessary or useful. Mr Tom completed the Strategic Engagement Checklist (see Appendix 1) to reflect on the family's treatment engagement. The checklist suggested that Mr Tom had neither a strong therapeutic alliance with the family nor a thorough understanding of how their identity, beliefs, and values related to their participation in treatment. Based on this information, Mr Tom created a plan to enhance engagement.

Cultural Acknowledgment

Mr Tom understood the impact of cultural values and beliefs on a family's engagement. He asked the family about their roles at home, and how race, ethnicity, age, and other aspects of culture affected their lives. In addition, he asked curious, open-ended questions to determine how these factors might influence treatment. He encouraged them to let him know if anything during treatment went against their beliefs. Mr Tom was aware of his own personal biases related to culture and race, particularly because Mr Tom and Jim's family were of different cultural and racial backgrounds.

Motivational Enhancement

Mr Tom knew that Jim in particular remained reluctant to enter treatment. To address this attitudinal barrier, Mr Tom avoided passing judgment about Jim's marijuana use. Instead of trying to persuade Jim that he should make better lifestyle choices, Mr Tom used an open and genuine approach to ask Jim what he found appealing about using marijuana.

Mr Tom enhanced Jim's motivation for change by helping him explore the benefits as well as the drawbacks of reducing his marijuana use. Mr Tom did not impose his own treatment goals on Jim; instead, Mr Tom emphasized the student's autonomy and used Socratic questioning to guide Jim toward small changes that he might consider making with regard to his marijuana use (eg, smoking only on the weekends as opposed to daily). Initially, Jim asserted that he was not ready to reduce his use, but he agreed to continue the conversation over the next few sessions. Through further motivational enhancement and Socratic questioning, Mr Tom helped Jim reflect on how marijuana use might affect his ability to achieve his life goals. Over the course of treatment, Mr Tom continued to use motivational enhancement along with goal setting and monitoring to empower Jim to make his desired changes, which were necessary for his success at home and school.

Goal Setting and Monitoring

As Mr Tom enhanced the family's motivation, he guided Jim and his grandfather to develop goals that were specific, measurable, attainable, relevant, and timely (ie, SMART goals) along with a method for measuring progress toward goals on a regular basis. Goal setting cemented the family's commitment to behavior change and provided a focus for treatment. During each meeting, they reviewed progress toward treatment goals. Through monitoring, Mr Tom used data to prompt reinforcement for treatment progress or modifications of the treatment plan in the absence of improvement.

Engagement Changes

Although Mr Tom developed a plan tailored to the family to foster their engagement, this plan would likely need to be updated throughout the course of treatment. Mr Tom knew that it was important for him to keep a watchful eye on the family's motivation for behavior change throughout treatment. It is common for youth and families to make progress but experience obstacles and setbacks along the way. Mr Tom realized that he must consistently monitor treatment progress, periodically reset goals, and continually assess new barriers to treatment. Mr Tom would readminister the BTPS in approximately 3 months to reassess for additional barriers and develop solutions to any new or continuing obstacles as well as when changes in treatment engagement were noted in terms of attendance, adherence, or attitudes (Box 3).[38]

Box 3
Tips for connecting and motivating to promote behavior change

- Assess for barriers to treatment
- Normalize and problem solve barriers
- Consider impact of culture, race, ethnicity, age, and so forth
- Be open and genuine when assessing current behaviors
- Use Socratic questioning
- Collaboratively set SMART goals
- Develop a method for measuring progress
- Reassess barriers later in treatment
- Maintain a positive attitude toward the family
- Send positive notes home or call caregivers to provide praise about their child

VIGNETTE 4: PROMOTING BEHAVIOR CHANGE THROUGH CONSISTENT PRACTICE
Case Background

Sam, a 10-year-old girl in fourth grade, was referred by her teacher for anxiety and mood dysregulation. Sam had been in treatment with Ms Smith for 3 months, and her parents attempted to attend a session at least once a month.

Facilitating Skill Mastery and Homework

Ms Smith wanted Sam to learn some social skills to reduce the anxiety she felt during social interactions. However, Ms Smith knew that it was difficult for someone to learn a new skill from just oral instruction. Thus, Ms Smith facilitated Sam's parents' mastery of skills through multiple avenues by (1) providing a rationale for exposure to clear up any misconceptions, (2) teaching them each step, (3) modeling each step, (4) eliciting the parents' perspective about the skills, (5) instructing them to practice the steps during the session, (6) eliciting their reactions to practice, (7) providing them with feedback, (8) collaborating with them to identify practice situations outside sessions (ie, homework), and (9) working to anticipate and resolve barriers to homework completion. Ms Smith always checked in regarding the use of the skill at subsequent sessions to reinforce participation and problem-solving issues that arose. She used these same steps for other skills (eg, behavior charts, effective instructions, labeled praises) to increase engagement and facilitate skill mastery.

Related to facilitating skill mastery for Sam, Ms Smith sent home handouts describing the skills that Sam was working on during therapy (eg, problem-solving skills). This strategy provided opportunity for the family to learn and reinforce the skills at home. Ms Smith strove to have a session with Sam's parents to review skills, but when face-to-face meetings were not possible, sending notes home or having brief telephone sessions were effective alternatives (Box 4).

Box 4
Tips for promoting behavior change through consistent practice

- Provide instruction and model new skills for caregivers during the session
- Allow caregivers time to practice the skills in session and provide feedback
- Discuss practicing skills at home and problem solve anticipated barriers
- Process experience with homework and problem solve challenges
- Praise caregivers for their participation, no matter how engaged they are
- Communicate with caregivers regularly via brief telephone calls, texts, or emails
- Send home information about topics covered during therapy

SUMMARY

Engaging youth and families in treatment is critical for providing effective mental health services and achieving successful treatment outcomes. Although SMH services significantly increase the accessibility of care and decrease the stigma associated with treatment, there are unique and significant barriers to engaging youth and families in care. The empirical literature has identified practices that might help enhance engagement in treatment. In this article, how the empirical literature laid the foundation for the development of resources to enhance provider reflection on and decision making about treatment engagement is described, and the application of these resources and practices is shown in a series of case vignettes. The relative contribution of these resources and individual practices to treatment engagement remains to be determined by future studies that examine providers' decision-making processes about levels of treatment engagement, selection of engagement strategies, and the impact of selected strategies on engagement. Until such research is conducted, weaving the science of engagement interventions with SMH care has the potential to enhance the treatment participation of youth and families in need.

APPENDIX 1: STRATEGIC ENGAGEMENT CHECKLIST

Ask Yourself	Answer		If "No," Try This
Do you regularly communicate and interact with youths and families (not enrolled in SMH services) in your school?	Yes	No	Rapport building Psychoeducation about services (school-wide activities)
Do you have a strong relationship with school staff/families/students?	Yes	No	
Do school staff/families/students recognize you as someone who can help?	Yes	No	
Do school staff/families/students understand the range of services you provide?	Yes	No	
Do school staff/families/students know how to identify a student in need and make a referral?	Yes	No	
Does your program have policies around scheduling, transportation, or childcare that aid families with getting to treatment?	Yes	No	Accessibility promotion
Does the youth/family display open body language?	Yes	No	Rapport building
Does the youth/family openly share information with you?	Yes	No	
Do you think you have a strong therapeutic alliance with the youth/family?	Yes	No	
Do you have a thorough understanding of all components of the youth/family's identity and how their beliefs influence treatment?	Yes	No	Cultural acknowledgment
Is the youth/family in agreement with all of the interventions you suggest?	Yes	No	
Do you have a clear idea of what needs to change for treatment to be successful?	Yes	No	Assessment
Have you provided the youth/family information about assessment results?	Yes	No	
Can the youth/family describe what treatment involves and how it will address their needs?	Yes	No	Psychoeducation about services
Can the youth/family describe their roles in treatment?	Yes	No	
Does the youth/family attend treatment consistently?	Yes	No	Assess barriers
Does the youth/family follow through with recommendations/homework?	Yes	No	Motivational enhancement
Has the youth/family identified the changes they need to make?	Yes	No	
Has the youth/family mentioned barriers to making changes?	Yes	No	
Does the youth/family believe that change is possible and that they have the capacity to change?	Yes	No	Instilling hope
Does the youth/family believe that others with similar problems have got better?	Yes	No	

(continued on next page)

Ask Yourself	Answer		If "No," Try This
Are there specific goals for treatment?	Yes	No	Goal setting
Did the youth/family help create treatment goals?	Yes	No	
Can the youth/family articulate those goals?	Yes	No	
Do you know if treatment is working?	Yes	No	Monitoring
Do you have a way of tracking goal progress and sharing that information with the youth/family?	Yes	No	
Has the youth/family recognized that they have made progress?	Yes	No	
Are you the only provider the youth/family is seeing for treatment?	Yes	No	Coordination
Does it seem like services in the youth/family's life complement, rather than compete with or duplicate, one another?	Yes	No	
Do the youth/family's problems involve academic issues?	Yes	No	
Does the youth/family easily implement the skills learned in session in other settings?	Yes	No	Skill mastery Homework
Has the family dropped out of treatment?	Yes	No	Reengage (positive notes/calls, assess barriers)
Has the family stopped answering your phone calls?	Yes	No	

REFERENCES

1. Costello E, Copeland W, Angold A. Trends in psychopathology across the adolescent years: what changes when children become adolescents, and when adolescents become adults? J Child Psychol Psychiatry 2011;52:1015–25.
2. Merikangas K, He J, Burstein M, et al. Service utilization for lifetime mental disorders in US adolescents: results of the National Comorbidity Survey-Adolescent supplement (NCS-A). J Am Acad Child Adolesc Psychiatr 2011; 50:32–45.
3. Ringel J, Sturm R. National estimates of mental health utilization and expenditures for children in 1998. J Behav Health Serv Res 2001;28:319–33.
4. Farmer E, Burns B, Phillips S, et al. Pathways into and through mental health services for children and adolescents. Psychiatr Serv 2003;54:60–6.
5. Burns B, Costello E, Erkanli A, et al. Children's mental health service use across service sectors. Health Aff 1995;14:147–59.
6. Guo S, Kataoka S, Bear L, et al. Differences in school-based referrals for mental health care: understanding racial/ethnic disparities between Asian American and Latino youth. School Mental Health 2014;6:27–39.
7. McKay M, McCadam K, Gonzales J. Addressing the barriers to mental health services for inner city children and their caretakers. Community Ment Health J 1996; 32:353–61.
8. Nock M, Kazdin A. Randomized controlled trial of a brief intervention for increasing participation in parent management training. J Consult Clin Psychol 2005;73:872–9.
9. Pellerin K, Costa N, Weems C, et al. An examination of treatment completers and non-completers at a child and adolescent community mental health clinic. Community Ment Health J 2010;46:273–81.
10. Ajzen I. The theory of planned behavior. Organ Behav Hum Decis Process 1991; 50:179–211.

11. Jaccard J, Dodge T, Dittus P. Parent-adolescent communication about sex and birth control: a conceptual framework. In: Feldman D, Rosenthal A, Damon W, editors. Talking sexuality: parent-adolescent communication. San Francisco (CA): Jossey-Bass; 2002. p. 9–41.
12. Morrissey-Kane E, Prinz R. Engagement in child and adolescent treatment: the role of parental cognitions and attributions. Clin Child Fam Psychol Rev 1999;2:183–98.
13. Staudt M. Treatment engagement with caregivers of at-risk children: gaps in research and conceptualization. J Child Fam Stud 2007;16:183–96.
14. Adelman H, Taylor L. Mental health in schools and system restructuring. Clin Psychol Rev 1999;19:137–63.
15. President's New Freedom Commission on Mental Health. Achieving the promise: transforming mental health care in America. Final Report for the President's New Freedom Commission on Mental Health (SMA Publication No. 03–3832). Rockville (MD): New Freedom Commission on Mental Health; 2003.
16. Weist M. Expanded school mental health services: a national movement in progress. Adv Clin Child Psychol 1997;19:319–52.
17. Catron T, Harris V, Weiss B. Posttreatment results after 2 years of services in the Vanderbilt School-Based Counseling project. In: Epstein MH, Kutash K, Duchnowski AJ, editors. Outcomes for children and youth with emotional and behavioral disorders and their families: programs and evaluation best practices. Austin (TX): PRO-ED; 1998. p. 633–56.
18. Catron T. The Vanderbilt School-based counseling program: an interagency, primary-care model of mental health care. J Emot Behav Disord 1994;2: 247–53.
19. Stephan S, Weist M, Kataoka S, et al. Transformation of children's mental health services: the role of school mental health. Psychiatr Serv 2007;58:1330–8.
20. Weist M. Challenges and opportunities in expanded school mental health. Clin Psychol Rev 1999;19:131–5.
21. Masia C, Klein R, Storch E, et al. School-based behavioral treatment for social anxiety disorder in adolescents: results of a pilot study. J Am Acad Child Adolesc Psychiatr 2001;40:780–6.
22. Lindsey M, Chambers K, Pohle C, et al. Understanding the behavioral determinants of mental health service use by urban, under-resourced black youth: adolescent and caregiver perspectives. J Child Fam Stud 2013;22:107–21.
23. Reinke WM, Stormont M, Herman KC, et al. Supporting children's mental health in schools: teacher perceptions of needs, roles, and barriers. Sch Psychol Q 2011; 26:1–13.
24. Thompson R, Dancy B, Knafl K, et al. African American families' expectations and intentions for mental health services. Adm Policy Ment Health 2013;40: 371–83.
25. Shucksmith J, Jones S, Summerbell C. The role of parental involvement in school-based mental health interventions at primary (elementary) school level. Adv Sch Ment Health Promot 2010;3:18–29.
26. Ceballo R, Maurizi L, Suarez G, et al. Gift and sacrifice: parental involvement in Latino adolescents' education. Cultur Divers Ethnic Minor Psychol 2014;20: 116–27.
27. DeMoss S, Vaughn C. Reflections on theory and practice in parent involvement from a phenomenological perspective. Sch Community J 2000;10:45–59.
28. Lindsey M, Brandt N, Becker K, et al. Identifying the common elements of treatment engagement interventions in children's mental health services. Clin Child Fam Psychol Rev 2014;17:283–98.

29. Becker KD, Lee B, Daleiden EL, et al. The common elements of engagement in children's mental health services: which elements for which outcomes? J Clin Child Adolesc Psychol 2013. [Epub ahead of print].
30. Gopalan G, Goldstein L, Klingenstein K, et al. Engaging families into child mental health treatment: updates and special considerations. J Can Acad Child Adolesc Psychiatry 2010;19:182–96.
31. Ingoldsby E. Review of interventions to improve family engagement and retention in parent and child mental health programs. J Child Fam Stud 2010;19:629–45.
32. Lefforge N, Donohue B, Strada M. Improving session attendance in mental health and substance abuse settings: a review of controlled studies. Behav Ther 2007; 38:1–22.
33. McKay M, Bannon W. Engaging families in child mental health services. Child Adolesc Psychiatr Clin N Am 2004;13:905–21.
34. Snell-Johns J, Mendez J, Smith B. Evidence-based solutions for overcoming access barriers, decreasing attrition, and promoting change with underserved families. J Fam Psychol 2004;18:19–35.
35. Chorpita B, Daleiden E, Weisz J. Identifying and selecting the common elements of evidence based intervention: a distillation and matching model. Ment Health Serv Res 2005;7:5–20.
36. Kazdin A. Perceived barriers to treatment participation and treatment acceptability among antisocial children and their families. J Child Fam Stud 2000;9: 157–74.
37. Kazdin A, Holland L, Crowley M. Family experience of barriers to treatment and premature termination from child therapy. J Consult Clin Psychol 1997;65: 453–63.
38. Kazdin A, Holland L, Crowley M, et al. Barriers to treatment participation scale: evaluation and validation in the context of child outpatient treatment. J Child Psychol Psychiatry 1997;38:1051–62.
39. Kazdin A, Wassell G. Barriers to treatment participation and therapeutic change among children referred for conduct disorder. J Clin Child Psychol 1999;28: 160–72.
40. Kazdin A, Wassell G. Therapeutic changes in children, parents, and families resulting from treatment of children with conduct problems. J Am Acad Child Adolesc Psychiatr 2000;39:414–20.
41. Becker KD, Mathis G, Mueller CW, et al. Barriers to treatment in an ethnically diverse sample of families enrolled in a community-based domestic violence intervention. J Aggress Maltreat Trauma 2012;21:829–50.

Implementing Clinical Outcomes Assessment in Everyday School Mental Health Practice

Jill Haak Bohnenkamp, PhD[a],*, Tracy Glascoe, LCSW[b],
Kathy A. Gracey, MEd[b], Richard A. Epstein, PhD, MPH[c],
Margaret M. Benningfield, MD, MSCI[d]

KEYWORDS

- Evidence-based assessment • School mental health
- Clinical outcomes assessment

KEY POINTS

- Evidence-based assessment (EBA) and outcomes monitoring can improve clinical care in school mental health.
- Several valid and reliable tools for EBA are available to clinicians at little or no cost.
- Many perceived barriers to implementation of EBA in school mental health settings can be overcome without significant burden on clinicians.

Evidence-based treatments have gained considerable attention in mental health and school mental health practice over the past decade, but less attention has been paid to the potential benefits of evidence-based assessment (EBA).[1,2] The American Psychological Association Task Force on Evidence-based Practice with Children and Adolescents defines EBA as "assessments shown to be psychometrically sound for the populations on whom they are used."[3(p.8)] EBA is critical to evidence-based practice because accurate assessment of a child and family's needs and strengths is essential to the identification of children's mental health concerns, selection of appropriate treatments, ongoing monitoring of children's response to interventions,

Disclosures: None.
[a] Division of Child and Adolescent Psychiatry, University of Maryland School of Medicine, 737 West Lombard Street, 4th Floor, Baltimore, MD 21201, USA; [b] Department of Pyschiatry, Vanderbilt University, 3841 Green Hills Village, Drive 3000-C, Nashville, TN 37215, USA; [c] Vanderbilt University School of Medicine, Department of Psychiatry, 1500 21st Avenue South, Village at Vanderbilt Suite 2200, Nashville, TN 37212, USA; [d] Vanderbilt University, Department of Psychiatry, 1601 23rd Avenue South, #3068C, Nashville, TN 37212, USA
* Corresponding author.
E-mail address: jbohnenk@psych.umaryland.edu

Child Adolesc Psychiatric Clin N Am 24 (2015) 399–413
http://dx.doi.org/10.1016/j.chc.2014.11.006
1056-4993/15/$ – see front matter © 2015 Elsevier Inc. All rights reserved.

childpsych.theclinics.com

Abbreviations	
ADHD	Attention Deficit Hyperactivity Disorder
CANS	Child and Adolescent Needs and Strengths
CBCL	Child Behavior Checklist
CSMH	Center for School Mental Health
DISC	Diagnostic Interview Schedule for Children
EBA	Evidence-based assessment
OMS	Outcomes Measurement System
SMHP	University of Maryland School Mental Health Program

and outcomes evaluation.[3] Assessment and ongoing progress monitoring are therefore an essential component of evidence-based clinical practice.[1,4] Despite consensus on the utility of EBA in improving care, however, it is not frequently implemented in routine clinical practice.[5] Even when there is agreement that accurate assessment is crucial to quality treatment, there may be questions regarding what to measure and how. Clinical outcomes measurements used in child and adolescent assessment may include self report, parent report, as well as direct observation of behavior. Clinician-administered instruments may be fully structured, semi-structured, or unstructured. Selection of the appropriate tool for assessment is essential for efficient data collection that informs quality treatment.[5]

This article reviews how potential barriers to implementation can be addressed and EBA can be integrated into clinical care without significant burden. This investment of time and energy has the potential to bring about significant improvement in clinical care. This article specifically focuses on the importance of and implementation considerations for EBA in school mental health practice. First, the background of EBA is reviewed, including use in research settings, and challenges and benefits associated with EBA instrument use in clinical practice. Examples of implementation of EBA in school mental health practice in two school mental health programs are also provided.

MAKING THE CASE FOR EVIDENCE-BASED ASSESSMENT IN SCHOOL MENTAL HEALTH PRACTICE: WHY IS IT IMPORTANT?

EBA can inform care at multiple stages of treatment and at multiple levels of service delivery. At the initial assessment stage of individual treatment, the use of standardized measures can increase the ease and accuracy of clinical diagnosis.[6,7] At the stage of ongoing progress monitoring, use of standardized measures may be even more critical because clinicians are often not able to accurately detect symptom change.[8] Finally, at the stage of discharge from services, results from these tools can be shared with patients and families to highlight successes in treatment and decide whether additional treatment goals need to be set.

The levels of service delivery informed by EBA include assessment of individual students, and evaluation of clinician caseload, clinical program, and systems of care considerations. At the individual student level, use of EBA can improve problem identification, diagnosis, treatment planning, and monitoring of progress.[9,10] Tracking of individual progress allows clinicians to know whether treatment goals have been met and highlights needs for adapting interventions to meet the needs of individual students. At the clinician level, assessment data can also be used in aggregate by the clinician to better understand the global needs of the clinician's caseload. At the program level, assessment tools inform decisions about staffing needs and provide data on clinician effectiveness and cost-benefit analyses of particular treatments used in a program.[2,11] Program administrators can use assessment data to address caseload balance based on acuity, identify and address clinical areas in need of improvement, and provide targeted training to clinical staff to meet the needs of the students in a program. Finally, at the system of care level, EBA can provide a common language to communicate the needs and strengths of a child across multiple child serving systems.[12] Given the multiple systems that serve children with mental health needs, including schools, child welfare, and juvenile justice, establishing a common language to be used across systems to identify strengths and needs is best practice.[13]

IMPLEMENTATION OF EVIDENCE-BASED ASSESSMENT IN CHILD AND ADOLESCENT MENTAL HEALTH RESEARCH

EBAs are routinely used in child and adolescent mental health research wherein data collection and treatment protocols are tightly controlled. Early examples of assessments of child and adolescent mental health can be found in epidemiologic research in the late 1980s. These studies used comprehensive diagnostic evaluations often performed by lay interviewers. For example, the Methods for the Epidemiology of Child and Adolescent Mental Disorders study established that lay interviewers could collect valid and reliable data in community samples.[14] This study used the National Institute of Mental Health Diagnostic Interview Schedule for Children (DISC), which took about 2 hours to administer and was reported to be tolerable to caregivers and youth.[14] Another large epidemiologic sample, the Great Smoky Mountains study, used the Child Behavior Checklist (CBCL)[15] as a screening questionnaire followed by the Child and Adolescent Psychiatric Assessment, a highly structured interview that uses computer-based algorithms for diagnostic classification.[16] Other structured diagnostic interviews have been described, including the Diagnostic Interview for Children and Adolescents (DICA),[17] the Children's Interview for Psychiatric Symptoms,[18] the Schedule for Affective Disorders and Schizophrenia for school-aged children,[19] and the Interview Schedule for Children and Adolescents.[20] Such instruments are valuable "gold standards" for diagnosis; however, the time pressures faced in routine clinical mental health practice, including school mental health practice, prohibit the use of most comprehensive semistructured clinical interviews. Therefore, school mental health clinicians seek assessment tools that are simple to administer reliably in a busy school mental health practice.[5]

In addition to the time constraints faced in school mental health clinical practice, the goals and methods of assessment often differ from those in research settings. For example, in research settings, assessment staff members often differ from treatment staff, whereas in clinical practice, the treating clinician is typically the person completing the assessment. Clinical trials for research typically focus on a specific target population rather than treating a heterogeneous client population as is typical in clinical practice. Therefore, in research settings, a primary purpose of assessment is often screening for strict inclusion and exclusion criteria that determine eligibility to participate further in clinical trials. In research settings, children and families are often paid to participate, a factor that may significantly increase parental involvement in assessment. Finally, in research settings, training on assessments is formalized and consistently evaluated for reliability and validity. Financing for training and assessment of reliability are built into the framework of the research study. In routine school mental health practice, it may be difficult to justify the needed investment in infrastructure required for training in a particular assessment method and evaluation of adherence to the assessment method. Thus, adaptations may be required of the clinical infrastructure to promote reliable implementation of EBA in school mental health clinical settings.

IMPLEMENTATION OF EVIDENCE-BASED ASSESSMENT IN SCHOOL MENTAL HEALTH CLINICAL PRACTICE

As described earlier, "real-world" clinical settings differ in significant ways from research settings, and significant challenges can threaten implementation of EBA in routine school mental health practice. Potential logistical barriers that frequently impact clinical outcome assessment include time to administer the measure, score, and interpret results; the need for additional training and monitoring of fidelity; and availability and cost of the measure.[5] In school mental health settings, access to teacher reports is often easier than in traditional clinic practice; however, access to parent respondents can present a significant challenge.[10] Clinician attitudes toward assessment also affect implementation. Clinicians have endorsed concerns about ease of use, purpose for collecting data, and fear of not having positive outcomes.[5,10,11,21] Clinicians' concerns may be associated with worries about how data may affect evaluation of their performance by supervisors or may be concerned about the time required to complete assessments given competing priorities. Some clinicians report thinking "clinical decision-making" is superior to more formal, structured assessment despite data that suggest otherwise.[10] Efforts to impact clinician views of outcome measurement may help facilitate successful implementation.[10,21] Data collection procedures that are manageable and user-friendly, provide immediate feedback to the clinician on client progress and utilize a larger data system that allows for individual and programmatic improvement tracking, can facilitate assessment usage.[10,22]

In the school mental health setting, several unique considerations deserve attention. One especially germane consideration is the type of outcomes that are most relevant and with whom these data may be shared. Schools have increasingly been recognized as an ideal place for mental health services across the public health continuum (including mental health promotion, prevention, and intervention) for several reasons, including the connection between mental health and school functioning.[23] This connection highlights the potential benefit of monitoring how services are impacting educational outcomes. Measurement of educational outcomes in addition to clinical outcomes may enhance the understanding of the impact of school mental health treatment on the student functioning.[24] Educational outcomes include a wide range of variables, including grades, achievement test scores, attendance, discipline reports, classroom behavior and functioning, school engagement, and social functioning. There is ongoing discussion in school mental health practice about which of these targets should be the focus of outcome measurement.[11,21,25] When data are shared between clinicians and school personnel, all parties must attend to the regulations regarding student privacy. Individually identifiable health information (including behavioral health information) is protected by federal HIPAA (Health Insurance Portability and Accountability Act) and student education records are protected under FERPA (Family Education Rights and Privacy Act). Clinicians must be aware of the regulations that govern their practice in their specific setting and within their organization. To comply with these regulations, parent consent should always be obtained to facilitate information sharing across entities.

Likely as a result of both the challenges and the unique considerations of EBA in the school setting, clinical outcomes assessment is highly variable in school mental health practice.[5,10,26,27] A multi-disciplinary survey on school-based mental health practice in Illinois found variation in EBA practice by clinician discipline.[21] This study found that school psychologists were more likely to use systematic data-collection methods or standardized measures to inform their practice compared to other providers.[21] This study also indicated that when clinicians do use data to inform clinical practice, preferences for the tool used also vary by discipline. For instance, school counselors and social workers have reported preference for teacher and student self-report measures; school nurses preferred student observation, and school psychologists preferred school data.[21] Interestingly, most school mental health clinicians who use assessment in their practice indicated using academic indicators more frequently than measures of clinical outcomes.[10] This preference may reflect school-employed professionals' mandate to address educational outcomes, in addition to being related to the logistical barriers in obtaining parent, student, and teacher reports.[10]

Despite the potential barriers to implementation, school-based clinicians do report using various assessment tools and methods.[25] Some of these measures are included in **Table 1**, which outlines the target population, cost, where the measure can be obtained, and some strengths and weaknesses of each. This list is not exhaustive but highlights instruments that have been successfully used in the school setting. The measures included were selected by the authors based on frequency of report in the literature and ease of implementation in school mental health programs. In addition to the measures included in **Table 1**, the national Center for School Mental Health (CSMH) has compiled a list of assessment measures by clinical indication that are available free of charge in the public domain. http://csmh.umaryland.edu/Resources/ClinicianTools/SummmaryofFreeAssessmentMeasures12.12.12.pdf.

Measures that are designed to detect change in children's emotional/behavioral functioning may be more helpful in school mental health practice than measures that are designed for diagnostic and screening purposes. Similarly, many school mental health programs are moving toward more frequent, briefer assessment measures to decrease administration and scoring time and increase ease of use in the fast-paced school environment. In addition, programs are using clinician-friendly data collection and monitoring procedures, such as clinical dashboards, to map interventions onto clinical and academic outcomes on a more frequent basis to inform practice decisions. The case studies discussed later describe examples of the use of EBA in school mental health practice in more detail. Before reviewing these examples, general guidelines for implementation are provided.

GENERAL STRATEGIES FOR SUSTAINABLE IMPLEMENTATION OF EVIDENCE-BASED ASSESSMENT IN SCHOOLS

Implementation of EBA begins with selection of the best tool for the clinical setting. Clinicians and program managers should begin with a review of several key questions that inform which instrument best suits the needs of patients and practitioners in a particular setting. The Substance Abuse and Mental Health Service Administration's National Registry of Evidence-Based Programs and Practices provided a useful summary of six recommended steps for identifying and selecting evidence-based practices, including detailed questions to use when selecting evidence-based practices (**Box 1**).[28]

In making programmatic decisions around EBA, administrators and clinicians should work together to identify assessment tools that both meet the programmatic and clinician needs and inform clinical practice and programmatic decision-making in a meaningful way. In addition, strategies that may improve clinician willingness to implement EBAs include clearly defining the reason for collecting the data, ensuring that the data collection procedures are manageable and user-friendly to school mental

Table 1
Sample clinical assessment tools and methods

Tool	Age	Cost	Strengths	Weaknesses
Achenbach System of Empirically Based Assessment CBCL Teacher's Report Form & Youth Self Report www.aseba.org Achenbach & Rescorla,[47] 2001	6–18	$25.00 for package of 50	Wide age range, option for multiple reporters, widely used in a variety of child serving systems. Strong psychometric properties	Time consuming for the informant to complete (more than 100 items). Variable sensitivity to change. Symptom focused
CANS www.praedfoundation.org Lyons et al,[13] 2004	0–18	$10.00 for initial training; no additional cost per use	Wide age range, measures strengths in addition to needs, widely used in US and other countries and developed in collaboration with several states' child service systems	Information is gathered through multiple sources, required certification training, not directly tied to DSM symptoms/diagnoses
Brief Problem Checklist http://www.childfirst.ucla.edu/Brief%20Problem%20 Checklist%20-%20Child.pdf; http://www.childfirst. ucla.edu/Brief Problem Checklist - Parent.pdf Chorpita et al,[42] 2010	7–18	Free	Brief (15 items). Tracks outcomes over time. Measures internalizing and externalizing problems	Does not evaluate for specific diagnoses
Strength and Difficulties Questionnaire www.sdqinfo.org Goodman,[41] 1997	3–16	Free	Wide age range, option for multiple reporters, available in many languages, measures strengths in addition to problems or concerns. Adequate internal consistency and validity	Does not evaluate for specific diagnoses
DISC-IV Shaffer et al,[48] 2000	6–18	Fee covers copying and mailing expenses. For information, contact: disc@worldnet.att.net	Wide age range, options for multiple reporters, relates directly to DSM-IV diagnostic categories	Complex and lengthy, approximately 90–120 min to administer. Requires significant training to administer

Instrument	Age	Cost	Features	Limitations
Conners Comprehensive Behavior Rating Scales (Conners) www.pearsonassessments.com Conners et al,[49] 2011	3–17	$60 for package of 25	Wide age range, option for multiple reporters, includes both screening and assessment	Focused only on ADHD
Child and Adolescent Functional Assessment Scale http://www.mhs.com Hodges,[50] 1990	4–18	$22 for package of 25 Training manual: $26 Consult Web site for current pricing	Wide age range and widely used in child service fields. Measures strengths in addition to problems or concerns	Measures functional impairment rather than the specific mental health concern underlying the impairment, does not include youth self-report for adolescents
NICHQ Vanderbilt Assessment Scales (ADHD) http://www.nichq.org/toolkits_publications/complete_adhd/04VanAssesScaleTeachInfor.pdf; http://www.nichq.org/toolkits_publications/complete_adhd/03VanAssesScaleParent%20Infor.pdf Wolraich et al,[51] 2003	6–12	Free	Option for multiple reporters. Screens for conduct and internalizing problems in addition to ADHD	Only measures symptoms related to ADHD
Impairment Rating Scale Fabiano et al,[45] 2006	4–12	Free	Multidimensional measure that assesses functioning across domains	Focused on assessing functioning, not for diagnostic purposes
Child and Adolescent Service Intensity Instrument http://www.aacap.org/AACAP/Member_Resources/Practice_Information/CASII.aspx Fallon et al,[52] 2006	6–18	Training and manual cost. See Web site for up-tc-date cost information	8-item instrument that assesses the service intensity needs of children and adolescents presenting with psychiatric, substance use, and/or developmental concerns	Focused on assessing service intensity needs, not for diagnostic purposes
Youth Top Problems http://csmh.umaryland.edu/Resources/Clinician Tools/ Weisz et al,[46] 2011	7–13	Free	Allows for problem specificity and is tailored to the individual report of the child and family	Does not evaluate for specific diagnoses

---

Box 1
Questions to consider when selecting a tool for evidence-based assessment

1. Outcome identification
   a. What issue is the tool intended to address?
   b. What outcomes are most relevant for the target population?
2. Identification of tools
   a. Have you reviewed available assessment tools?
   b. Have you discussed the tool with others who are familiar with its use?
   c. Have you considered how the tool fits with your clinical setting?
3. Consideration of evidence supporting the tool
   a. What are the measures of validity?
   b. What are the measures of reliability?
4. Organizational and community fit
   a. Is the measure feasible?
   b. Do you have adequate support from leadership?
   c. Are there political priorities that require consideration?
5. Capacity and resources needed to effectively implement the tool
   a. What are the training needs?
   b. How will you conduct ongoing assessment of reliable delivery?
6. Monitoring and sustainability over time
   a. How will you measure fidelity?
   b. How will you measure quality of data collection?

Adapted from SAMHSA. Identifying and selecting evidence-based programs and practices: questions to consider. 2014. Available at: http://nrepp.samhsa.gov/pdfs/identifyingand selecting.pdf. Accessed November 01, 2014.

---

health professionals, and establishing a system to use data for continuous improvement at the individual student and school-wide level.[29]

Once an instrument has been selected, program administrators must ensure that clinicians are trained to administer the tool reliably and measure fidelity on an ongoing basis. Research regarding best practice for implementation suggests several steps to ensure delivery with fidelity to the tool.[30] Trainees must be clear about the objectives, purpose, and intended outcomes of the training. The content of the training must be relevant for the particular practice setting. Training aids should be provided to assist trainees in learning, organizing, and recalling content. The training should offer opportunities to practice skills. Feedback should be provided to trainees on skills practiced. Training should offer the opportunity to observe and interact with peers. Finally, trainers should provide effective coordination of the programming with integration into clinical practice. Ongoing implementation fidelity monitoring and skill review is essential for sustained long-term implementation of EBA. The following case examples describe two school mental health programs' experiences with clinical and educational outcomes assessment in school mental health programs in Tennessee and Maryland.

Case 1: Vanderbilt School Mental Health Program

The Vanderbilt School Mental Health Program has served students in the Metropolitan Nashville Public School System in Nashville, Tennessee for more than 20 years, but the implementation of EBA in this program has occurred only quite recently. Currently serving students in 38 schools, the program began using the Child and Adolescent Needs and Strengths (CANS)[31] in 2010. Implementation of standardized assessment in this program had two primary goals: measurement of clinical outcomes at the child, family, and program level, and facilitation of communication across child serving systems.[12,13] The CANS was chosen to meet these goals because it is a reliable and valid assessment tool[32–37] that has been used to facilitate service planning at the child and family level, and to measure and manage program and system level outcomes.[38–40] Improved communication across systems was particularly important for this program because of its engagement with other child serving agencies, for example, local child welfare and juvenile justice systems. Feasibility of implementation was another important factor in the choice of this tool—leadership in the school mental health program works closely with members of the team that had implemented training and delivery of the CANS with fidelity by child protective service workers. In Tennessee, the child welfare and juvenile justice systems are both part of the Department of Children's Services, which had adopted use of the CANS for all children over the age of 5 years in 2006. Training to use the instrument is the only cost associated with the CANS, which is freely available online (www.praedfoundation.org). School mental health clinicians were trained to rate a case vignette with at least 70% reliability in comparison with the gold standard. Remedial training is provided for clinicians who do not pass the certification test and clinicians recertify annually.

One benefit of the CANS is its reliability and validity at the single-item level,[32] allowing clinicians to tailor the tool to fit the needs of their practice. Several clinicians in the Vanderbilt program volunteered to participate on a committee to review the items that were most relevant for their practice and customize the tool based on their analysis. The items selected by school mental health clinicians for inclusion are listed in **Box 2**. Clinicians in this program use the CANS to rate child and family needs and strengths for each child on their caseload at least 2 times per year: once at the beginning of treatment and again at the close of each school year or when significant changes occur. The CANS incorporates information from multiple reporters including parents, teachers, administrators, and any other individuals involved in the care of the child. Academic indicators are included as one domain in the measure, allowing for assessment of the impact of mental health needs on academic functioning.

A few limitations related to use of the CANS are worth noting. First, the CANS is not a diagnostic tool and therefore does not provide the clinician with information about particular clinical syndromes. Instead, the items assess child and family needs and strengths from a more general perspective. The benefit of this approach is the tool's utility in providing a common language across child serving systems, but it could be viewed as a limitation of its utility in clinical care. In addition, depending on the number of items selected for inclusion, the tool can become lengthy. Even so, the identification of particular needs and strengths that stand out among the items can be very helpful in selecting initial treatment targets. Recently, the Vanderbilt program has implemented a graphic presentation of CANS data that will assist clinicians in identifying particular needs and strengths that can be identified as targets for treatment and monitored for change over time. Scores from each item are plotted on a chart including up to three time points for evaluation of change with treatment. Finally, the CANS is not intended for monitoring of change in clinical symptoms from visit to visit, but instead to assess

Box 2
Child and Adolescent Needs and Strengths items selected for use in Vanderbilt school mental health assessment

Child

Strengths	Risk Factors	Emotional/behavioral needs
Interpersonal Adult	Suicide risk	Impulsivity/hyperactivity
Interpersonal Peer	Self-mutilation	Oppositional
Resiliency	Other self-harm	Conduct
Educational	Danger to others	Anger control
Vocational	Bullying others	Emotional control
Talents/interests	Bullying victim	Depression
Spiritual/religious	Runaway	Anxiety
Life domain Functioning	Sanction seeking	Trauma experience
Safety	Sexuality	Trauma module (if indicated)
Social functioning	Sexually reactive behavior	Sexual abuse
Sleep	Sexual aggression	Physical abuse
School attendance	Delinquency	Neglect
School behavior	Substance use	Emotional abuse
School achievement	Gang involvement	Medical trauma
Family	Medication compliance	Natural disaster
Living situation		Witness family violence
Legal		Witness community violence
Identity		Witness/victim of criminal act
		Re-experiencing
		Avoidance
		Numbing
		Dissociation

Caregiver

Needs
  Involvement
  Social resources
  Residential stability
Life domain functioning
  Physical
  Mental health
Risk factors
  Supervision
  Substance abuse

progress over longer time spans. For this reason, clinicians complete the CANS once at the beginning of treatment and again at the close of the school year or when significant changes in the clinical needs occur, such as at transitions in care.

The idea of using an EBA in general and use of the CANS in particular has generally been well accepted by the program's clinicians. Although formal monitoring of academic data has not up to this point been included in outcomes measurement in this program, a data-sharing agreement was recently established with the school system that will allow for collection of attendance, discipline, and academic achievement indicators to complement measurement of clinical outcomes. Detailed analyses of these data are forthcoming.

Case 2: University of Maryland Center for School Mental Health

The national CSMH at the University of Maryland is affiliated with five school mental health programs serving the diverse needs of schools and students across the state. Each program has unique program goals and objectives that meet the targeted needs of the communities they serve, and thus, some of the specific assessment practices within each program vary. Across all programs, there is a focus on collecting both academic and clinical outcomes. All programs use report card data as part of their assessment process, in addition to using the state's public mental health clinical outcome measurement tool, the Outcomes Measurement System (OMS). The OMS is a survey measure that parents (in conjunction with the student, depending on age) complete with their mental health clinician at intake and every 6 months to monitor progress. The OMS includes questions covering a range of topics including symptom assessment and school and community functioning and support.

The University of Maryland School Mental Health Program (SMHP) serves 27 schools in Baltimore City and is the largest program affiliated with CSMH. This program serves children in regular education and supplements existing school resources by providing a full continuum of mental health supports, including mental health promotion, prevention, and intervention. Clinicians within SMHP receive yearly training in clinical assessment and are provided with a tool kit of EBA measures to use in their clinical practice. Assessment measures included in the tool kit are all available in the public domain and include general measures of symptoms and functioning, such as the Strengths and Difficulties Questionnaire[41] and Brief Problems Checklist,[42] in addition to disorder-specific assessment measures, such as the Revised Children's Anxiety and Depression Scale[43] and the Vanderbilt Attention Deficit Hyperactivity Disorder (ADHD) Diagnostic Rating Scales.[44] Clinicians are encouraged to use EBA measures at intake and to administer follow-up measures across treatment to monitor progress. Given the variability in measure utilization across clinicians, this information is solely used by the clinician to inform clinical decision-making and is not collected in aggregate. This year the program is piloting the use of a modified version of the Impairment Rating Scale[45] to assess the impact of problem behaviors on academic and classroom functioning on intake and at the end of treatment across all participants, to supplement report card and OMS data and better understand the impact of treatment on academic functioning.

The other four school mental health programs affiliated with CSMH are smaller programs serving approximately 3 to 15 schools each. Their program goals and objectives are targeted at supplementing school mental health services for a subset of students. For instance, two of the programs specifically serve students in special education who are at risk for more restrictive educational placements. These programs use the Youth Top Problems[46] and Brief Problems Checklist[42] assessment measures across all clients to measure student clinical outcomes. The Youth Top Problems[46] measure is collected at intake and monthly for every client to monitor progress and inform treatment planning. The Brief Problems Checklist (teacher, parent, and student versions)[42] are collected at intake and on a quarterly basis for every client to monitor progress and inform treatment planning. In addition, these data are used to monitor overall program outcomes and inform programmatic planning.

Clinicians within these programs are consulted regularly to better understand their satisfaction with and challenges to programmatic EBA policies and procedures. Current policies and procedures reflect a balance of clinician and program goals and objectives with most clinicians reporting that the costs and benefits of the current assessment procedures are manageable within their practice. Reported challenges with the current procedures include difficulty obtaining school-level academic data, which requires access from school office staff, and difficulty with respondent completion of parent and teacher report measures. On-going supervision on how to address barriers to data access and how to best use required assessment measures to inform clinical practice has been useful to increase clinician satisfaction.

SUMMARY

The literature highlights several advantages to assessment and ongoing progress monitoring in children's mental health care, including providing accurate diagnosis and data-driven clinical decision-making. Despite consensus in children's mental health that EBA is critical to quality treatment, there are significant challenges to successful implementation of EBA in routine clinical practice. School mental health programs must address additional considerations, including access to parents and the importance of including academic indicators in outcomes assessment. Several free or low-cost, user-friendly assessment measures are available and are currently being used in school mental health services across the country—many of these are listed here. School mental health programs should be thoughtful around selecting measures that are tailored to their specific clinical populations that serve their individual clinician and programmatic needs; providing high-quality training on the proper use of the tools; and supporting clinicians in their efforts to implement these measures consistently with fidelity over time. Increased utilization of EBA within the school mental health programming requires effort, but has the potential to significantly increase the quality of school mental health services that are provided to youth and families.

REFERENCES

1. Hunsley J, Mash EJ. Evidence-based assessment. Annu Rev Clin Psychol 2007; 3:29–51. http://dx.doi.org/10.1146/annurev.clinpsy.3.022806.091419.
2. Lyon AR, Dorsey S, Pullmann M, et al. Clinician use of standardized assessments following a common elements psychotherapy training and consultation program. Adm Policy Ment Health 2014. http://dx.doi.org/10.1007/s10488-014-0543-7.
3. American Psychological Association Task Force on Evidence-Based Practice for Children and Adolescents. Disseminating evidence-based practice for children and adolescents: a systems approach to enhancing care. Washington, DC: American Psychological Association; 2008.
4. Weist MD, Youngstrom EA, Stephan S, et al. Challenges and ideas from a research program on high-quality, evidence-based practice in school mental health. J Clin Child Adolesc Psychol 2014;43(2):244–55. http://dx.doi.org/10. 1080/15374416.2013.833097.

5. Hatfield DR, Ogles BM. Why some clinicians use outcome measures and others do not. Adm Policy Ment Health 2007;34(3):283–91. http://dx.doi.org/10.1007/s10488-006-0110-y.
6. Jenkins MM, Youngstrom EA, Washburn JJ, et al. Evidence-based strategies improve assessment of pediatric bipolar disorder by community practitioners. Prof Psychol Res Pr 2011;42(2):121–9. http://dx.doi.org/10.1037/a0022506.
7. Youngstrom EA, Choukas-Bradley S, Calhoun CD, et al. Clinical guide to the evidence-based assessment approach to diagnosis and treatment. Cogn Behav Pract 2014. http://dx.doi.org/10.1016/j.cbpra.2013.12.005.
8. Hannan C, Lambert MJ, Harmon C, et al. A lab test and algorithms for identifying clients at risk for treatment failure. J Clin Psychol 2005;61(2):155–63. http://dx.doi.org/10.1002/jclp.20108.
9. Groth-Marnat G. Handbook of psychological assessment. Hoboken, NJ: Wiley; 2009.
10. Connors EH, Arora P, Curtis L, et al. Evidence-based assessment in school mental health. Cogn Behav Pract 2014. http://dx.doi.org/10.1016/j.cbpra.2014.03.008.
11. Sander M, Everts J, Johnson J. Using data to inform program design and implementation and make the case for school mental health. Adv Sch Ment Health Promot 2011;4(4):13–21.
12. Lyons JS, Epstein RA, Jordan N. Evolving systems of care with total clinical outcomes management. Eval Program Plann 2010;33:53–5. http://dx.doi.org/10.1016/j.evalprogplan.2009.05.015.
13. Lyons JS, Weiner DA, Lyons MB, et al. Measurement as communication in outcomes management: the Child and Adolescent Needs and Strengths (CANS). In: Maruish ME, editor. The use of psychological testing for treatment planning and outcomes assessment. Mahwah, NJ: Lawrence Erlbaum Associates; 2004. p. 461–76.
14. Lahey BB, Flagg EW, Bird HR, et al. The NIMH Methods for the Epidemiology of Child and Adolescent Mental Disorders (MECA) study: background and methodology. J Am Acad Child Adolesc Psychiatry 1996;35(7):855–64. http://dx.doi.org/10.1097/00004583-199607000-00011.
15. The Child Behavior Checklist and related instruments. In: Achenbach TM, Maruish ME, editors. The use of psychological testing for treatment planning and outcomes assessment. 2nd edition. Mahwah, NJ: Lawrence Erlbaum Associates; 1999. p. 429–66.
16. Costello EJ, Angold A, Burns BJ, et al. The Great Smoky Mountains Study of Youth. Goals, design, methods, and the prevalence of DSM-III-R disorders. Arch Gen Psychiatry 1996;53(12):1129–36.
17. Reich W. Diagnostic interview for children and adolescents (DICA). J Am Acad Child Adolesc Psychiatry 2000;39(1):59–66. http://dx.doi.org/10.1097/00004583-200001000-00017.
18. Weller EB, Weller RA, Fristad MA, et al. Children's Interview for Psychiatric Syndromes (ChIPS). J Am Acad Child Adolesc Psychiatry 2000;39(1):76–84. http://dx.doi.org/10.1097/00004583-200001000-00019.
19. Kaufman J, Birmaher B, Brent D, et al. Schedule for Affective Disorders and Schizophrenia for School-Age Children-Present and Lifetime Version (K-SADS-PL): initial reliability and validity data. J Am Acad Child Adolesc Psychiatry 1997;36(7):980–8. http://dx.doi.org/10.1097/00004583-199707000-00021.
20. Sherrill JT, Kovacs M. Interview schedule for children and adolescents (ISCA). J Am Acad Child Adolesc Psychiatry 2000;39(1):67–75. http://dx.doi.org/10.1097/00004583-200001000-00018.

21. Kelly M, Lueck C. Adopting a data-driven public health framework in schools: results from a multi-disciplinary survey on school-based mental health practice. Adv Sch Ment Health Promot 2011;4(4):5–12.
22. Kelly M. Data-driven decision making in school-based mental health: (how) is it possible? Adv Sch Ment Health Promot 2011;4(4):2–4.
23. Committee on School Health. School-based mental health services. Pediatrics 2004;113(6):1839–45.
24. Becker KD, Brandt NE, Stephan SH, et al. A review of educational outcomes in the children's mental health treatment literature. Adv Sch Ment Health Promot 2013;7(1):5–23. http://dx.doi.org/10.1080/1754730X.2013.851980.
25. Lyon A, McCauley E, Vander Stoep A. Toward successful implementation of evidence-based practices: characterizing the intervention context of counselors in school-based health centerstle. Emot Behav Disord Youth 2011;11:19–25. Available at: http://www.civicresearchinstitute.com/online/article_abstract.php?pid=5&aid=1745&iid=255. Accessed November 18, 2014.
26. Jensen-Doss A, Hawley KM. Understanding clinicians' diagnostic practices: attitudes toward the utility of diagnosis and standardized diagnostic tools. Adm Policy Ment Health 2011;38(6):476–85. http://dx.doi.org/10.1007/s10488-011-0334-3.
27. Palmiter DJ. A survey of the assessment practices of child and adolescent clinicians. Am J Orthopsychiatry 2004;74(2):122–8. http://dx.doi.org/10.1037/0002-9432.74.2.122.
28. SAMHSA. Identifying and selecting evidence-based programs and practices: questions to consider. 2014. Available at: http://www.nrepp.samhsa.gov/pdfs/Questions_To_Ask_Developers.pdf. Accessed Noverber 18, 2014.
29. Poston JM, Hanson WE. Meta-analysis of psychological assessment as a therapeutic intervention. Psychol Assess 2010;22(2):203–12. http://dx.doi.org/10.1037/a0018679.
30. Salas E, Tannenbaum SI, Kraiger K, et al. The science of training and development in organizations: what matters in practice. Psychol Sci Public Interest 2012;13(2):74–101. http://dx.doi.org/10.1177/1529100612436661.
31. Lyons JS. Knowledge creation through total clinical outcomes management: a practice-based evidence solution to address some of the challenges of knowledge translation. J Can Acad Child Adolesc Psychiatry 2009;18(1):38–45.
32. Anderson RL, Lyons JS, Giles DM, et al. Reliability of the Child and Adolescent Needs and Strengths-Mental Health (CANS-MH) Scale. Journal of Child and Family Studies 2003;12(3):279–89.
33. Anderson R, Estle G. Predicting level of mental health care among children served in a delivery system in a rural state. J Rural Health 2001;17(3):259–65.
34. Epstein RA, Jordan N, Rhee YJ, et al. The relationship between caregiver capacity and intensive community treatment for children with a mental health crisis. J Child Fam Stud 2008;18(3):303–11. http://dx.doi.org/10.1007/s10826-008-9231-0.
35. He X, Lyons J, Heinemann A. Modeling crisis decision-making for children in state custody. Gen Hosp Psychiatry 2004;26(5):378–83.
36. Lyons J, Uziel-Miller N, Reyes F, et al. Strengths of children and adolescents in residential settings: prevalence and associations with psychopathology and discharge placement. J Am Acad Child Adolesc Psychiatry 2000;39(2):176–81.
37. Lyons J, Griffin G, Quintenz S, et al. Clinical and forensic outcomes from the Illinois mental health juvenile justice initiative. Psychiatr Serv 2003;54(12):1629–34.
38. Lyons J. Communimetrics: a measurement theory for human service enterprises. New York: Springer; 2009.

39. Lyons J, Weiner D, editors. Strategies in behavioral healthcare: total clinical outcomes management. New York: Civic Research Institute; 2008.
40. Lyons JS. Redressing the emperor: improving our children's public mental health system. Westport, CT: Greenwood Publishing Group; 2004.
41. Goodman R. The strengths and difficulties questionnaire: a research note. J Child Psychol Psychiatry 1997;38:581–6. http://dx.doi.org/10.1111/j.1469-7610.1997.tb01545.x.
42. Chorpita BF, Reise S, Weisz JR, et al. Evaluation of the brief problem checklist: child and caregiver interviews to measure clinical progress. J Consult Clin Psychol 2010;78(4):526–36. http://dx.doi.org/10.1037/a0019602.
43. Brown TA, Chorpita BF, Korotitsch W, et al. Psychometric properties of the Depression Anxiety Stress Scales (DASS) in clinical samples. Behav Res Ther 1997;35(1):79–89.
44. Wolraich ML, Feurer ID, Hannah JN, et al. Obtaining systematic teacher reports of disruptive behavior disorders utilizing DSM-IV. J Abnorm Child Psychol 1998; 26(2):141–52.
45. Fabiano GA, Pelham WE, Waschbusch D, et al. A practical impairment measure: psychometric properties of the impairment rating scale in samples of children with attention-deficit/hyperactivity disorder and two school-based samples. J Clin Child Adolesc Psychol 2006;35:369–85. http://dx.doi.org/10.1207/s15374424jccp3503.
46. Weisz JR, Chorpita BF, Frye A, et al. Youth top problems: using idiographic, consumer-guided assessment to identify treatment needs and to track change during psychotherapy. J Consult Clin Psychol 2011;79:369–80. http://dx.doi.org/10.1037/a0023307.
47. Achenbach TM, Rescorla L. ASEBA school-age forms & profiles. Burlington (VT): Aseba; 2001.
48. Shaffer D, Fisher P, Lucas CP, et al. NIMH Diagnostic Interview Schedule for Children Version IV (NIMH DISC-IV): description, differences from previous versions, and reliability of some common diagnoses. J Am Acad Child Adolesc Psychiatry 2000;39(1):28–38.
49. Conners CK, Pitkanen J, Rzepa SR. Conners comprehensive behavior rating scale. In: Kreutzer J, DeLuca J, et al, editors. Encyclopedia of clinical neuropsychology. New York: Springer; 2011. p. 678–80.
50. Hodges K. Child and Adolescent Functional Assessment Scale (CAFAS). In: Maruish ME, editor. The Use of Psychological Testing for Treatment Planning and Outcome Assessment. Mahwah, NJ: Lawrence Erlbaum Associates; 1999. p. 631–64.
51. Wolraich ML, Lambert W, Doffing MA, et al. Psychometric properties of the Vanderbilt ADHD diagnostic parent rating scale in a referred population. J Pediatr Psychol 2003;28(8):559–68.
52. Fallon T Jr, Pumariega A, Sowers W, et al. A level of care instrument for children's systems of care: construction, reliability and validity. J Child Fam Stud 2006; 15(2):140–52.

The Evolution of a School Behavioral Health Model in the US Army

Michael E. Faran, MD, PhD[a],*, Patti L. Johnson, PhD[a], Paul Ban, PhD[a],
Tracy Shue, MS[a], Mark D. Weist, PhD[b]

KEYWORDS

- School behavioral health • US Army • Child and family behavioral health system
- Military children

KEY POINTS

- The US Army has developed an innovative School Behavioral Health (SBH) program, which was initiated by Tripler Army Medical Center at schools on Schofield Barracks in Hawaii in the late 1990s and has since expanded to 7 additional installations in the United States and Germany.
- Expansion of the SBH program has been associated with the establishment in 2009 of the Child, Adolescent and Family Behavioral Health Office at Joint Base Lewis-McChord, Washington State, and the increasing prioritization of behavioral health care tailored to meet the needs of this population.
- The SBH program is expanding to be part of a broader effort referred to as the Child and Family Behavioral Health System, a collaborative, consultative behavioral health care model that includes SBH, standardized training of primary care providers in treatment of common behavioral health problems, use of tele-consultation/tele-behavioral health, optimizing community outreach services, and integration with other related behavioral health services.

UNIQUE NEEDS OF MILITARY CHILDREN AND FAMILIES

Military families experience increased stress associated with aspects of military life, including moving frequently, being separated from family, experiencing deployment, and for those in combat, confronting violence and trauma.[1] During the last 13 years, the stresses experienced by military youth have intensified, associated with parental combat deployments in support of the wars in Iraq and Afghanistan. Research

Funding sources: none.
Conflicts of interest: none.
[a] Child and Family Behavioral Health Office, United States Army Medical Command, 9913-A Madigan Annex, Tacoma, WA 98431, USA; [b] Department of Psychology, University of South Carolina, 1512 Pendleton Street, Barnwell 237D, Columbia, SC 29208, USA
* Corresponding author.
E-mail address: michael.e.faran.civ@mail.mil

Child Adolesc Psychiatric Clin N Am 24 (2015) 415–428
http://dx.doi.org/10.1016/j.chc.2014.11.008
1056-4993/15/$ – see front matter Published by Elsevier Inc.

childpsych.theclinics.com

Abbreviations	
AMEDD	Army Medical Department
BH	Behavioral health
CAFBHO	Child, Adolescent, and Family Behavioral Health Office
CAFBHS	Child and Family Behavioral Health System
CAPS	Child and Adolescent Psychiatry Service
DoE	Department of Education
EBP	Evidence-based practices
JBLM	Joint Base Lewis-McChord
PCM	Primary care manager
PCMH	Patient-Centered Medical Home
SBH	School Behavioral Health
TAMC	Tripler Army Medical Center

indicates that parental deployment increases the risk of concerning emotional/behavioral problems for military youth across all age groups.[2-5] During deployment, children and adolescents show poorer peer and family relationships,[2,6] as well as experiencing decreases in school engagement and academic performance.[2,6-8] Several large statewide self-report surveys of middle school and high school students have shown that there is an increased risk of alcohol and drug use,[9,10] increased feelings of sadness, depression, and suicidal ideation,[11,12] and increased fighting and weapons carrying[13] for youth of a currently or recently deployed parent. Moreover, rates of diagnosed mental health disorders,[14] rates of behavioral and mental health visits,[15] prescriptions for psychotropic medication,[16] and rates of psychiatric hospitalizations[17] increase for military-connected youth who have experienced a parental deployment.

Several indicators suggest that adult family members have also not coped well with service member deployment. Rates of screening positive for depression, both during pregnancy and at postpartum, are higher for women whose spouse is deployed than for those whose spouse is nondeployed,[18,19] and mental health diagnoses are higher for wives of deployed soldiers than wives of nondeployed soldiers.[20] Perhaps even more concerning, child maltreatment in Army families has been shown to increase during combat-related deployments.[21,22]

Although clearly in need, military families may be especially unlikely to seek mental health services, related to barriers that operate for all families (eg, stress, poor knowledge of mental health, transportation, and financial barriers[23]) and stigma, which is even more intense for them relating to the culture in the armed services, and perceptions that mental health problems are a sign of weakness and may likely interfere with military career advancement.[1] In addition, military-connected children move 6 to 9 times during their K-12 education; they change schools 3 times more often than their civilian peers.[24]

These findings underscore the intensified need for accessible and effective mental health services for military children and families, an increased need that will not be significantly reduced in the years to come, even with wars in Iraq and Afghanistan ending. The psychological impact of experiencing a parental combat deployment seems to continue for some time, even after the parent returns.[2,5,7] As of August, 2014, 6815 service members had died while deployed to war zones,[25] leaving behind about 4900 children and adolescents who had lost a parent.[26] Moreover, military children may likely have soldier parents with mental health problems and other invisible wounds of war,[27] including posttraumatic stress disorder (PTSD), depression, anxiety, substance abuse, and traumatic head injury. Such parental challenges are established risk factors for negative emotional and behavioral outcomes in children and adolescents. **Box 1** presents some tips that may be useful in working with children and adolescents affected by military stressors.

The US Army is responding to the identified mental health needs of this patient population. By building an initiative to assist military children and families through school behavioral health (SBH) and related service strategies that reduce the stigma of and barriers to care, the Army is focusing on improving the functioning, wellness, and resiliency of this vulnerable population. In the following sections, the development of this initiative, named the Child and Family Behavioral Health System (CAFBHS), in which the SBH program plays a foundational role, is described.

EARLY DEVELOPMENT OF THE US ARMY'S SCHOOL BEHAVIORAL HEALTH PROGRAM

Before 2000, the Child and Adolescent Psychiatry Service (CAPS) at Tripler Army Medical Center (TAMC) provided mental health services at Solomon Elementary School located on Schofield Barracks, an Army installation on Oahu, Hawaii. These services were in the form of a traditional school consultation model, with child psychiatry fellows consulting with administrative staff (eg, assistant principal, principal) and school-employed mental health staff (eg, counselors, psychologists) and occasionally providing some direct intervention to children identified with challenging problems.

In 2000, the services provided by TAMC CAPS to Solomon Elementary transformed from a traditional consultative model with occasional direct interventions provided at

---

Box 1
Tips for behavioral health (BH) clinicians working with military/veteran children and families

- Ask about Active Duty/National Guard/Reserve/Veteran status

- Ask about deployment history: when, how often, how long

- Ask about parental functioning and mental health history, marital relationship, and other family issues related to military experiences and challenges

- Explore impact of military-related stressors on current functioning, and diagnostic and treatment implications

- Consider comprehensive treatment approaches, including evidence-based psychosocial interventions and medication management as indicated

- Establish strategies to systematically communicate/partner/collaborate with patient's primary care provider and with school-based resources and personnel

- Educate school personnel, especially in schools that are geographically disparate from military bases, to be sensitive of the impact of military stressors (eg, deployment, postdeployment, invisible wounds of war) on children and families

- Increase your own awareness of military support services (eg, Family Readiness Groups, Exceptional Family Member Program, Army Community Services, Child and Youth School Services, military chaplains, Families Overcoming Under Stress Program, Military One Source, Military Kids Connect), as well as community-based/state/national resources (eg, Military Child Education Coalition, Operation Military Kids, National Child Traumatic Stress Network, American Academy of Child and Adolescent Psychiatry, American Psychological Association, American Academy of Pediatrics)

- Encourage patients to use the resources listed above

the school to an embedded SBH model. By embedding the BH provider directly in the school, the providers are integrated into the school environment, culture, and community, providing a continuum of services (eg, education, prevention, early intervention, assessment, and treatment) within the student's natural environment: the school.[28] This transformation occurred in partnership with an innovative principal, who was willing to try this relatively new approach to improve the lives of students and benefit the school as a whole.[29] Because of the success at Solomon Elementary and the positive response of the school staff, parents, and community, over the next several years the SBH program obtained funding to expand this embedded BH model to 3 additional schools on Schofield Barracks and 1 elementary school at the Kaneohe Marine Corps Air Station on Oahu, Hawaii. Through this experience, a framework for high-quality SBH services developed. Key elements include: (1) interdisciplinary collaboration among the Army SBH team (child and adolescent psychiatrists, psychologists, and social workers) and school staff; (2) a full continuum of care in the schools, including school-wide training and education (eg, on resilience in the context of frequent deployment); (3) early identification and intervention for youth presenting with more challenging needs; and (4) on-site treatment of students and families, including youth with more serious disorders, involving combined psychotherapy and psychopharmacologic approaches.[29]

One of the truly unique features of the evolution of this embedded SBH program was the consistent and intensive involvement of mental health providers, in this case, child and adolescent psychiatrists, during all phases of the development and implementation of the program. The traditional psychiatric clinic-centric model transformed into a comprehensive embedded SBH model, in which psychological health is viewed as integral to the academic experience of the students. For example, providers met with the school officials (principals, local district superintendents and staff, and the state superintendent and staff) to promote the SBH program and to develop a memorandum of agreement with the Hawaii Department of Education (DoE); they met with Army and civilian leaders to establish a District Advisory Council, which provided oversight to the SBH program; they provided education and training to the school staff on the impact of deployment and other military stressors on military-connected children and families; they hired and trained the BH providers in the embedded BH model; and they provided direct treatment and medication management to child and adolescent patients at the 5 on-post schools.

During this same time frame, as the Army transformed their school service delivery model, the leaders of the Army SBH program established formal connections with leaders in school mental health from the University of Maryland, Center for School Mental Health. The relationship led to the development of specific standards for improving the quality and use of evidence-based practices (EBP) in the SBH program. This development included ensuring that the program adhered to principles of best practice,[28] assessing the overall organization and effectiveness of SBH programming through regular quality assessment, improving the functioning of teams, and increasing training and implementation support for EBP. Within several years, this effort began to attain national visibility, through participation in partnerships with organizations like the IDEA Partnership (coordinated by the National Association of State Directors of Special Education) and by presentations at key national conferences and meetings. Involvement of national partners shaped and improved the SBH program for military families. As a result of this success, SBH gained recognition within the Army as an effective intervention to improve the lives of soldiers' children and adolescents, leading to the Army Medical Command funding 2 additional SBH programs at Fort Campbell, Kentucky and Fort Meade, Maryland.

ESTABLISHMENT OF THE CHILD AND FAMILY BEHAVIORAL HEALTH OFFICE AND FURTHER ADVANCEMENT OF SCHOOL BEHAVIORAL HEALTH

The Child and Family Behavioral Health Office (CAFBHO) was established in 2009, at Joint Base Lewis-McChord (JBLM) in Washington State, as a coordinating center for SBH and other efforts of the Army focused on military child and family BH. At that time, funds were allocated for program expansion, and the 3 extant SBH programs grew into 8 managed by the CAFBHO. The program at TAMC continued to serve as a model and developed into a training site for SBH. The 5 new locations included JBLM, WA; Fort Carson, Colorado; Fort Bliss, Texas; Landstuhl Regional Army Medical Center, Germany; and Bavaria Medical Department Activity, Germany.

The CAFBHO, in collaboration with a leader from the University of Maryland Center for School Mental Health (M. Weist) developed an operations guide for army SBH,[30] which established guidelines to systematize the implementation process, increasing standardization of programs promoting high-quality practices along several dimensions.[31] These guidelines ensured (1) the establishment of school-level and installation-level advisory groups made up of diverse stakeholders (including families, Army and education system leaders); (2) implementation of a continuum of school-wide BH promotion, prevention, early intervention, and treatment [32]; (3) adoption of a collaborative and supportive style with students and families to promote their active engagement and empowerment; (4) use of EBPs for the most common childhood disorders of depression, anxiety, attention-deficit/hyperactivity disorder, conduct problems, and trauma-related problems; (5) ongoing quality assessment and improvement; and (6) evaluation of impacts of the program on student emotional/behavioral and school functioning.[33]

Site visits at each of these installations were conducted to train staff and ensure consistency and standardization in implementation of practices as delineated in the operations guide. In addition, the CAFBHO, through collaboration with the Center for School Mental Health and the IDEA Partnership, established a practice group on military families as part of a National Community of Practice on Collaborative SBH. This group helped raise awareness of the critical BH needs of military families and the benefits of SBH in meeting these needs and assisted in development of collaborative relationships among the 8 installations connected to the CAFBHO and with other interested stakeholders from numerous US states and other national organizations (eg, Military Child Education Coalition; Military Interstate Children's Compact Commission; Specialized Training of Military Parents), which have a specific mission to support military-connected children and families, with their unique educational needs and frequent moves. The spirit of collaboration and innovation among agencies has proved instrumental in supporting the Army SBH program.

A foundational component of the SBH program is embedding BH providers (psychologists, social workers, and on some installations, child and adolescent psychiatrists) into the natural environment of schools, augmenting programs and services of school-employed providers, and enhancing the depth and quality of BH services. Based on principles of high-quality SBH,[28] the program also coordinates its work within and across schools on installations, and participates in partnerships with other service systems within the US Army (eg, Army Community Services, School Liaison Office), the local education system, the local mental health system, and other youth serving systems (eg, Child Welfare, Juvenile Justice). Consistent with the broader literature on school mental health, embedding BH resources significantly improves access to care[34] for students and also provides a less stigmatizing entry point to care for family members. Services focus on reducing and removing barriers to student learning, improving emotional/behavioral functioning and academic achievement, improving wellness and resilience for students and families, and contributing to soldier readiness, or the ability of soldiers to focus on the mission at hand without distraction or worry about emotional/behavioral challenges experienced by children and other family members.[34] An example of how this model works effectively is given in the following vignette.

VIGNETTE

The 16-year-old daughter of an active duty Army father and working mother with 2 younger siblings.

A teacher referred this student to the SBH program because her grades had decreased, she had ongoing peer problems, appeared sad and angry, and reported suicidal ideation. This student disclosed a long history of depression with suicidal thoughts to her primary care manager (PCM) and SBH therapist, which she attributed to significant absences of her father throughout her life (multiple deployments) and father's recent diagnosis of PTSD, which affected his emotional connection with the family, and led to marital conflict and family discord. In collaboration, the PCM and SBH therapist instituted a safety plan. The PCM referred the patient to a child and adolescent psychiatrist for medication management, because of her long history of depression, suicidal ideation, and complicated psychosocial situation. The psychiatrist maintained close communication with her PCM and SBH therapist to coordinate treatment. Because her therapist was available at school, the student was able to seek help whenever she felt overwhelmed or depressed during the day. This rapid access to care prevented self-harm on multiple occasions and subsequently led to resolution of her suicidal ideation. Both parents participated in treatment with the patient at the school, focused on improving their relationship with the patient. Her parents were also referred for marital therapy through the military chaplains. The patient's father was able to fulfill his ongoing military duties, including brief absences from the family because of training requirements. The student's depression resolved, with no recurrence of suicidal thinking. The teacher reported that the student was doing well after treatment. Her grades had improved. She no longer appeared sad and angry, and her interactions with peers were appropriate.

At the time of submission of this article, across the 8 installations, SBH programs have been implemented in 46 schools (34 elementary schools, 8 middle/junior high schools, 1 middle/high school combined, and 3 high schools); with the exception of 1 elementary school in Hawaii, all of the other 45 schools are on post (ie, on the installations). In Hawaii, a partnership SBH pilot was established in 2012 at an elementary school located just off the Schofield Barracks installation in the town of Wahiawa (Albert Saito, MD, and Stan Whitsett, PhD, personal communication, 2012). The partnership brings together the resources of the TAMC SBH program to address the BH needs of the military students with the resources of the Hawaii DoE and the Queen's Medical Center (a local private health care delivery system) to address the BH needs of the nonmilitary students. The TAMC SBH embeds a part-time team consisting of a clinical psychologist, licensed clinical social worker and part-time child and adolescent psychiatrist, who provide on-site psychological/psychiatric services to the military students and their families. With shared funding from the Hawaii DoE, the Queen's Medical Center provides comparable personnel and services to nonmilitary students and their families at the school. Staff from both programs work together as a team to deliver collaborative and integrative BH care in a seamless and blended fashion to all the students in this off-post school. This pilot SBH partnership expanded to the neighboring off-post middle school when the new school year began in August, 2014.

Notwithstanding this innovative partnership involving an Army medical center, a local health care system, and a local school district, a major limitation, related to insufficient resources, has been the inability to provide a coordinated continuum of BH services to military-connected children and families in schools off the installation (off post). Most military-connected school-age students live off post, attend public or private schools, or are homeschooled. The implication is that most military-connected school-age students are likely to experience limited mental health services available to them through school-employed mental health professionals (eg, school psychologists, counselors, and social workers); at levels lower than recommended ratios, contending with position constraints[35]; or are referred either to BH services through the local Military Treatment Facility or to a TRICARE network provider, funded through the military health care system. The following section describes the Army's partial solution to the need for universal SBH.

EXPANSION OF THE INITIATIVE AND THE CHILD AND FAMILY BEHAVIORAL HEALTH SYSTEM (CAFBHS)

"A first major challenge for the next decade is to integrate basic mental health care into primary care, which could be a core element of getting mental health parity right.[36]"

Because of limited BH resources, particularly child and adolescent psychiatrists, limited access to care, and fiscal constraints, the US Army Medical Department (AMEDD) Behavioral Health Service Line is implementing the CAFBHS, which partners and collaborates with the Army's Patient-Centered Medical Home (PCMH) model to meet the needs of the military families. The PCMH model emphasizes a team approach to medical care, which focuses on the whole person concept, in which the primary care practice is responsible for all of the patient's health care needs, including providing/integrating/coordinating specialty care services (see Patient-Centered Primary Care Collaborative, http://www.pcpcc.net, for more detail). In this context, the medical literature supports maximizing the role of the PCM in addressing common BH disorders within the primary care setting, and children and families are willing to be treated by the PCM for their BH needs.[37] The CAFBHS is a comprehensive BH model that aligns and collaborates with the PCMH and other primary care family member–oriented clinics in the Military Treatment Facility. The CAFBHS model blends best practices in consultation, collaboration, and integration of BH care in primary care settings.[38] The AMEDD issued an operations order (OPORD 14–44) in March, 2014 that mandates the establishment of the CAFBHS Army-wide, over a 3-year period, to meet the BH needs of the Army family member population centered on the PCMH model.

This comprehensive initiative integrates several interrelated components to expand accessibility and availability of BH for Army children and families across the military health care system. With respect to the SBH program, the operations order directs expansion of the SBH program from the current 8 installations to 18 and from 46 to potentially 107 on-post schools.

The 7 goals of the CAFBHS are to:

1. Implement a consultative/collaborative BH care model for Army children and families, with the objective of promoting optimal soldier readiness through Army family wellness and resilience
2. Provide BH services through the BH service line, including oversight, resourcing, and service delivery, ensuring that all installations throughout a region are supported in their consultation and coordination of BH services for Army children and families

3. Increase access to care by providing an easily accessible and coordinated BH consultative and collaborative care model that sufficiently supports identified population needs
4. Implement standardized BH consultative and collaborative care services using the Military Treatment Facility's Department of Behavioral Health, and regional tele-consultation and tele-BH services to ensure efficiency and effective use of resources
5. Implement standardized training programs for PCMs (pediatricians and family practitioners) and BH specialty clinicians to ensure use of best practices across the enterprise
6. Promote excellence in BH care delivery through the use of EBPs and ongoing performance improvement processes, which include quantitative and qualitative outcome measures
7. Implement BH services supporting the Army Family Covenant: "The strength of the Nation is our Army; the strength of our Army is the Soldier; the strength of the Soldier is the Family."

Fig. 1 presents core structure and functions within the CAFBHS. The figure shows key functions of consultation, collaboration, and service integration, combining to contribute to enhanced efficiency and effectiveness of linked service lines, including SBH, services within a multidisciplinary BH center, community outreach, tele-consultation and tele-BH, and training and supporting of PCMs within the PCMH model.

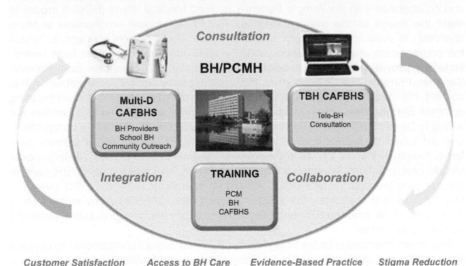

Fig. 1. Core functions/units of the CAFBHS.

CAFBHS care, including SBH, directly supports the PCMH, in which the PCM takes the lead for integrating and coordinating patients' care. The entire system is designed to adopt a holistic approach to health care, improve customer satisfaction, increase access to needed BH care, reduce stigma, and strengthen family wellness and resiliency.

Fig. 2 shows the importance of systemic transformation from a silo approach of BH care (ie, multiple clinical settings providing BH care with minimal communication among them) to an interconnected systems partnership approach in which the patient's health and well-being are a shared responsibility among BH providers in

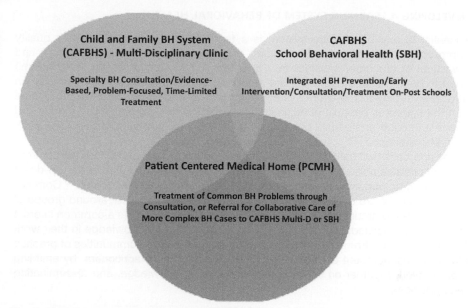

Fig. 2. BH interconnected systems partnerships.

the clinical setting (Multidisciplinary CAFBHS), BH providers in the school setting (SBH), and the PCMs in the PCMHs. In the pre-CAFBHS iteration of the SBH program, SBH providers had incidental consultations with the student's PCM. In the CAFBHS model, as shown in **Fig. 2**, the relationship is an overt partnership, in which consultation about patients and collaborative care is intentional.

"Do School mental health right."[36]

As the SBH program expands and transforms, challenges with integrating SBH into the overall CAFBHS model must be identified to develop potential solutions to optimize success of the program. Some of these challenges are already apparent, whereas others will likely emerge as the program expands to additional installations. Challenges identified include:

1. How can SBH providers and PCMs effectively engage in a consultative, collaborative care approach? How will patients flow between these 2 components of the health care delivery system? What are the most efficient means of communication?
2. How can the mental health care culture best integrate with the medical care culture? How can these 2 professional cultures adapt to this new model, both independently, as well as part of an interconnected system of care?
3. How can such a large enterprise-wide system of care ensure fidelity to the model as it is disseminated across the Army? What core components are necessary? To what degree can individual SBH programs make adaptations based on their installation needs and still maintain the integrity of the model?
4. How to recruit and hire the right people with these relatively novel job skills, particularly at remote or overseas locations?

Strategies adopted by the CAFBHO to address these potential challenges, identify others as they arise, and promote best practices across the enterprise are discussed in the following sections.

DEVELOPING A LEARNING SYSTEM OF BEHAVIORAL HEALTH

Essential to any health care system is a feedback process that provides quality improvement efforts, outcome metrics, ongoing performance improvement, and measures of customer satisfaction. For a learning system of health, mechanisms need to be in place to guarantee that health care data and experience gathered on a local level benefit the entire system. That is, there needs to be a way to ensure that the system is capable of adjusting to circumstances, so that it can modify and improve through an iterative process of collecting and studying data and feedback from stakeholders.[31,39]

The approach that the CAFBHS uses for its learning system of health is the communities of practice approach of knowledge management, which combines a top-down and bottom-up ongoing review of its programs, strategies, and outcomes.[40] Communities of practice are really learning systems. This approach is built around groups of practitioners (communities), who individually and collectively have a common interest in an area of knowledge (shared agenda) and who use that knowledge in their work (practice), to learn from and build on each other's expertise. Communities of practice place the management of knowledge in the hands of the practitioners, by enabling them to work together on solving problems, sharing knowledge, and disseminating best practices.

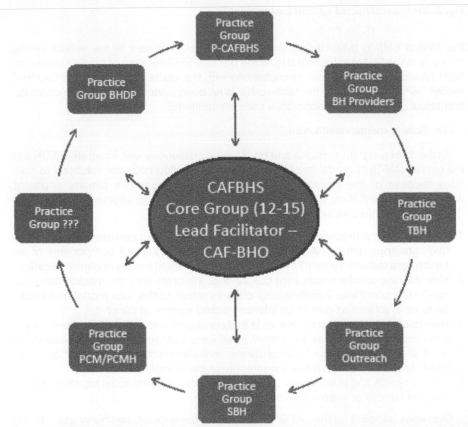

Fig. 3. CAFBHS communities of practice model. BHDP, Behavioral health data portal; P-CAFBHS, Prototype child and family behavioral health system.

The formal top-down component of the communities of practice typically uses traditional metrics to measure outcomes, in the case of the CAFBHS metrics, such as access to care, provider productivity, proportion of clients seen within the Military Treatment Facility compared with the TRICARE Network, and customer satisfaction. The less formal bottom-up communities of practice strategy includes the establishment of organizational structures known as practice groups, which convene practitioners who share and examine their work and then communicate with others in a core group what they have learned (**Fig. 3**). Practice groups identify and work on common issues, new solutions, and best practices, and advise and assist the core group in identifying systemic threats to implementation fidelity, as well as making recommendations that may lead to enterprise-wide improvements or revisions of policies, and so forth. The communities of practice approach pulls together the knowledge (eg, experiences, expertise, and practices) from across the enterprise to continually improve the system. It facilitates the learning from within, leading to better outcomes and healthier communities.

SUMMARY

The US Army is providing innovative health care to meet the BH needs of military children and families. The SBH program has had a foundational role in this effort, expanding from 1 installation serving 4 schools to 8 installations and 45 on-post schools and 1 off-post school, with plans to include 18 installations and 107 on-post schools. SBH is an integral part of the enterprise-wide CAFBHS. Implementation of CAFBHS in support of the PCMH model addresses the health and well-being of Army children and families through a comprehensive BH model that blends best practices in consultation, collaboration, and integration of BH care with primary care.

With Army-wide implementation, scheduled to occur over the next 3 years, the CAFBHS faces many present and future challenges. The paucity of highly skilled BH providers in many geographically isolated Army installations, both within the continental United States and overseas, is a major hurdle already affecting military communities. Recruiting and retaining the best possible personnel are imperative to quality BH care delivery and the long-term success of CAFBHS programs. Another challenge facing implementation is the cultural change inherent in the CAFBHS and PCMH model, which requires practice modification of both the PCM and the BH provider. Sederer wrote, in an opinion about implementing BH care within primary care, "Changing medical practices gives new meaning to the word difficult.[41]" He stated that perhaps the greatest difficulties were cultural and attitudinal and that the focus should be on behavioral change. Facilitating the process of adoption of new practices through training, coaching, and experience will be a major focus throughout the implementation phases of the CAFBHS. A learning system of health, aided through the communities of practice framework,[35] will be critical in sharing of lessons learned and promoting best practices across all installations.

REFERENCES

1. Faran ME, Weist MD, Faran DA, et al. Promoting resilience in military children and adolescents. In: Clauss-Ehlers C, Weist MD, editors. Community planning to foster resilience in children. New York: Springer; 2004. p. 233–48.
2. Chandra A, Lara-Cinisomo S, Jaycox LH, et al. Children on the homefront: the experience of children from military families. Pediatrics 2010;125:16–25.

3. Chartrand MM, Frank DA, White LF, et al. Effect of parents' wartime deployment on the behavior of young children in military families. Arch Pediatr Adolesc Med 2008;162:1009–14.
4. Flake EM, Davis BE, Johnson PL, et al. The psychosocial effects of deployment on military children. J Dev Behav Pediatr 2009;30:271–8.
5. Lester P, Peterson K, Reeves J, et al. The long war and parental combat deployment: effects on military children and at-home spouses. J Am Acad Child Adolesc Psychiatry 2010;49:310–20.
6. Richardson A, Chandra A, Martin LT, et al. Effects of soldiers' deployment on children's academic performance and behavioral health. Santa Monica (CA): RAND Corporation; 2011. MG-1095-A.
7. Engel RC, Gallagher LB, Lyle DS. Military deployments and children's academic achievement: evidence from Department of Defense Education Activity Schools. Econ Educ Rev 2010;29:73–82.
8. Lyle DS. Using military deployments and job assignments to estimate the effect of parental absences and household relocations on children's academics. J Labor Econ 2006;24:319–50.
9. Acion L, Ramirez MR, Jorge RE, et al. Increased risk of alcohol and drug use among children from deployed military families. Addiction 2013;108:1418–25.
10. Gilreath TD, Cederbaum JA, Astor RA, et al. Substance use among military-connected youth: the California Healthy Kids Survey. Am J Prev Med 2013;44: 150–3.
11. Cederbaum JA, Gilreath TD, Benbenishty R, et al. Well-being and suicidal ideation of secondary school students from military families. J Adolesc Health 2014; 54:672–7.
12. Reed SC, Bell JF, Edwards TC. Adolescent well-being in Washington State military families. Am J Public Health 2011;101:1676–82.
13. Reed SC, Bell JF, Edwards TC. Weapon carrying, physical fighting and gang membership among youth in Washington State military families. Matern Child Health J 2014;18(8):1863–72.
14. Mansfield AJ, Kaufman JS, Engel CC, et al. Deployment and mental health diagnoses among children of US Army personnel. Arch Pediatr Adolesc Med 2011; 165:999–1005.
15. Gorman LA, Eide M, Hisle-Gorman E. Wartime military deployment and increased pediatric mental and behavioral health complaints. Pediatrics 2010;126:1058–66.
16. Larson MJ, Mohr BA, Adams RS, et al. Association of military deployment of a parent or spouse and changes in dependent use of health care services. Med Care 2012;50:821–8.
17. Millegan J, Engel C, Liu X, et al. Parental Iraq/Afghanistan deployment and child psychiatric hospitalization in the US Military. Gen Hosp Psychiatry 2013;35: 556–60.
18. Smith DC, Munroe ML, Foglia LM. Effects of deployment on depression screening scores in pregnancy at an army military treatment facility. Obstet Gynecol 2010; 116:679–84.
19. Spooner S, Rastle M, Elmore K. Maternal depression screening during prenatal and postpartum care at a Navy and Marine Corps military treatment facility. Mil Med 2012;177:1208–11.
20. Mansfield AJ, Kaufman JS, Marshall SW, et al. Deployment and the use of mental health services among US Army wives. N Engl J Med 2010;362:101–9.
21. Gibbs DA, Martin SL, Kupper LL, et al. Child maltreatment in enlisted soldiers' families during combat related deployments. J Am Med Assoc 2007;298:528–35.

22. Rentz ED, Marshall SW, Loomis D, et al. Effect of deployment on the occurrence of child maltreatment in military and nonmilitary families. Am J Epidemiol 2007; 165:1199–206.

23. Weist MD. Expanded school mental health services: a national movement in progress. In: Ollendick TH, Prinz RJ, editors. Advances in clinical child psychology. New York: Plenum Press; 1997. p. 319–52.

24. Military Child Education Coalition. Facts about military-connected children. Move 2014;8:40–1.

25. Department of Defense (DoD). In: Casualty data [pdf]. 2014. Available at: www.defense.gov/news/casualty.pdf. Accessed August 08, 2014.

26. Tragedy Assistance Program for Survivors (TAPS). In: TAPS fact sheet and statistics on families of the fallen tragedy assistance program for survivors (TAPS) [pdf]. n.d. Available at: www.taps.org/uploadedFiles/TAPS/RESOURCES/Documents/FactSheet.pdf. Accessed August 1, 2014.

27. Department of Defense (DoD). In: Report on the impact of deployment of members of the armed forces on their dependent children [pdf]. Military OneSource online. Available at: http://www.militaryonesource.mil/12038/MOS/Reports/Report_to_Congress_on_Impact_of_Deployment_on_Military_Children.pdf. Accessed July 15, 2014.

28. Weist MD, Sander MA, Walrath C, et al. Developing principles for best practice in expanded school mental health. J Youth Adolesc 2005;34:7–13.

29. Faran ME, Weist MD, Saito AY, et al. School-based mental health on a United States Army installation. In: Weist MD, Evans SW, Lever NA, editors. Handbook of school mental health: advancing practice and research. New York: Kluwer Academic/Plenum Publishers; 2003. p. 191–202.

30. United States Army Medical Command. School Behavioral Health Program: Operations Manual. Washington: Office of the Surgeon General, Joint Base Lewis McChord; 2011.

31. Fixen DL, Naoom SF, Blasé KA, et al. Implementation research: a synthesis of the literature (FMHI Publication #231). Tampa (FL): University of South Florida: National Implementation Research Network; 2005.

32. Barrett S, Eber L, Weist MD. Advancing education effectiveness: an interconnected systems framework for Positive Behavioral Interventions and Supports (PBIS) and school mental health. Center for Positive Behavioral Interventions and Supports (funded by the Office of Special Education Programs, U.S. Department of Education). Eugene (OR): University of Oregon Press; 2013.

33. Whitsett SA, Saito AY. Integrating mental health care into military-connected school systems: essential components of effective service delivery. Paper presented at the 121st Annual Convention of the American Psychological Association. Honolulu (HI), July 31 – August 4, 2013.

34. Weist MD, Lever N, Bradshaw C, et al. Handbook of school mental health: research, training, practice, and policy. 2nd edition. New York: Springer; 2014.

35. Weist MD, Evans SW, Lever N. Handbook of school mental health: advancing practice and research. New York: Springer; 2003.

36. Joshi PT. Presidential address: partnering for the world's children. J Am Acad Child Adolesc Psychiatry 2014;1:3–8.

37. Kolko DJ, Campo J, Kilbourne AM, et al. Collaborative care outcomes for pediatric behavioral health problems: a cluster randomized trial. Pediatrics 2014;133: e981–92.

38. Collins C, Hewson DL, Munger R, et al. Evolving models of behavioral health integration in primary care. New York: Milbank Memorial Fund; 2010.

39. Cashman J, Linehan P, Purcell L, et al. Leading by convening: a blueprint for authentic engagement. Alexandria (VA): National Association of State Directors of Special Education; 2014.
40. Wenger E. Knowledge management is a donut: shaping your knowledge strategy with communities of practice. Ivey Business Journal 2004;68:1–8.
41. Sederer LI. What does it take for primary care practices to truly deliver behavioral health care? JAMA Psychiatry 2014;71:485–6.

Index

Note: Page numbers of article titles are in **boldface** type.

Child Adolesc Psychiatric Clin N Am 24 (2015) 429–438
http://dx.doi.org/10.1016/S1056-4993(15)00009-7
1056-4993/15/$ – see front matter © 2015 Elsevier Inc. All rights reserved.

childpsych.theclinics.com

Moving?

Make sure your subscription moves with you!

To notify us of your new address, find your **Clinics Account Number** (located on your mailing label above your name), and contact customer service at:

Email: journalscustomerservice-usa@elsevier.com

800-654-2452 (subscribers in the U.S. & Canada)
314-447-8871 (subscribers outside of the U.S. & Canada)

Fax number: 314-447-8029

Elsevier Health Sciences Division
Subscription Customer Service
3251 Riverport Lane
Maryland Heights, MO 63043

*To ensure uninterrupted delivery of your subscription, please notify us at least 4 weeks in advance of move.

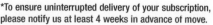

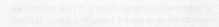

Printed and bound by CPI Group (UK) Ltd, Croydon, CR0 4YY

03/10/2024

01040495-0003